TRIGEMINAL NEURALGIA

Volume 28 in the Series

Major Problems in Neurology
PROFESSOR CP WARLOW, BA, MB, BChir, MD, FRCP
PROFESSOR J VAN GIJN, MD, FRCPE
Consulting Editors

OTHER MONOGRAPHS IN THE SERIES

TRIGEMINAL NEURALGIA

JOANNA M. ZAKRZEWSKA
Consultant Oral Physician
Eastman Dental and University College Hospitals
Honorary Consultant
The National Hospital for Neurology and Neurosurgery
Honorary Senior Lecturer
Eastman Dental Institute for Oral Health Care Sciences
London, UK

with a contribution by

P.N. PATSALOS
Senior Lecturer and Head of Pharmacology and Therapeutics Unit
University Department of Clinical Neurology
Institute of Neurology
The National Hospital for Neurology and Neurosurgery
Queen Square, London, UK

W. B. Saunders Company Ltd
London · Philadelphia · Toronto · Sydney · Tokyo

W. B. Saunders Company Ltd   24–28 Oval Road
London NW1 7DX

The Curtis Center
Independence Square West
Philadelphia, PA 19106–3399, USA

Harcourt Brace & Company
55 Horner Avenue
Toronto, Ontario M8Z 4X6, Canada

Harcourt Brace & Company, Australia
30–52 Smidmore Street
Marrickville, NSW 2204, Australia

Harcourt Brace & Company, Japan
Ichibancho Central Building, 22–1 Ichibancho
Chiyoda-ku, Tokyo 102, Japan

A catalogue record for this book is available from the British Library

ISBN 0–7020–1696–9

Typeset by Phoenix Photosetting, Chatham, Kent
Printed and bound in Great Britain by The University Press, Cambridge

Contents

Dedication

To the many patients who made this book possible and to my family for their patience and understanding.

Foreword

Trigeminal neuralgia is a mysterious disorder which, although not life threatening, can be extraordinarily debilitating. It may present to – and be managed by – dentists, neurologists, neurosurgeons, oral surgeons and ear, nose and throat surgeons. So, no one specialist can hope to see trigeminal neuralgia in all its aspects. However, there are occasional exceptions to this rule, and Joanna Zakrzewska is one of them. Not only is she a trained dentist, as well as a doctor, and is presently a Consultant and Honorary Senior Lecturer in Oral Medicine at the Eastman Dental Institute and an NHS Consultant at University College Hospital London, but – in collaboration with neurosurgeons and others – she has been studying patients with trigeminal neuralgia for over a decade. Her vast experience in diagnosing and managing patients with this condition shines through every chapter in this book, which is hardly surprising since she sees more patients in a year than most other specialists will see in a lifetime. Moreover, she follows her patients up so is in a unique position to write about the long term complications of treatment, a topic which is so often ignored by the protagonists for the vast array of treatments that have been suggested. Finally, Dr Zakrzewska is an enthusiast for her subject. Not only is this enthusiasm good for her patients but it is an essential ingredient of this excellent account of her subject.

Preface

This book is, I hope, a practical one which should be of interest not only to the specialist, but also to those clinicians who treat patients with trigeminal neuralgia on an occasional basis and may not be aware of the latest advances in management.

My own interest in this group of patients arose as a result of our Institute's research into facial pain. Among the many patients with facial pain I was particularly struck by those with trigeminal neuralgia who received such very varied treatment. It occurred to me that not a single randomized control trial had been done on the surgical management of these patients and that assessment of outcome of treatment has rarely been done by an independent observer who takes into account not only physical outcome but also psychological and behavioural factors. My own attempt to evaluate surgical procedures in an independent way brought me into contact with over 500 patients and so began my long-term involvement in the management of patients with trigeminal neuralgia.

It was, therefore, with enthusiasm but great trepidation that I approached the writing of this book. As well as including the traditional chapters on historical review, clinical features, aetiology, differential diagnosis and medical and surgical management I have also included a chapter on pain—its measurement and effect on the quality of life—and one on postoperative complications.

The clinical history is the basis for the diagnosis of trigeminal neuralgia but other investigations are currently being evaluated and these are discussed in Chapter 2. There is ever increasing research into our understanding of chronic pain and the effect pain has on the quality of life. These issues are rarely discussed in the context of patients with trigeminal neuralgia and so I have devoted Chapter 3 to this subject. Chapter 4 is a synopsis of the aetiology and pathophysiology of the condition: it may help clinicians to appreciate the complexity of the disease and explain how various treatments have evolved through the years.

My training in both dentistry and medicine has given me an unusually extensive knowledge of facial and dental pain which I have tried to reflect in Chapter 5 on the differential diagnosis of trigeminal neuralgia.

Over the years I have worked closely with Dr Philip Patsalos, a clinical pharmacologist, in evaluating a variety of drugs used in the management of patients with trigeminal neuralgia. This expertise is reflected in Chapter 6 which Philip Patsalos has written.

I have given only a broad outline of the surgical techniques used in this group of patients in Chapters 7, 8 and 9 and referred the interested reader to the many excellent texts dealing with the minutiae of the surgical procedures. I have attempted to summarize all the results in tables which highlight the problems associated with the lack of good prospective data collection.

In my post-operative outpatient clinics I deal with a wide range of complications and realized that these were rarely mentioned in the literature. I have, therefore, devoted Chapter 10 to the management of these complications.

Finally, in Chapter 11, I have tried to provide an overview of the management of the patient with trigeminal neuralgia in the light of my personal experience.

No book of this type can be written without immense input from numerous colleagues in a wide range of specialities and I am grateful to all who helped me. I am particularly indebted to Professor Malcolm Harris who sparked off my interest in this group of patients and to Dr Stephen Flint who provided me with a vast amount of literature and ideas on the topic. Dr Fergal Nally, a pioneer in the use of cryotherapy, not only taught me the technique but also showed me the importance of treating the whole patient and ensuring good communication between patient and clinician. Dr Lesley Fallowfield convinced me of the necessity of including quality of life measures in assessment of treatment outcomes. Professor David G. Thomas provided continuous encouragement and unlimited access to his extensive group of patients. The surgical chapters were read with great care by Mr Robin Illingworth who also gave me access to his patients with trigeminal neuralgia and allowed me to report on their outcome. Drs John Scadding and John Wade provided me with a firm neurological background. The chapter on the aetiological aspects of the condition was enhanced by Dr Scaddings' helpful comments. A former medical school classmate, Mr Ray Brown, gave me useful comments on the care of the eyes after surgery. Without Dr Charlotte Feinmann's continual expert help both in the writing of this book and in the management of many of the patients with complex conditions of facial pain, this book may never have been written. I am also very grateful to her for her critical appraisal of the chapter on pain assessment. Professor Charles Warlow, the instigator of this book, had the patience to sit and read the whole book. His highly positive critical evaluation was greatly appreciated and has enhanced the text. Barbara Cumbers, our librarian at the Eastman Dental Institute, and Janet Payne, her assistant, were a constant source of support. Their ingenuity in tracking down the most obscure references is greatly appreciated.

Not least I would like to thank Graham O'Brien and Beth Lawton for their extremely professional secretarial assistance, a task neither do for their daily living. They were able to decipher the most intricate of my footnotes and provide useful and, at times, amusing feedback.

Throughout the writing of this book, my whole family have shown remarkable forbearance and deserve my deepest thanks.

This book would not, however, have been possible without the help of innumerable patients. They were always willing to help me with the evaluations of new therapies. They would be willing to come frequently for drug assessments, fill in volumes of questionnaires, keep daily or even hourly diaries and comment on any information leaflets that I wrote. I am extremely grateful to them all for this and hope that this book will, in turn, help them. It may also be a stimulus to start a trigeminal neuralgia association in the UK, similar to the one in the USA (details of which are included in the appendix).

I am also grateful to the staff of W.B. Saunders for their patience with me and for their considerable help in preparing the illustrations.

I would like to acknowledge the financial assistance I received from the Welton Foundation while a trainee, which enabled me to write my thesis and so develop my interest in trigeminal neuralgia.

We must all die. But that I can save [a person] from days of torture, that is what I feel as my great and ever new privilege. Pain is a more terrible lord of mankind then even death himself.
                                                        Albert Schweitzer, 1953

Joanna M. Zakrzewska

1

History

Trigeminal neuralgia is not a new disease. It was probably recognized by the Greeks and Romans but, owing to the short life expectancy in those days, was extremely rare (Penman, 1968; Wilkins, 1990).

Jujani's writings (1066–1136) describe a unilateral facial pain that causes spasms and anxiety (Wilkins, 1990). However, the first clear descriptions of trigeminal neuralgia originate in the seventeenth century (Ameli, 1965). The original classical descriptions of trigeminal neuralgia were by Locke in 1677, André in 1756, Fothergill in 1773 and Pujol in 1787 (Terrence, 1987a).

These early descriptions are the more remarkable when one considers that the fifth cranial nerve was not identified as a distinct nerve till 1829. Although Fallopius recognized the trigeminal nerve in the sixteenth century and Vieussons identified the semilunar ganglion, most considered the trigeminal nerve to be part of the seventh cranial nerve. Hirsch of Vienna named the ganglion the Gasserian ganglion after his teacher Ludwig Gasser, and Meckel in 1748 described its dural coverings. It was, however, Bell in 1829 who confirmed that the fifth nerve had sensory and motor components that were distinct from those of the seventh nerve. He demonstrated that cutting the infraorbital nerve resulted in loss of sensation but not paralysis. Bell wrote in 1829, 'the fifth nerve is usually called trigeminus, from piercing the skull in three grand divisions'.

The clinical features described by these early workers have remained, for the most part, accurate to this day. However, the paroxysmal nature of the disease with its long remissions was not recognized for many decades. Patrick in 1914 named the areas in which pain arose the dolorgenetic zones or trigger areas. He pointed out that these zones could be in another division from where the pain was experienced, and stressed that peripheral surgery should be carried out on the trigger areas, not the radiation area.

DEFINITIONS AND DIFFERENTIAL DIAGNOSIS

The word trigeminal derives from two words: *tres* (Latin for three) and *geminus* (Latin for twin). Neuralgia derives from two Greek words: *neuro* (nerve) and *algia* (pain). Dorland (1974) defines neuralgia as paroxysmal pain extending along the course of one or more nerves. Despite this definition, paroxysmal is also often added to the name to indicate the intermittent nature of the attacks.

Over the centuries trigeminal neuralgia has been called by a variety of names, including painful affliction of the face, dolor faciei Fothergillii, trisma dolorificans, epileptiform neuralgia and trifacial neuralgia. One of the earliest names still in use is *tic douleureux*, used by André, but, strictly, the words mean only painful spasmodic movement or twitching and so could be applied to any part of the body. Aretaeus called it cephalalgia (Rohrer and Burchiel, 1993).

Since the beginning of this century it has been recognized that trigeminal neuralgia must be distinguished from other forms of facial pain. Harris (1926) quoted pain of dental origin as being the commonest cause of trigeminal neuralgia-like pain. Lewy and Grant (1938) made the distinction between typical and atypical trigeminal neuralgia. They considered that patients with true trigeminal neuralgia were all characteristically extrovert, sociable, talkative and good humoured whereas the atypical group were introverts continually engrossed in their pain, a finding also reported by Loeser (1984). Stookey and Ransohoff (1959) referred to similar patients with facial pain and suggested that the latter group should be investigated by a psychiatrist. They stressed that surgery does nothing to help and can even make matters worse in those with atypical features. These observations led Frazier and Russell (1924) to coin the term atypical facial neuralgia and refer to major trigeminal neuralgia as the classical trigeminal neuralgia. Glaser (1928) then went on to expand this and differentiated between trigeminal neuralgia and atypical facial neuralgia. Glaser's classification, which includes more than 15 conditions such as 'trigeminal ghosts', 'senile neuralgia' and a variety of other systematic and organic lesions including psychoneurosis, highlights the problems of any attempt to classify these various facial pains.

As Stookey and Ransohoff (1959) pointed out, this classification becomes too broad and they suggested three disorders: painful cephalic vascular disorders, atypical trigeminal neuralgia and prosopalagia, the last of which encompasses other pains in the face. This classification, however, does not distinguish between local and central pain states, which need entirely different management (Loeser, 1984). Despite its extremely broad use the term atypical facial neuralgia remains in use and Terrence (1987) used it synonymously with atypical facial pain. Atypical neuralgia was described by Rohrer and Burchiel (1993) as typical trigeminal neuralgia but with a constant dull background of aching pain. They considered atypical facial pain to be a pain of psychological origin. This adds to the confusion.

Loeser (1984) warned against dividing trigeminal neuralgia into symptomatic or idiopathic trigeminal neuralgia. It has been erroneously assumed that, even if no neurological symptoms are present, there is no underlying structural lesion. In 57 cases reviewed by Abbott and Killeffer (1970) five patients had tumours. Three patients had no historical or physical signs of neurological disease and one had even responded to medical management. Terrence (1987b) quoted examples of his own patients and those in the literature which show the danger of this classification.

Trigeminal neuralgia is, therefore, not as easy to diagnose as appears at first glance (Loeser, 1984). Many clinicians in reporting patients do not quote the diagnostic criteria used to make the diagnosis, which makes comparison between different authors difficult.

Wartenberg (1958) stated that the following five features should be present before a diagnosis of trigeminal neuralgia can be made:

1. paroxysmal pains with free intervals;
2. no objective clinical findings;
3. no pathological findings at postmortem;
4. trigger zones;
5. pain restricted to the area of the trigeminal nerve.

Wartenberg stressed that only half the patients have trigger zones and so this is not essential for the diagnosis. The restriction of the pain to the trigeminal area is not pathognomonic.

Rohrer and Burchiel (1993) use the term symptomatic trigeminal neuralgia for those patients who have multiple sclerosis and secondary trigeminal neuralgia, and for those with tumours or compressions who have neurological signs. Post-traumatic trigeminal neuralgia or trigeminal neuropathic pain occur after facial trauma or surgery, and may represent neuroma or deafferentation pain (Rohrer and Burchiel, 1993).

TREATMENT

It is against this background of possible misdiagnosis that the different treatments used for trigeminal neuralgia must be evaluated (Loeser, 1984). Criteria for success have become stricter and the use of controls and sophisticated statistics have improved the reliability of recent results. Owing to the paroxysmal nature of the condition, evaluation of different treatments is extremely difficult. It is probably the natural remission of the conditions that enabled success to be claimed for so many different types of therapy.

The range of treatments used for trigeminal neuralgia is vast, and Penman (1968) pointed out that, in the early days, many new neurosurgical treatments and drugs were tried out on patients with trigeminal neuralgia. This resulted in such bizarre treatments as local galvanic stimulation, diathermy and appendicectomy, radiation therapy, mastoidectomy, desensitization to allergy and artificial pyrexia (Penman, 1968). A wide variety of drugs has also been used, ranging from poisons such as arsenic, strychnine, *Gelsemium* and bee venom to metals, analgesics, vitamin B and vasodilators. Carbamazepine, introduced by Blom in 1962, was a major landmark in the treatment of trigeminal neuralgia.

While all these therapies were being attempted, surgery on the trigeminal nerve was also being undertaken and André performed one of the earliest procedures—neurectomy. A very detailed account of the historical evolution of neurosurgery for the trigeminal nerve is provided by Sweet (1985) in a paper entitled 'The history of the development of treatment for trigeminal neuralgia'.

In the early days neurectomy was performed not just on the trigeminal but also on the facial nerve. Later, various substances were injected peripherally, for example alcohol and chloroform. However, surgeons realized that to achieve more long-term effects, surgery needed to be carried out further up the nerve. The first operation on the gasserian ganglion was by Rose in 1890. Soon afterwards, further middle fossa surgery was reported by Horsley *et al.* (1891), who used an intradural approach, and by Hartley (1892) and Krause (1892), who performed extradural operations. These were technically difficult and the extradural rhizotomy procedure as described by Spiller and Frazier (1901) became very popular despite the high risk of complications. However, the procedure that is now most frequently used worldwide is that of radiofrequency thermocoagulation as described by Sweet and Wepsic in 1974.

The next major advance was by Dandy (1925), who divided the sensory root at the pons via a lateral suboccipital exposure. Although few surgeons followed his lead, Dandy's technique paved the way for microvascular decompression of the trigeminal nerve.

While the aetiology of trigeminal neuralgia remains unknown, new treatments will continually be evolving in the search for total and permanent pain relief with no associated mortality and morbidity.

2

Clinical Features

INTRODUCTION

At first glance it seems easy to make a diagnosis of trigeminal neuralgia; however, the more patients one sees, the more complex the diagnosis becomes. Loeser's statement (1994) that 'the patient has not often read the textbook and the differential diagnosis may not be as easy in the examining room as in the literature' is very apt. The clinical history is crucial for a correct diagnosis and time has to be taken over this aspect as there are no diagnostic tests. If the patient is in too much pain to give a good history, then I give a local anaesthetic injection into the trigger site. This provides immediate relief of pain and enables the patient to talk easily. Witnessing such an attack of pain, of course, makes diagnosis very much easier.

EPIDEMIOLOGY

INCIDENCE

Figures on the incidence and prevalence of this disease are difficult to obtain; there have been no studies to determine prevalence. Penman (1968) estimated an annual prevalence of trigeminal neuralgia of 4.7 per 1 000 000 males and 7.2 per 1 000 000 females. These estimates were based on the known association of trigeminal neuralgia with multiple sclerosis (MS), a disease of known prevalence. From published reports, the prevalence of MS in the general population, the prevalence of trigeminal neuralgia among patients with MS and of MS among patients with trigeminal neuralgia was used to determine the annual incidence of trigeminal neuralgia.

Although a debilitating disease, trigeminal neuralgia rarely leads to death. Death occurs only as a result of treatment or suicide (committed because of severe pain). The diagnosis, therefore, rarely appears on death certificates, a major method of epidemiological data collection. It is not a notifiable disease and no registers of its incidence are kept. The diagnosis would also have to be made by a skilled clinician, who could differentiate trigeminal neuralgia from other forms of facial pain. Data regarding prevalence cannot be collected from census forms as patients cannot make the diagnosis themselves.

In an attempt to ascertain incidence and prevalence, an epidemiological comparison of pain complaints in a city in the USA showed that 12% had suffered facial pain in the last 6 months (von Korff *et al.*, 1988). Life-table estimates showed that 34% of the population will experience facial pain by the age of 70 years. From the postal questionnaire it was impossible to make a more specific diagnosis. Only 14% of the patients with facial pain reported that they were unable to carry out daily activities. Only patients with severe trigeminal neuralgia are likely to be unable to carry out daily activities, so it is likely that many of the reported facial pains were stress-related and not due to trigeminal neuralgia. Kurland (1958) found 28 patients in whom the diagnosis of trigeminal neuralgia had been considered, but after careful assessment nine were found to have atypical facial pain.

Kurland (1958), using the population of Rochester, Minnesota, estimated 6800 new cases of trigeminal neuralgia per year in the USA, based on a rate of four new cases per 100 000 population per year in the period 1945–1956. Yoshimasu *et al.* (1972), using the same Rochester population as Kurland (1958), estimated the incidence as 4.3 per 100 000 population per year (age-adjusted) using data from 1945 to 1969. Over a 25-year period they identified 36 patients diagnosed in the Mayo Clinic and its affiliated hospitals. There was a predominance of females (5.0 per 100 000 per annum) over males (2.7 per 100 000 per annum). If one extrapolates the Rochester results to apply to the rest of the USA, an estimate of 5000–10 000 new cases per year is obtained. Katusic *et al.* (1990) also from Rochester, gave a crude incidence rate of 4.3 per 100 000 based on data collected between 1945 and 1984, from 75 patients attending the Mayo Clinic. The age-adjusted rate for women was 5.9 per 100 000 per annum and that for men 3.4 per 100 000 per annum. Thus, the incidence has not changed at a statistically significant level (Table 2.1).

The only estimate made outside the USA is a small study in the UK. Brewis *et al.* (1966) gave an annual incidence of 2.1 cases per 100 000 based on ten cases reported between 1955 and 1961 in Carlisle residents. They specified that this was a conservative estimate, as they did not examine the records of the ear, nose and throat department at the City Hospital.

Table 2.1 Incidence of trigeminal neuralgia based on the population in Rochester, Minnesota

| Reference | Time period | Incidence per 100 000 population per year | | |
		New cases	Females	Males
Kurland (1958)	1945–1956	4.0	—	—
Yoshimasu *et al.* (1972)	1945–1969	4.3	5.0	2.7
Katusic *et al.* (1990)	1945–1984	4.3	5.9	3.4

These figures suggest that general medical practitioners may expect to see about one 'new' case of trigeminal neuralgia in their working lifetime. However, none of these studies takes into account the fact that many patients are satisfactorily controlled medically or die before the need to attend hospital arises. Many patients, at least in my experience in the UK, go to their dental practitioners for primary diagnosis and initial treatment. Jannetta (1977) has reported that, of his first 100 patients with microvascular decompression, 80 had first been seen by a dentist. Many, however, failed to recognize the condition and so patients had unnecessary tooth extractions.

SEX

The few epidemiological studies that have been performed show a female predominance. Rothman and Monson (1973), using data on 526 hospitalized patients with trigeminal neuralgia in Massachusetts, gave a female:male ratio of 1.17:1. They based this on a case–control study matching the 526 patients with trigeminal neuralgia with 528 with cervical spondylosis or arthritis. Their study, therefore, took into consideration the fact that the sex ratio in the population at risk (the elderly) has a predominance of females.

AGE

Although a disease of the elderly, patients as young as 12 years have been recorded (Harris, 1926) and trigeminal neuralgia recently has been described in a 13-month-old girl, although the diagnosis was not made until she was around 7 years old (Mason *et al.* 1991).

In a survey of the literature involving 8124 patients between 1940 and 1969, White and Sweet (1969) showed the distribution for age of onset of the disease in decades (Fig. 2.1).

TRIGEMINAL NEURALGIA AND MULTIPLE SCLEROSIS

Multiple sclerosis is the disease most clearly linked with trigeminal neuralgia. Harris (1950) reported that 64 (4%) of 1622 patients with MS also had trigeminal neuralgia. In 3880 patients with MS, Rushton and Olafson (1965) reported a prevalence of trigeminal neuralgia of 0.9%, but they suggested that it could be higher. White and Sweet (1969), in a review of the literature (1934–1969) on 10 220 patients with trigeminal neuralgia, found that 172 patients (1.7%) also had MS. A similar frequency was reported by Jenson *et al.* (1982): 2.4% in 900 Danish patients. Other workers have, however, reported a higher frequency. Brisman (1987), in a group of 235 patients in the USA with trigeminal neuralgia reported a 7.2% frequency of MS, which is in agreement with Chakravorty's (1966) findings of an 8% frequency in 124 Irish patients with trigeminal neuralgia, and those of Yoshimasu *et al.* (1972) in the USA of 7% in 36 patients with trigeminal neuralgia.

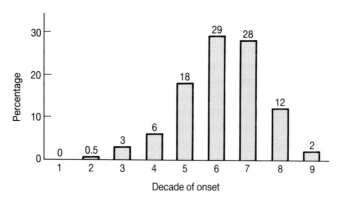

Figure 2.1   Distribution of age of onset of trigeminal neuralgia, based on a review of the literature. (Data from White and Sweet, 1969.)

Pain often starts at an earlier age in patients with MS (Rushton and Olafson, 1965; Jenson *et al.*, 1982; Brisman, 1987). Those with multiple sclerosis are also more liable to develop bilateral facial pain (Harris, 1950; Jenson *et al.*, 1982; Brisman, 1987). Eleven percent of patients with MS and trigeminal neuralgia had bilateral pain, as opposed to 4% in the idiopathic group (Rushton and Olafson, 1965).

Jenson and colleagues (1982) reported that, of 22 patients with MS, trigeminal neuralgia was the presenting symptom in only 3, whereas in the others it occurred on average 12 years after the appearance of MS. This is in agreement with the findings of Rushton and Olafson (1965), who described 30 patients with MS (out of 369) who first presented with trigeminal neuralgia. Not all patients present with facial sensory deficits (Harris, 1950; Chakravorty, 1966).

The presence of an MS plaque in the root entry zone in a patient with both trigeminal neuralgia and MS has been shown by electron microscopy (Olafson *et al.* 1966).

There is, however, still insufficient evidence to link MS directly with trigeminal neuralgia. In my experience, patients with concurrent MS are more difficult to manage: they cannot tolerate high doses of anticonvulsant drugs and have a higher recurrence rate after surgery. Brisman (1987) has made a similar comment, but has not proven the link with MS statistically. Most surgeons are reluctant to perform microvascular decompression in patients with MS as there is a higher risk of recurrence (Brisman, 1987).

OTHER RISK FACTORS AND DISEASES

Probable risk factors identified in a case–control study of 526 patients with trigeminal neuralgia were non-Jewish religion and birth in the USA (Rothman and Monson, 1973). Other factors assessed, such as handedness, alcohol, coffee and cigarette consumption, and also diseases such as stroke, heart attacks, gallstones, asthma, MS, tonsillectomy and sore throats, have not been linked (Rothman and Monson, 1973). The only possible risk factors are non-smoking, non-drinking and the presence of tonsils (Rothman and Monson, 1973). No links between herpes simplex and trigeminal neuralgia have been found, although herpes eruptions are common after operation (Rothman and Monson, 1973). There may be a link with hypertension (Lewy and Grant, 1938; Katusic *et al.* 1990). Zhang *et al.* (1990) reported that 91 of 200 patients undergoing microvascular decompression had mild hypertension, and 82% had arteriosclerosis. Dental causes have always been suspected, and Harris (1926) stated that he had seen many patients with trigeminal neuralgia following a difficult dental extraction. Tew and van Loveren (1988) reported that 4% of patients develop trigeminal neuralgia after dental extractions. My own clinical observations would support Harris's views in part. I have not seen trigeminal neuralgia in a person with complete dentition and no history of any dental disease or treatment—although there are very few elderly people with an intact dentition. It is also very rare to see patients with trigeminal neuralgia affecting only the ophthalmic division. Although many of the patients I have seen link the onset of disease with an actual dental treatment, I think that—although treatment can have a long-term effect—there must be some other factor that makes some people susceptible to the development of trigeminal neuralgia.

Syringobulbia, old pontomedullary infarction, vascular compression, aneurysm, arachnoiditis and basilar impressions have all been reported in patients with trigeminal neuralgia (Terrence, 1987). Acoustic neuromas, epidermoids and meningiomas, schwanomas and cholesteatomas appear to be the most frequently associated tumours (White and Sweet, 1969; van Loveren *et al.*, 1982; Bederson and Wilson, 1989). The frequency of a posterior fossa tumour is variable 1 of 500 patients (Penman, 1968), 7 of 252 (Bederson and Wilson, 1989) and as high as 3 of 52 (Richards *et al.*, 1983).

HEREDITY

Harris (1926) described several families with trigeminal neuralgia, including one in which nine members were sufferers. He noted that in familial cases there was a tendency for the disease to present earlier in each successive generation. Since then, several other authors have reported single families in which the disease has a hereditary basis (White and Sweet, 1969).

These patients are the exception rather than the rule, and the evidence for a hereditary component is not strong at present. Pollack *et al.* (1988) in their series of 699 patients with trigeminal neuralgia found that 35 patients had bilateral disease, of which six cases (17%) were hereditary; of the 664 patients with unilateral neuralgia, only 27 (4%) had a family history. The difference was statistically significant. Yoshimasu *et al.* (1972), in an epidemiological series of 36 patients in Rochester, Minnesota, had one patient with a family history.

In most of the familial cases, there is a clustering in the fourth and fifth decades of life. Kirkpatrick (1989) described a family in which three of six sisters had trigeminal neuralgia, and also one paternal aunt. Based on this and other evidence in the literature, he suggested a dominant pattern of genetic inheritance. However, it remains unclear as to what it may be that is inherited.

HISTORY

Any patient in pain must be assessed fully, as discussed in Chapter 3. The specific features of trigeminal neuralgia discussed here are: character, site, type, periodicity, duration, radiation, provoking, relieving and associated factors, a classification suggested by Ryle in 1936 and summarized in Table 2.2.

Table 2.2   Clinical features of idiopathic trigeminal neuralgia

Character of pain	Sharp, shooting
Site	Distribution of the trigeminal nerve
Radiation	Trigeminal area, unilateral; 3% bilateral
Periodicity	Paroxysmal
Duration	With remission, many years
Severity	Extremely severe
Provoking factors	Light touch
Relieving factors	Anticonvulsants, local anaesthetic agent
Associated factors	Trigger points, weight loss
Examination	Nil, but objective sensory loss in a small proportion

CHARACTER

The pain of trigeminal neuralgia is classically described as a sharp, shooting pain, like lightning or an electric shock. Many patients, however, also have a dull, burning, throbbing pain between attacks, which can be severe (Henderson, 1967; Loeser, 1984). Szapiro *et al.* (1985), in a review of patients undergoing microvascular compression, found a division into two groups: those with paroxysmal pain only and those with a superimposed dull ache. This latter group had a significantly lower 'cure' rate than the first group: 58% compared with 95% in those with only paroxysmal pain.

I believe that patients with superimposed dull pain have mixed pain, a mixture of trigeminal neuralgia and atypical facial pain, which we have tried to define using the McGill Pain Questionnaire (Melzack *et al.*, 1986; J.M. Zakrzewska and C. Feinmann, unpublished data). Most of the surgical treatments are aimed at relieving only the sharp, shooting component of the pain. Patients with mixed pain, therefore, do badly after surgery, as they are left with a dull ache that is unmasked by the surgery. In a postoperative review, we found that facial pain (other than trigeminal neuralgia), was present in 37% of patients who had received radiofrequency thermocoagulation (Zakrzewska and Thomas, 1993). A further 3-year follow-up prospective study has shown that those patients diagnosed as having mixed pain before operation with radiofrequency thermocoagulation not only continued to have background pain but also complained more of side-effects and were less keen to undergo further surgery (Jassim, 1994). Careful selection of patients for surgery may prevent these patients from being operated on, especially if the pain is predominantly atypical facial pain. Explanation of the effect of surgery on the pain may also reduce the disappointment that occurs when patients still have pain after operation.

I have found the McGill Pain Questionnaire indispensable in assessing patients in pain, and use it routinely. Its use is explained in Chapter 3; Fig. 5.1 illustrates its use.

SITE AND RADIATION

Trigeminal neuralgia must, by definition, occur in the distribution of the trigeminal nerve, and it is nearly always unilateral. True trigeminal neuralgia never spreads across the midline, yet the nerves on both sides may be affected, so that the disease becomes bilateral (Harris, 1926). There is often a gap of several years before the other side is affected. In one series this was an average of 8.9 years later; only one of 35 patients had pain bilaterally simultaneously (Pollack *et al.*, 1988). There was a greater number of females, a greater percentage of familial cases and increased frequency of additional cranial nerve dysfunction and hypertension in the bilateral cases. Pollack *et al.* (1988) suggested that there may be a predisposition in certain families to neurovascular compression, as they found a higher frequency of arterial and venous compression in these patients at operation.

White and Sweet (1969), in a review of the literature, showed that trigeminal neuralgia was noted to be right-sided in 61% of patients, left-sided in 36% and bilateral in 4%. Rothman and Wepsic (1974) looked for factors to explain this consistent distribution of pain. In a study of 508 patients with unilateral trigeminal neuralgia, they found no association between side of pain and handedness. Left-sided trigeminal neuralgia was present in 38% of patients, and did not correlate with age or sex. Of this group, 46 patients had skull radiography; no correlation was found between elevation of the petrous apex and the side of the pain.

The pain may affect all three divisions or only a very specific nerve ending. White and Sweet (1969) reviewed the literature on 8124 patients; the results are illustrated in Fig. 2.2. Harris (1926) stressed the rarity of pain occurring only in the first division and also pointed out that, if present in that division, it always affects the supraorbital nerve. The site of pain is not constant; it migrates to other branches and divisions. Henderson (1967) has called this 'displaced pain', and points out that it may occur months or years after the initial pain. He suggests that displaced pain is the reason for failure after operation or injection. I found this in patients who had undergone cryotherapy to peripheral nerve branches. In 38% of patients, pain recurrence was in a different nerve branch (Zakrzewska and Nally, 1988).

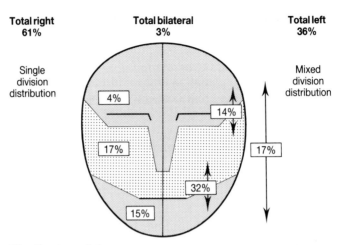

Figure 2.2 Distribution of divisions affected in patients with trigeminal neuralgia. (Data from White and Sweet, 1969.)

Henderson (1967) preferred to describe the site of pain not in terms of divisions, but of 'zones'. Pain is either in the mouth-to-ear zone (ear, upper and lower gums) or in the nose-to-orbit zone (eye, nose, cheek). He was able to assign all but 5% of 650 patients to one or other of these groups: 33% nose-to-orbit and 62% mouth-to-ear. In the remaining 5% of patients, the pain moved from one zone to the next at some stage.

PERIODICITY AND DURATION

Patients are often very clear about the timing of the first attack (Jannetta, 1977). By definition, trigeminal neuralgia is paroxysmal and there are periods of complete freedom from pain. Penman (1968) made a distinction between: (a) 'paroxysms' or short periods when pain is continuous; (b) 'runs' when there are only brief periods of relief between paroxysms; (c) 'bouts' when there are longer periods of pain relief but some pain can still occur; and (d) 'remissions' when there is no pain at all. The paroxysms of pain last for only a few minutes or even seconds. They rarely occur at night, and Jannetta (1977) postulated that this is because the compressing artery moves away from the root entry zone when the patient is in the lateral position.

Each attack of pain reaches maximum intensity fairly rapidly, then becomes stable before finally subsiding (Kugelberg and Lindblom, 1959). The pain spreads rapidly at the beginning of the attack and then recedes more slowly. The attack is followed by a refractory period whose length is related to the intensity and duration of the pain and not to the stimulus. Attacks that occur within the refractory period are of decreased duration and intensity (Kugelberg and Lindblom, 1959).

Most clinicians would agree that successive bouts tend to be worse and occur more frequently (White and Sweet, 1969). Patients would like to know how long a remission or relapse they can expect after the first bout of pain. Rushton and MacDonald (1957) attempted to answer this question after assessing 155 patients. They reported that 78 had one or more spontaneous remissions for 6 months or longer, and 38 had natural remissions for 12 months or more. They suggested that the time of onset of the disease, first presentation for treatment and duration of the longest spontaneous remission could give a clue as to the future course of the disease. Kurland (1958), in an epidemiological study, noted that 58% of patients had long spontaneous remissions, many occurring soon after diagnosis. I have found it difficult to predict the length of remission periods, but have no doubt that they gradually get shorter.

SEVERITY OF PAIN

The severity of pain can range from mild to extremely severe in the same patient. Some patients never have more than mild pain, whereas others have varying degrees of severity. In general, the intensity of the pain increases with time (Penman, 1968; White and Sweet, 1969). At the beginning of a severe attack of pain, the patient 'freezes'. Often the hand rises to the face, but rarely is the face touched. The face contorts (hence the term 'tic') and some patients remain in this position until the pain eases, whereas others may cry out in pain. Anyone witnessing such a severe attack is also very upset. Severe pain will stop patients eating, shaving, washing their face or brushing their teeth, as shown in Fig. 2.3.

Before effective means of pain control became available, suicide was sometimes the only way out (Harris, 1926; Loeser, 1990). The severity of the pain also affects the patient's choice of treatment (Penman, 1968). When patients have severe attacks, I have found that they will accept any form of treatment, whatever the potential complications. These same patients when in remission, however, are much more critical of the different forms of treatment. It is important, therefore, to discuss different types of management at times when the pain is less severe, so that patients know that other forms of treatment are available. They can then make a more rational decision about further management. Many

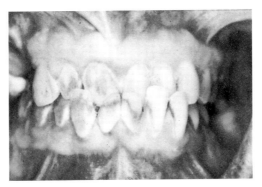

Figure 2.3   Poor oral hygiene as a result of severe trigeminal neuralgia.

of my patients say that knowing they can have an immediate appointment for treatment when the pain is severe helps to allay anxiety. For this reason I do not discharge patients from my care, but try to keep them under review by means of an annual questionnaire.

PROVOKING FACTORS

Touch, draught of air and movement of the face can elicit an outburst of pain. Eating, talking and washing become very painful activities, as they immediately elicit pain (Rasmussen, 1991). Kugelberg and Lindblom (1959) found that pain is not provoked directly by thermal stimuli, which suggests that the largest touch fibres are not involved. They also showed that, in some cases, rapid displacement of a single fine hair was sufficient to trigger an attack, although, in most cases, larger spatial summation of afferent impulses was necessary. Most patients will protect their face from winds as they stimulate the fine hairs on the face and so provoke an attack (White and Sweet, 1969; Rasmussen, 1991).

It has also been recognized that emotional disturbances can bring on an attack (Henderson, 1967; Penman, 1968). I have several patients in whom severe attacks of trigeminal neuralgia are related to stress factors. Several of my patients are, therefore, taking tricyclic antidepressants as well as antineuralgic therapy.

Henderson (1967) suggested that auditory stimuli, acute infection and trauma can, in rare cases, provoke an attack. I have a few female patients who develop more severe pain in the premenstrual period.

RELIEVING FACTORS

Patients learn to avoid those activities that bring on pain, which can lead to weight loss and poor hygiene. Weight loss of 15 lb may occur within 2–3 weeks in patients with severe trigeminal neuralgia (Peet and Schneider, 1952). The inability to eat also means patients are less willing to socialize, with its consequent effect on quality of life. This is discussed more fully in Chapter 3. For some patients, sleep is the only relieving factor, probably related to the lack of continually changing touch stimuli (Harris, 1926).

Only drugs and surgery provide relief from trigeminal neuralgia unless spontaneous remission occurs.

ASSOCIATED FACTORS

The manner in which the patient describes the pain is very characteristic, and witnessing an attack of pain is diagnostic.

Patrick in 1914 first wrote about trigger zones as areas where a slight irritation could start the pain. This low-intensity mechanical stimulation is mediated through the large myelinated Aβ fibres (Hampf *et al.*, 1990). These areas can, at times, be no larger than a fingernail. In some patients the trigger zone is no larger than 1 or 2 mm², but in others it is diffuse and large (Kugelberg & Lindblom 1959). There appears to be no relationship between the size of the trigger area and the severity of the attack (Kugelberg and Lindblom, 1959). In most patients the pain starts in the trigger zone, but in 5–9% the trigger zone may be outside the pain area (Rasmussen, 1991). Dental pathology can also be a trigger for trigeminal neuralgia in some patients (Loeser, 1990).

Trigger areas are very characteristic of trigeminal neuralgia, and I always ask patients whether they can point with one finger to this area. A local anaesthetic given into a trigger area should, if it is a localized point, abolish all pain.

Lewy and Grant (1938) studied 40 patients with trigeminal neuralgia anthropologically and observed that they were of short, thick build and had a tendency to be extrovert, and so differed from other patients with facial pain. They suggested that these findings correlate well with clinicians' intuitive 'feel' for which patients have real trigeminal neuralgia and so would benefit from surgery.

EXAMINATION

Clinical examination is in most cases negative (Editorial, 1988). Lewy and Grant (1938) were the first to show, in a study of 50 patients with trigeminal neuralgia, that 25% had some sensory loss. They stressed that examination with a pin and cotton wool might be negative, but that the use of graduated hairs would show up defects. Between 15% and 25% of patients may have sensory changes that are not noticed by the patient (Jannetta, 1976; Lazar, 1980; Szapiro *et al.*, 1985). Often methods used to detect these changes are not specified. Mingrino and Salar (1981) studied 14 patients and found that four (29%) had altered sensation on routine examination, but that this rose to eight (57%) on instrumental examination, using specially adapted von Frey's hairs.

In a small series of patients studied by Terrence (1987), 20% were found to have an abnormal area of decreased sensation. He used an aesthesiometer for these assessments. Hariz and Laitinen (1986) observed no sensory deficits in the 19 patients they tested with electrical stimulation before and after surgery.

The areas of sensory loss may be very small and hence not noticed by the patient. Both large- and small-diameter fibres show increased thresholds for sensation (Nurmikko, 1991). There may also be some loss of sensation in divisions not directly affected by disease, the so-called 'silent' branch (Nurmikko, 1991). Hampf *et al.* (1990) carried out quantitative somatosensory testing in 24 patients with trigeminal neuralgia and showed no difference between the affected and normal sides. They did, however, find a reduction in the skin temperature around the foramen of the affected nerve. This was lost after the patients had undergone radiofrequency thermocoagulation. Nurmikko (1991) tested 26 patients with trigeminal neuralgia and matched controls for sensory perception (thermal, pinprick, tactile and two-point discrimination) and found that 15 of the patients had at least one abnormal measure of sensation, not only in the trigger zone division, but also in adjacent divisions as compared with the opposite side or healthy controls. There were no temperature asymmetries. Apart from the observation of Szapiro *et al.* (1985) that patients with sensory loss do less well after surgery, it is not really known what the clinical significance of these findings is in individual patients. There is no evidence to support the statement that abnormal neurological examination denotes a structural lesion and hence requires further investigation. I believe that, unless the sensory loss is marked and progressive, and noticed by the patient, it does not affect clinical management.

A thorough oral examination should be carried out to exclude dental causes of pain. Many patients with trigeminal neuralgia present first to a dental surgeon as they believe the pain to be dental in origin. In a study of 25 patients Siegfried (1981) found that 115 unnecessary dental extractions had been performed, and Tew and van Loveren (1988) reported that, of 1100 patients, one-third had had unnecessary extractions after the onset of trigeminal neuralgia.

INVESTIGATIONS

There is no investigation that can, as yet, confirm the diagnosis of trigeminal neuralgia. Investigations are, however, useful to detect symptomatic trigeminal neuralgia; these are summarized in Table 2.3.

RADIOLOGICAL

Radiography

If there is any evidence in the history or examination that the cause may be oral, radiographs should be taken, to include intraoral views, orthopantomograms and occipitomental views. Dental problems can give rise to symptoms similar to trigeminal neuralgia, or even play a part in its development (Blair and Gordon, 1973). Patients should, therefore, be encouraged to have a full dental and oral examination.

Table 2.3   Investigations used in patients with trigeminal neuralgia

Investigation	Value
Dental radiography	Exclude dental causes
Skull radiography	Little value
CT of posterior fossa	Useful but misses lesions
MRI	Very useful
Sensory testing	Significance of abnormalities unknown
Visual evoked potentials	Identify patients with MS
Trigeminal sensory evoked potentials	Research tool only
Thermography	Still being evaluated

Computerised Tomograms

Skull radiography is of little value, but computed tomography (CT) can be useful (Sobel *et al.*, 1980). Terrence (1987) suggested that only patients with neurological deficits, or those who subsequently develop them, should undergo CT. The use of CT is limited, as it may not reveal small tumours, preganglionic segments and plaques of MS (Richards *et al.*, 1983). Even with contrast enhancement, the images are not very good. Sobel *et al.* (1980) assessed 61 patients with trigeminal neuralgia using pre- and post-contrast CT. Vascular abnormalities were found in six patients and tumours in two. In most patients the vessel responsible was not identified with CT, but the aneurysms and tumours were found.

Magnetic resonance imaging

Magnetic resonance imaging (MRI) overcomes many of the problems of CT as the full course of the trigeminal nerve can be traced and even small tumours detected (Daniels *et al.*, 1986; Hutchins *et al.*, 1989; Darlow *et al.*, 1992). The resolution of MRI, especially of soft tissue, is far higher than that of CT, and the procedure can be combined with contrast (Darlow *et al.*, 1992).

Tash and colleagues (1989) used MRI to assess whether compression was present at the root entry zone in six patients with trigeminal neuralgia and in 85 asymptomatic subjects with no trigeminal neuralgia. In the six patients, a vascular structure was noted, and vessels were found in the three who subsequently had surgery. In the 85 asymptomatic subjects, 30% of the 170 trigeminal nerves had contact with a vascular structure, but in only 2% was actual deformity noted. These results suggest that compression does not always lead to symptoms but that, if compression is found in patients with trigeminal neuralgia, microvascular decompression may be the treatment of choice. If no compression is found, more peripheral surgery could be indicated. MRI is twice as expensive as CT, but it does offer better visualization and is equally non-invasive (Darlow *et al.*, 1992). It will detect plaques of MS, and is not affected by bony structures.

MRI angiography enables the relationship between the nerve and blood vessels to be established. This MRI can be further enhanced by a 3D gradient-echo FLASH sequence which can assess the relationship between the trigeminal nerve and blood vessels; this has been described in five patients (Sens and Higer, 1991). These findings, however, have still to be correlated with surgical findings.

Patients with atypical symptoms, unusual pain distribution or duration, or who are not responding to medication, should undergo MRI. Other indications include a young age of onset, especially if there are few periods of remission, and objective changes in sensation. It must, however, also be remembered that classical trigeminal neuralgia with few or no abnormal signs may occasionally be symptomatic of a posterior fossa tumour (Darlow *et al.*, 1992). As more centres acquire the facilities for MRI, this may become an important investigation, as it will identify patients who need surgical treatment. It is a non-invasive procedure and well tolerated by patients.

Angiography

Angiography should not be performed routinely. Sobel *et al.* (1980) suggested that it should be used only in patients in whom CT identified the presence of a tumour or aneurysm. Of seven patients they studied, only two were found to have abnormalities. Since compression of the trigeminal nerve has been postulated as a cause for trigeminal neuralgia, methods have been looked for that would confirm the finding before surgery. Angiography is one technique that has been used, and de Lange *et al.* (1986) have attempted to evaluate its use. Using 159 controls (patients with no trigeminal neuralgia), they showed that trigeminal looping occurred in 36%, and so could not be used as a diagnostic test. They defined looping as: 'elongation of an artery to the part where the trigeminal nerve root is located and intimate relationship between the two structures may be expected'. They pointed out, however, that the structures may touch without the occurrence of compression. When arteries do compress the nerve, they show a very characteristic pattern. Venous compression is not as convincing. Using intra-arterial digital subtraction angiography, de Lange *et al.* (1986) attempted to predict those patients who would subsequently be found to have compression. They predicted that 20 patients would have arterial compression, and two others venous compression.

Angiography can thus be more accurate than CT, but it cannot demonstrate the exact relationship between the vertebrobasilar vascular system and the trigeminal nerve, as the latter cannot be visualized (de Lange *et al.*, 1986). It is an invasive procedure and therefore carries more risk to the patient than CT or MRI, and some neurosurgeons do not find it helpful (Richards *et al.*, 1983).

Neurosurgeons would, however, like to know before operation whether compression is present, and new investigations are continually being evaluated.

Positron Emission Tomography (PET)

This technique involves imaging the biodistribution and tissue localization of small amounts of radiolabelled biomolecules or drugs. It was used in five patients with trigeminal neuralgia before and after surgery (radiofrequency thermocoagulation) and showed increased binding of [^{11}C]diprenorphine when pain free, which suggests that endogenous opiates are no longer filling receptor sites (N. Kitchen, personal communication). At present, PET is very expensive and used only as a research tool, but it may in the future become a useful investigation.

SENSORY TESTING

At present, sophisticated sensory testing does not form part of the routine investigation of patients with trigeminal neuralgia.

EVOKED POTENTIALS

Cerebral evoked potentials have been recorded for many years. The introduction of digital computers for signal averaging made it possible to record smaller and faster-occurring evoked potentials.

Measurement of visual evoked responses (VERs) is a well-established aid in the diagnosis of multiple sclerosis, although MRI is now often used. Before microvascular decompression is performed, many patients undergo investigations with the aim of excluding a diagnosis of MS. However, as Loeser (1990) has pointed out, one does 'the patient a disservice to invoke the terrors of such a diagnosis when the only finding is tic pain'.

I restrict the use of this investigation to patients with other features suggestive of MS in the medical histories.

When Larssen and Previc first recorded somatosensory evoked potentials (SEPs) from the second and third divisions of the trigeminal nerve in 1970, it appeared that this could become the diagnostic investigation. They examined 20 patients with trigeminal neuralgia and found increased latency in 17. There were no significant differences in amplitude. However, no controls were used and no comparison was made with other painful facial conditions. Subsequently, Singh *et al.* (1982) recorded SEPs in 25 patients with a wide variety of disorders and found increased latency in all of them. Bremerich *et al.* (1991) similarly found increased latency in all patients with pain, of whom ten had trigeminal neuralgia, 21 atypical facial pain and 12 pain due to carcinoma; the study included 100 healthy controls. They also noted that 35% of patients had altered latency in the corresponding healthy branches. Patients with pain show amplitude changes, but these appear to be more notable in those with trigeminal neuralgia. Bennett and Jannetta (1983), however, showed that SEPs are significantly different in patients with classical trigeminal neuralgia compared with other patients with pain and in controls. They obtained SEPs from 36 patients with classical trigeminal neuralgia, 15 with atypical trigeminal neuralgia, 15 with other facial pain and from 18 volunteer controls. Poor outcome after microvascular decompression was correlated with less abnormal SEPs, and the authors suggested that only those with abnormal SEPs should undergo microvascular decompression. All the patients with pain also had raised thresholds.

Further studies performed on patients undergoing retrogasserian glycerol rhizotomy (Bennett and Lunsford, 1984) have added to the controversy. Of the 22 patients studied, ten had had some other surgery and so the abnormal SEPs found before operation could have been related to that rather than to the disease itself. After operation six patients who had pain relief continued to have abnormal SEPs (four of these had not had previous surgery).

SEPs are relatively easy to obtain, but careful calibration of the stimulating and recording equipment is essential if consistent results are to be obtained. The procedure is non-invasive, but can be affected by the presence of pain. Bremerich *et al.* (1991) also suggested that the effect of age, sex and drugs on SEPs needs to be evaluated before too many conclusions can be drawn.

I found that the stimulus required to produce an adequate response is large enough to be painful. Patients, who already have pain, may therefore find the whole procedure difficult to tolerate. At present recording of SEPs remains more of a research procedure than an essential investigation for trigeminal neuralgia.

Stimulation of auditory evoked potentials is often performed by neurosurgeons before microvascular decompression to assess hearing function, as hearing can be lost, mostly on the ipsilateral side, after this procedure (Piatt and Wilkins, 1984; Pollack *et al.*, 1988).

THERMOGRAPHY

Thermography has been used in neurological, vascular, inflammatory and painful conditions as a non-invasive diagnostic test. Mumford and Miles (1977) reported its use in patients with orofacial pain, but found it useful only in anaesthesia dolorosa. They found no changes in patients with trigeminal neuralgia both before and immediately after the pain.

Hardy and Bowsher (1989) studied 15 patients with trigeminal neuralgia using liquid crystal thermography and found a lower skin temperature on the affected side in 14 patients, suggesting increased sympathetic activity.

Using ten healthy controls and 17 patients with craniofacial pain, Mongini *et al.* (1990) analysed thermographic findings. The effect of teeth-clenching for 3 minutes was also assessed. The majority of patients showed thermal alterations and asymmetry, but the results were not consistent. Of the seven patients with trigeminal neuralgia, only three showed marked asymmetry, and in two it corresponded with the painful area. Prolonged teeth-clenching also produced thermographic changes, and all patients with trigeminal neuralgia showed localized hyperthermic areas. In atypical facial pain, five of 14 patients showed hyperthermic spots.

To achieve consistent results, certain conditions must be adhered to. The patients must sit for at least 15 minutes in a room that has a constant temperature of 21°C. They must not have smoked for several hours or put anything on their face. The results are obtained immediately, and can be recorded on Polaroid film for interpretation at leisure. It is not easy to perform the test when patients are in pain, as they may not tolerate the plate against the face. As yet, the results are not diagnostic and do not help to differentiate trigeminal neuralgia from atypical facial pain. Although non-invasive, thermography in its present format is not useful in the diagnosis of trigeminal neuralgia.

CONCLUSION

At present there are no reliable tests for the diagnosis of trigeminal neuralgia, so diagnosis must therefore rest entirely on the history. It is essential to take the history carefully to ensure that all the symptoms are elicited and that the correct diagnosis has been made. Clinicians need to be aware that trigeminal neuralgia can exist with other forms of facial pain and that such patients are often the hardest to treat. Careful psychological and behavioural assessment, as described in Chapter 5, is extremely important if these patients are to be well managed over the years of pain that they will inevitably face.

3

Pain: Its Assessment and Effect on the Quality of Life

INTRODUCTION

This chapter aims to highlight research carried out in the field of pain that may be of importance in managing patients with trigeminal neuralgia. The general principles underlying the taking of any pain history are discussed here. The specific features of trigeminal neuralgia have been described in Chapter 2.

There is a vast amount of literature in this field and two excellent textbooks are those edited by Wall and Melzack (1994) and Bonica (1990). The treatment of most chronic pain is multidisciplinary in specialized pain clinics, and this sort of pain management may be appropriate for patients with trigeminal neuralgia (Bonica, 1974).

Trigeminal neuralgia is an episodic disorder with a stereotypical presentation and management is normally carried out in specialized neurological units. However, trigeminal neuralgia is not only a physical complaint with a physical treatment but a complex experience, and patients should be assessed in the same way as others with chronic pain. Improved psychological and behavioural management may change the treatment outcome. Figure 3.1 summarizes an ideal management programme for patients with trigeminal neuralgia.

Relatively little work has been done on the influence of multiple social, cultural, psychological and clinical variables on the reporting of patients with facial pain. The largest groups of patients studied have been those with idiopathic facial pain and relatively little work has been performed on patients with trigeminal neuralgia.

Patients with trigeminal neuralgia have often had inappropriate medical treatment in the past, which leads them to be wary of clinicians. However, at the same time, they live in constant fear that the pain will return and may not be controllable. It is, therefore, of great importance that they be given a definitive diagnosis and the reassurance that the pain is real and not imaginary.

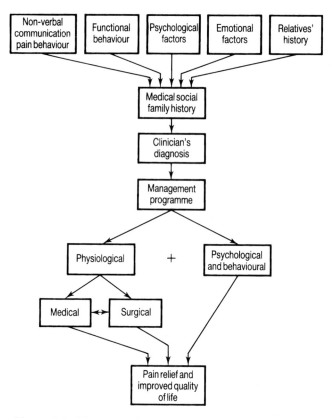

Figure 3.1   Elements of trigeminal neuralgia management.

DEFINITIONS

Pain can be defined in many different ways depending on one's profession and circumstances. Degenaar (1979) in a paper 'Some philosophical considerations on pain', pointed out that pain is defined by 'neurologists in terms of nerve impulses, psychologists in terms of emotional qualities, philosophers in terms of sensations, feeling, suffering and meaning, and theologians in terms of guilt and punishment'. Each group may change its definition as more knowledge is acquired.

In recent years it has been realized that any definition of pain must be psychological and take into account the individual experiencing it (Merskey, 1983). The International Association for the Study of Pain (IASP, 1986) has defined pain as 'an unpleasant sensory and emotional experience associated with actual and potential tissue damage or described in terms of such damage'. This definition stresses the fact that pain does not always have a physical cause and that all pain results in an emotional experience. Pain can be purely psychological provided it is reported in the same way as that caused by tissue damage. It is not just a simple neurophysiological signal but is modified by psychological, ethnic, social and environmental factors, which must be taken into account when assessing any patient with pain (Bond, 1979).

Chronic pain was once considered to be merely a prolongation of the acute mechanisms, but it is now recognized as an entity in its own right (Wall, 1984). The IASP (1986) has defined it as 'pain which persists past the normal time of healing'. One to three months is used as the point of division between acute and chronic pain. Whereas acute pain is a protective mechanism, chronic pain no longer signals real or impending tissue damage and, as such, is of no biological value. Relief of chronic pain is no longer achieved only by opioids or non-steroidal anti-inflammatory analgesics, which suggests that the pain mechanisms are different. Pain relief, however, can be obtained by tricyclic antidepressants (Feinmann, 1985).

The pathophysiological basis of pain, and especially of trigeminal neuralgia, is discussed in more detail in Chapter 4.

ASSESSMENT OF PAIN

GENERAL PRINCIPLES

Pain is a totally subjective experience and so can be reported only by the individual experiencing it. As Gracely (1980) has stated: 'Man's unique verbal abilities open a window to private experience and only through such experience is pain defined'. It is always 'felt' in some part or parts of the body and, although its description must be accepted by the clinician, an in-depth interpretation is required (Lipton and Marbach, 1983). It is also important to distinguish between what patients say and what they do about the pain (Fordyce, 1983). Patients with atypical facial pain often say the pain is severe and yet it does not interfere with their lives, whereas those with severe trigeminal neuralgia find their lives disrupted by the pain.

A careful history is essential in any patient with pain, not just at the first visit but also in subsequent acute exacerbation. Adequate time must be set aside for history-taking in a relaxed atmosphere, so that good rapport is established.

Clinicians should be skilled not only in history-taking but must also possess good communication skills. They must be aware that the patient's reported distress and related emotions will affect their own approach to that patient. It is well known that patients who show little distress are assumed to have little pain, and so are undertreated (Pilowsky and Bond, 1969). Patients sometimes find it difficult to communicate their experiences of pain, as the clinician may use a different language and have different experiences and expectations.

The sensory component of pain must be evaluated as well as the patient's response to it, including coping strategies that have evolved, the impact of the pain on their life and on the people they live with. In chronic pain, psychosocial and behavioural factors are of great importance as these influence the nature, severity and persistence of pain and disability (McCreary *et al.*, 1981; Lipton and Marbach, 1983). For research purposes more detailed assessments are often required.

PATIENT'S PAIN HISTORY

The patient must first be given a chance to describe the pain in their own words. This gives the clinician insight not only into the physical characteristics of the pain but also the patient's response to it. Patients may use words that are pathognomonic of certain conditions. Studies have shown that the severity of pain is highly associated with particular adjectives (Lipton and Marbach, 1983). This is especially true in patients with trigeminal neuralgia, who use words such as electric shock-like and lightning pains. The variation of the pain over time and its relationship to activities needs to be evaluated. Some measure of pain intensity can be obtained using a variety of measures that are discussed below.

Patients should also be asked whether they are experiencing pain anywhere else in the body, and how it relates to the trigeminal neuralgia. Sometimes previous episodes of pain are forgotten about—or even concealed. Patients should be asked about medication: what and how they take it. Some patients take antineuralgic medication as an analgesic, i.e. only when they have acute pain; others take it only after meals, as the instructions given with the medication state that this is the preferred timing. This may be correct for patients with epilepsy but for those with trigeminal neuralgia mealtimes are periods of severe exacerbation of pain, so they should take the medication before meals and wait for it to become active.

FUNCTIONAL ACTIVITIES

Patients' ability to perform various activities can be severely affected by the pain and may be the reason for them seeking help (Lipton and Marbach, 1983). Patients with trigeminal neuralgia are unable to eat, talk, shave and brush their teeth, but many will continue to work. Some activities may be restricted, not because of the demands they place on the patient but because they are found to be a chore, whereas others are performed because they are pleasurable (Turner and Romano, 1990). Many patients are reluctant to go out in the cold if winds are known to trigger the pain. Social functions are avoided, especially if they involve eating or excessive talking.

The extent of the disability will give an indirect indication of the severity of the pain.

NON-VERBAL COMMUNICATION/PAIN BEHAVIOUR

Non-verbal communication is of crucial importance and the clinician must be on the look out for it (Craig and Prkachin, 1983). It is often not recorded in the patient's notes and yet will influence the clinician's assessment. Overt expression of pain provides a method of making the pain observable. Once pain is observable, people around either do or do not react. It is important to understand what response the pain elicits. These social reinforcers of pain can play a significant role in maintaining pain behaviour (Turner and Romano, 1990). Pain behaviour (summarized in Table 3.1) includes vocalizations, e.g. moans and sighs, and abnormal facial expressions such as grimacing. Patients with trigeminal neuralgia are reluctant to touch their face or even put up their hands in a protective way in front of the pain area. Those with orofacial pain have been shown to exhibit a variety of facial expressions, often linked with high levels of tension (LeResche and Dworkin, 1984).

It is important to determine what patients do to reduce the pain as this can give invaluable insight into their evaluation of the pain and ability to cope. In an attempt to find a cure, many patients will report seeking opinions from a wide variety of health-care professionals, as well as from practitioners of alternative medicine (Heaton *et al.*, 1982). Their attitude to health-care professionals will vary from aggression and resentment to blind acceptance (Merskey, 1983). Many may feel frustrated by the lack of information and conflicting advice they have received.

It is therefore important to determine what expectations the patient has from the consultation. Do they want an instant 'cure' or better control and coping strategies?

Table 3.1   Pain behaviour in patients with trigeminal neuralgia

Facial expressions	Distortion, crying
Motor activity	Reduced facial movements, immobility
Body gestures	Guarded posture—face protected
Behaviour to reduce pain	Covering the face outdoors Decreased socializing Medication Multiple medical opinions
Functional limitations	Reluctance to talk Inability to eat Inability to brush teeth, shave or wash

PSYCHOLOGICAL AND COGNITIVE/BEHAVIOURAL FACTORS AFFECTING PAIN

Any chronic pain will lead to psychological and behavioural changes (Fordyce, 1976; Keefe *et al.*, 1978). Personality traits and unresolved conflicts may play a role in predisposing patients to chronic pain and affecting their behaviour towards it (Pilowsky and Spence, 1976). Anxiousness, depressiveness and hysterical, hypochondriacal and obsessive traits are especially likely to influence a patient's response to pain (Bond, 1979). Patients' beliefs, expectations and coping strategies will influence the pain (Turk *et al.*, 1983). It can also be argued that chronic pain itself alters emotions and mood (Merskey, 1986).

The psychological conditions linked most closely with pain are anxiety and depression, but it is extremely difficult to validate the connection. It seems logical that chronic pain, like other chronic diseases, should result in depression but it is equally true that depression can occur completely independently in patients who have pain (Fields, 1987).

This relationship between pain and depression has been well reviewed by Romano and Turner (1985). They noted that any conclusions drawn can be only tentative, owing to variables in methodology and analysis.

Patients with trigeminal neuralgia are more likely to have anhedonia (decreased pleasure in life) than diurnal depression (Marbach and Lund, 1981).

Psychological and behavioural assessments can be done either by the use of questionnaires or by interview; these are discussed later.

SOCIAL AND EMOTIONAL FACTORS

A full family and social history is essential if the patient rather than just the pain is to be assessed.

Social class and ethnicity should be ascertained. Pain perception and neuroticism have been shown to be the same in all social classes, and the concept that it is higher in lower social classes is a result of poor communication (Larson and Marcer, 1984). Patients in lower social classes may be less articulate and physicians are less likely to discuss the condition with them. This leads to poorer outcome and accentuation of pain (Larson and Marcer, 1984). Cultural factors, however, have been shown to affect both somatic complaints and pain behaviour (Turner and Romano, 1990).

The family history, including that of the siblings, parents, spouse and children, provides important insight into how patients cope with illness. A personal history, including the patient's upbringing and their enjoyment of childhood and school, should be enquired into. Parental style renders children vulnerable to psychosomatic disorders. If attention and sympathy was given by the parents only when the child was ill, the patient is likely to have poor coping behaviour (Lloyd, 1991). Details of past and present partners and relationships, dates of separation, divorce and bereavement need to be elicited as these can coincide with pain episodes.

The patient's education, work record and financial status may identify stress areas. The way in which the pain has changed the patient's ability to work and pursue leisure activities needs evaluation. Loss of a job or reduced earning power and lower levels of responsibility nearly always result in reduced status, which alters the power that the patient can exert on relatives and may therefore result in manipulative illness behaviour (Lloyd, 1991). Many patients with trigeminal neuralgia can continue to work, especially if their work is not socially interactive. This may help in ensuring that the quality of life remains adequate.

Life events and stresses affect pain: they not only cause pain but may prolong it (Williams, 1988). Many patients with psychogenic facial pain have reported an adverse life event in the 6 months before the onset of pain (Feinmann *et al.*, 1984). Pain can leave patients more vulnerable to other ordinary adverse life events, and repeated pain episodes increase vulnerability (Lennon *et al.*, 1990).

RELATIVES' HISTORY

Spouses and other people (so-called significant others) who live and work with the patient provide useful insight. 'How much is the patient's and spouse's life affected by the condition?'; 'how do they respond?'; and 'what effect does it have on marital, sexual and family relationships?' are questions that need to be answered (Turk *et al.*, 1983). Recent life stresses as perceived by relatives can be ascertained, as these could be different from the patient's perception (Williams, 1988).

The patient's use of medication, and even alcohol abuse, may be enquired about, as the relative is often in control of the medication. Spouses themselves may be ill or have chronic pain, which in turn will affect the patient. These evaluations enable the clinician to assess the support or lack of support the patient has in coping with the pain. Highly protective responses by partners to a patient with chronic pain have been shown to result in increased perceived pain and decreased activity (Flor *et al.*, 1987). Shifts can also occur in family members' roles and responsibilities, which may reinforce illness behaviour. It may be difficult to change these later unless the family is involved.

MEASUREMENTS

INTRODUCTION

Over the years a wide range of instruments have been developed to assess pain severity, psychological distress, patients' coping behaviours, attitudes and impact of the pain on quality of life. Some of them are extremely complex and time consuming in use and so of value only in research work; others are fairly simple. Some basic measure, such as a questionnaire or structured interview, should be used in all patients as it has been shown consistently that physicians fail to identify patients with depression, stressful life events and psychiatric disturbance (Brody, 1980; Nielsen and Williams, 1980; Hanks *et al.*, 1985). These measures are useful not only in identifying the initial problem but also for a variety of other reasons (Table 3.2).

With the increasing use of computers some of the instruments could be completed by patients on the computers, which would ensure rapid and reliable scoring and storage for future analysis (Hanks *et al.*, 1985).

The choice of instrument, be it questionnaire or interview, ultimately depends on the clinician, but will probably involve at least two as no one

Table 3.2   Value of measurements in pain assessment

1. Identify presenting problem
2. Identify controlling variables
3. Match treatment to individual patient
4. Assess ongoing treatment
5. Assess long-term prognosis
6. Compare responses to different forms of treatment in both individuals and groups

instrument fulfils all the requirements. The differences between a questionnaire and interview are summarized in Table 3.3.

Questionnaires are frequently used in clinical trials but, unless used correctly, the information gained from them will not be useful. The clinician must be convinced of their use and ensure that they are completely filled in. They should not be treated as just a bit of paper and given out casually by the nurse. Clinicians' interest in them will ensure that the patient fills them in with the correct attitude. If they are too long or complex they will not be completed accurately unless the patient is given sufficient time. Complex questionnaires should not be completed in busy waiting rooms where concentration may be poor. It is important to know whether the patient filled them in himself/herself or whether someone was helping. If someone was helping it should be ascertained who it was—a relative or a member of the health-care team. It is also important to establish the frequency with which the same questionnaire is to be used, as patients may or may not remember previous answers.

The goals of the assessment must be clear in the clinician's mind, as only then will the best instruments be chosen for the required information. The clinician must be sure that he or she can answer the questions in Table 3.4. The goals will vary depending on whether the instrument is being used solely for clinical use or for research purposes. Once the instruments have been chosen, it is important for the forms and scoring procedures to be readily available to all staff. It is essential to check that all self-report instruments have been completed fully.

An extensive review of reliable and valid measures for assessing patients

Table 3.3   Questionnaire versus interview for pain assessment

	Questionnaire	Interview
Administration	Easy	Complex, needs training
Time for completion	Quick	Time consuming
Data Collection	May include somatic symptoms	Selective, establishes relationship of symptoms to physical illness
Patient acceptability	Moderate	Good
Evaluation	Varies	Easy
Quantifiable measure	Yes	No
Establishes diagnosis	No	Yes
Types available	Many	Depends on clinician

Table 3.4   Questions to ask when choosing an instrument for use in patients with trigeminal neuralgia

---

1. Is the measure relevant to trigeminal neuralgia and its treatment?
2. Is it a reliable and valid instrument?
3. What is its previous history; how does it compare?
4. Will it be sensitive to changes resulting from a particular treatment?
5. Will patients find it acceptable?
6. Who will score, code and analyse the date?
7. Will it answer the question?

---

with chronic pain has been provided by Williams (1988). He divided his measures into physical, functional, behavioural and cognitive, emotional, economic and sociocultural.

PAIN MEASUREMENT

Single-dimension rating scales

These are used most commonly and are illustrated in Fig. 3.2.

Verbal Rating Scale
Instruction: Choose the word that best describes your present pain.

      nil   mild   moderate   severe

Numerical Rating Scale
Instruction: Choose the number that best describes your present pain.

no pain = 0   1   2   3   4   5   6   7   8   9   10 = worst possible pain

Visual Analogue Scale
Instruction: Mark with a verticle line how much pain you have at present.

no pain   worst possible pain

Visual Analogue Scale
Instruction: Mark with a horizontal line how much relief you have had from your pain in comparison to yesterday.

                         0% relief

                         Complete 100% relief

Figure 3.2   Single-dimension rating scales.

Verbal rating scale. The oldest methods for assessing pain were purely descriptive (Keele, 1948). Pain is defined as nil, mild, moderate or severe. Alternatively the words can be replaced by numbers, fractions or percentages to make a numerical rating scale. Although simple, these verbal rating scales (VRSs) are insensitive as small changes are not picked up.

Visual analogue scale. The visual analogue scale (VAS) is based on a 10-cm line that has anchors at each end, at right angles to the line to limit the distribution of results (Scott and Huskisson, 1976). A variety of descriptions are put at the end of each anchor, beyond the stops. It does not matter which end is made the severe end. Descriptions should not be added along the line as this affects the distribution of results and turns the scale into a VRS (Scott and Huskisson, 1976). The patient is asked to mark the line to indicate intensity. Variations on this scale are in use, such as light analogue pain scores, electronic analogue scales and pain slide ruler scorers (Smith and Covino, 1985).

To be reliable the patient must understand the instructions; some patients find the scale impossible to complete (Kremer *et al.*, 1980). Opinions are divided as to the reliability of the VAS in patients with chronic pain (Ohnhaus and Adler, 1975; Carlsson, 1983). Although reasonably reproducible, there are problems at the centre of the scale (Dixon and Bird, 1981). The other problem common to all scales with extremes is that, if the patient has previously labelled the top of the scale and the pain then becomes worse, this increased severity cannot be recorded. It has been suggested that the extremes could be labelled 'no relief' and 'complete relief' to overcome this problem (Reading, 1984).

Another simple source of error occurs in the production of the VAS: repeated photocopying results in lengthening of the line. Although a single dimension of scale, the technique can be made more versatile by using more than one, with different descriptions.

The VAS is good for clinical trials, especially those of cross-over design. It is useful to allow patients to look at previous results, as they tend to overestimate their pain with time and what is really being assessed is change (Scott and Huskisson, 1979a).

Multidimensional rating scale

Memorial Pain Assessment Card (Fishmann *et al.*, 1986). This scale combines the VRS and VAS and makes it into a repeated-use VAS, but in this way it becomes multidimensional. There are eight words to choose from, ranging from nil, weak and just noticeable to severe, strong and excruciating. On three separate VASs (horizontal scales), pain, pain relief and mood are scored. The card is folded over so the patient sees only one scale at a time—otherwise they could compare previous results. This scale still needs to be validated and is used only in the USA.

McGill Pain Questionnaire (MPQ) (Melzack, 1975). This is undoubtedly the most extensively used and tested multidimensional scale in use at the present time

WHAT DOES YOUR PAIN FEEL LIKE?

Some of the words I will read to you describe your present pain. Tell me which words best describe it. Leave out any word-group that is not suitable. Use only a single word in each appropriate group—the one that applied *best*.

1		**2**		**3**		**4**
1 Flickering	1	Jumping	1	Pricking	1	Sharp
2 Quivering	2	Flashing	2	Boring	2	Cutting
3 Pulsing	3	Shooting	3	Drilling	3	Lacerating
4 Throbbing			4	Stabbing		
5 Beating			5	Lancinating		
6 Pounding						

5		**6**		**7**		**8**
1 Pinching	1	Tugging	1	Hot	1	Tingling
2 Pressing	2	Pulling	2	Burning	2	Itchy
3 Gnawing	3	Wrenching	3	Scalding	3	Smarting
4 Cramping			4	Searing	4	Stinging
5 Crushing						

9		**10**		**11**		**12**
1 Dull	1	Tender	1	Tiring	1	Sickening
2 Sore	2	Taut	2	Exhausting	2	Suffocating
3 Hurting	3	Rasping				
4 Aching	4	Splitting				
5 Heavy						

13		**14**		**15**		**16**
1 Fearful	1	Punishing	1	Wretched	1	Annoying
2 Frightful	2	Gruelling	2	Blinding	2	Troublesome
3 Terrifying	3	Cruel			3	Miserable
	4	Vicious			4	Intense
	5	Killing			5	Unbearable

17		**18**		**19**		**20**
1 Spreading	1	Tight	1	Cool	1	Nagging
2 Radiating	2	Numb	2	Cold	2	Nauseating
3 Penetrating	3	Drawing	3	Freezing	3	Agonizing
4 Piercing	4	Squeezing			4	Dreadful
	5	Tearing			5	Torturing

Figure 3.3 Part of the McGill Pain Questionnaire.

(Fig. 3.3). Melzack (1975) asked patients to specify the pain in terms of sensory, affective and evaluative descriptors, and then organized the pain adjectives in such a way as to make them quantifiable.

The questionnaire consists of 78 words arranged in 20 groups, of which groups 1–10 are sensory, 11–15 affective and 16 evaluative; the remaining three are miscellaneous. A pain rating index (PRI) is obtained on the scale values attached to each word and can be calculated as a total or for each subscale individually. The number of words chosen (NWC) reflects the PRI index. A present pain intensity score is obtained based on five scaled words. It takes 5–15 minutes to complete, and a shortened form has also been proposed (Melzack, 1987).

The scale can be administered both orally and in the written form, but differences are obtained, so if the scores are to be compared it is important to keep to only one format (Klepac *et al.*, 1981). The reliability of the scale has been examined by a variety of workers and found to be good (Reading, 1983).

The construct, concurrent, predictive and discriminative validity of the MPQ have been studied by many workers; they are extremely complex to interpret (Reading, 1984). Some studies have confirmed the discriminative capacity of the questionnaire (Grushka and Sessle, 1984; Chen and Treede, 1985), whereas others have found that particularly severe pain may obscure this ability (Kremer *et al.*, 1983; Turk *et al.*, 1985).

It has also been suggested that the MPQ provides a good measure of affective distress and may be useful in those patients who do not want to complete more psychologically based questionnaires (Melzack, 1986).

As a clinical tool the MPQ remains the most widely used. It has been used in a variety of facial and dental settings, such as dental pain (Grushka and Sessle, 1984; Hall *et al.*, 1986), burning mouth syndrome (Grushka *et al.*, 1987), facial pain and headaches (Melzack *et al.*, 1986; Jerome *et al.*, 1988). It has been used on 73 patients with facial pain to differentiate between atypical facial pain and trigeminal neuralgia, and the workers were able to classify 91% of the patients correctly on the basis of seven descriptors (Melzack *et al.*, 1986). It can also be adapted for facial pain (Melzack *et al.*, 1986), as has been done for headache (Hunter, 1983). I use it routinely in all patients with facial pain, and find the descriptors of greatest value, whereas scores from the different subgroups are not so useful in diagnosis but are helpful in monitoring treatment outcome (see Fig. 5.1).

Multidimensional Pain Inventory (MPI).
This questionnaire was designed by Kerns *et al.* (1985) to measure not just pain but patients' response to it. It consists of three parts. Part I assesses pain severity and its effect on the patient's life; part II assesses the patient's reports of behavioural responses by other close people; and part III is a checklist of activities that are affected by the pain. The MPI has been used to assess the treatment of patients with temporomandibular joint pain but no other type of orofacial pain (Rudy *et al.*, 1995).

Other pain measures. Other instruments that are being evaluated include cross-modality matching, which is a psychophysical technique (Gracely, 1980), descriptor differential scales (Gracely and Dubner, 1981), pain perception profile (Tursky *et al.*, 1982) and card-sort methods (Reading and Newton, 1978). The West Haven–Yale Multidimensional Pain Inventory (Kerns *et al.*, 1985) and Brief Pain Inventory (Daut *et al.*, 1983) are attempts to design questionnaires that are briefer but broader than the MPQ.

The latest pain assessment instrument is one developed in Dundee by Swanston *et al.* (1993), which makes use of 'interactive computer-generated animations of symbolic visual representations of various categories of pain experience'. This can translate patients' qualitative descriptions into quantitative data, and puts less emphasis on the use of language.

Pain diaries. A diary kept by the patient can provide extremely useful data and be used as a form of therapy. Diaries can be kept not only of pain episodes but also of pain behaviour (Fig. 3.4). Although patients may not complete them, or do so only retrospectively (Epstein and Abel, 1977), a diary can be more accurate than questionnaires filled in at the clinic (Andrasik and Holyroyd, 1980).

PSYCHIATRIC AND BEHAVIOURAL ASSESSMENTS

All patients with chronic pain must have some form of psychiatric and behavioural assessment, and this can be in the form of an interview or questionnaire. These assessments may need to be repeated at intervals, as it has been well documented that pain behaviour may persist for different reasons and may also change with time (Fordyce, 1983).

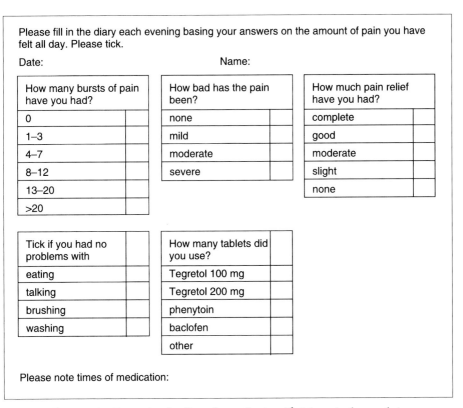

Figure 3.4   Example of a diary for patients with trigeminal neuralgia.

The MPQ, although primarily a tool for pain assessment, does include some measure of affective distress. In the same way, some of the instruments used for psychological assessment incorporate pain measures.

Psychological instruments

General Health Questionnaire (GHQ) (Goldberg, 1972). This questionnaire may be used in its entirety (60 items) or in shortened versions that exclude somatic symptoms (Goldberg and Hillier, 1979). A high score indicates the probability of psychiatric illness, and the patient's need to be fully assessed.

The questionnaire has been used in patients with temporomandibular joint dysfunction, and showed that these patients have little psychological disturbance (Salter *et al.*, 1983).

Beck Depression Inventory (BDI) (Beck *et al.*, 1961). This is a 21-item self-report measure in which patients select one of four or five statements ranked in order of severity. Scores range from 0 to 63. The higher the score, the greater the depression, scores 13–21 indicate mild to moderate depression. There are a few somatic items that in some patients may lead to a false-positive result, especially if lower scores are used to diagnose depression. The inventory takes only a few minutes to complete and score.

The instrument is widely used clinically and in research (Turner and Romano, 1984). Although it is highly suitable for use in patients with trigeminal neuralgia, this has not yet been reported.

Hospital Anxiety and Depression Scale (HAD) (Zigmond and Snaith, 1983). This is a short questionnaire with seven items, each for anxiety and depression, rated on a scale of 1–4. It was developed specifically for use in non-psychiatric patients to assess the impact of physical illness on psychological well-being. It does not contain somatic items and attempts to assess the anhedonic state (lowered ability to experience pleasure). A total score over 11 in either of the subscales indicates the presence of anxiety or depression, a score between 8 and 10 is borderline, and one of 7 or less is normal.

The questionnaire is very quick to complete and score, and few patients have problems with it. It has recently been validated against the Irritability Depression and Anxiety Scale and two subscales of the General Health Questionnaire, and found to be a useful instrument as a preliminary screening for anxiety and depression in a clinical setting (Aylard *et al.*, 1987).

Its ease of use has led to its routine use in all our facial pain clinics, together with the MPQ. It has been used before and after operation in patients with trigeminal neuralgia, and has shown that treatment results in improvement of symptoms (Zakrzewska and Thomas, 1993).

Other Instruments for Depression and Anxiety. Many of these measures have been reviewed by Kellner (1986). Scales used include the Hamilton Depression Scale

(Hamilton, 1960), the Zung Self-Rating Depression Scale (Zung, 1965) and the Montgomery–Asberg Depression Rating Scale (Montgomery and Asberg, 1979), the last of which was used in patients with atypical facial pain both before and after treatment (Feinmann *et al.*, 1984).

The State–Trait Anxiety Test (Speilberger *et al.*, 1970) has been used in two groups of patients with facial pain. It did not differentiate between myofacial pain dysfunction syndrome, arthritis of the temporomandibular joint and trigeminal neuralgia (Marbach and Lund, 1981). A small group (19) of patients with trigeminal neuralgia have been investigated with the State–Trait Anxiety Test and shown to have slightly higher anxiety levels than controls (Campbell *et al.*, 1990). Some include somatic items, and reliability and validity have not been tested in patients with chronic pain.

Illness Behaviour Questionnaire (IBQ) (Pilowsky and Spence, 1975). This 62-item questionnaire is based on the concept described by Mechanic (1962), who defined illness behaviour as the ways in which 'symptoms may be differentially perceived, evaluated and acted (or not acted) upon by the individual'. The seven areas measured using Yes/No replies are general hypochondriasis, disease conviction, psychological or somatic perception of illness, affective inhibition, affective disturbance, denial and irritability. The questionnaire assesses these factors in greater depth than the Minnesota Multiphasic Personality Inventory (Hathaway and McKinley, 1967) (see below). Some workers have found it useful in identifying abnormal pain behaviour and hence a poorer response to treatment (Speculand *et al.*, 1983), whereas others have not found it so useful in pain clinics (Tyrer *et al.*, 1989).

This scale has been used in two studies involving patients with trigeminal neuralgia, although both groups were small—32 and 19 patients (Gordon and Hitchcock, 1983; Campbell *et al.*, 1990). Gordon and Hitchcock (1983) showed that patients with trigeminal neuralgia had a higher score on denial than those with other types of facial pain but Campbell *et al.* (1990) found that patients who underwent microvascular decompression exhibited less denial than those having more peripheral surgery. Patients with trigeminal neuralgia have a normal score with regard to hypochondriasis and irritability, but they score low on effective inhibition (Campbell *et al.*, 1990). Gordon and Hitchcock (1983) showed that patients with trigeminal neuralgia were less convinced that there was a physical cause for their disease than others with atypical facial pain, but this was not confirmed in a study by Campbell and colleagues (1990).

Personality Measurements

Eysenck Personality Inventory (Eysenck and Eysenck, 1969). This is a well-established questionnaire that measures stability/neuroticism (N) and introversion/extraversion (E). The former gives an estimate of emotional vulnerability. The higher the N score the more neuroticism is displayed, denoting a higher susceptibility to breakdown. The higher the E score, the more extrovert the individual. Extrovert individuals are cheerful, energetic personalities who complain more freely than introverts who, by contrast, tend to be solitary, seriously minded and relatively uncommunicative.

Patients with psychogenic atypical facial pain and trigeminal neuralgia tend to score lower on the neuroticism scale than those with other types of facial pain (Gordon and Hitchcock, 1983).

The Minnesota Multiphasic Personality Inventory (MMPI). This is a very lengthy questionnaire (566 items) that is particularly suited to English-speaking Americans, and has been used widely in research. It measures, among other items, hypochondriasis, depression, hysteria, mania, agitation and self-confidence. Age, sex and cultural, educational and social background must be taken into account when interpreting it. The MMPI has been well reviewed by Turner and Romano (1990). It has been used in patients with the burning mouth syndrome. These patients have features similar to those of other patients with chronic pain (Grushka *et al.*, 1987). Hypochondriasis, depression and hysteria have also been shown to be high in patients with atypical facial pain or myogenic facial pain (Eversole *et al.*, 1985).

Behavioural questionnaires

A cognitive analysis investigates how a patient thinks about pain and how verbalized reactions to it may account for difficulty in coping with the pain.

A coping strategies questionnaire is a highly specialized behavioural instrument to assess the patient's use of cognitive and behavioural strategies to cope with pain. The Pain Beliefs and Apperceptions Inventory attempts to assess pain beliefs and shows that patients who view the pain as enduring and a mystery are less likely to comply with treatment (Williams and Thorn, 1989).

Keefe and Beckham (1990) are developing a Behavioural Analysis Questionnaire that will analyse behavioural patterns in patients with pain.

Patients' conception about the pain may be crucial to long-term outcome (Edwards *et al.*, 1992); two questionnaires can be used: the Patient Pain Belief Questionnaire (S. Pearce, personal communication) and the Pain Cognitions Questionnaire (Boston *et al.*, 1989). Both of these are undergoing evaluation in patients with atypical facial pain.

Behavioural diaries. These are similar to pain diaries but a record is kept of the type and level of activity, including rest periods, stress, anxiety or social events in relation to time and day. They may be used to record the frequency of use of coping skills, negative thoughts and response of those around the patient to the pain (Keefe and Beckham, 1990). Patients must learn to distinguish between events, thoughts and feelings (Turner and Romano, 1990). These are not easy diaries to keep and patients may persist reliably for periods of only 1–2 weeks (Horowitz *et al.*, 1979). The diary may be filled in retrospectively with help from a partner.

QUALITY OF LIFE

In a paper reviewing their failed cases of microvascular decompression for patients with trigeminal neuralgia, Jannetta and Bissonette (1985) commented: 'the quality of life as affected by the primary problem as well as results and side effects of treatment should be studied and may be meaningful in future decision making'.

The increasing awareness of the need to measure end results of health-care has led to the development of measures to assess the quality of life. However, the major problem in trying to measure health or quality of life lies in the definitions. The World Health Organization (1978) has defined health as a state of physical, medical and social well-being, and this has been used as a basis for the definition of the quality of life.

Some form of health or quality-of-life measure in patients with trigeminal neuralgia is essential, for the same reasons that pain assessment is necessary. Information about the pretreatment status of the patient is important in order to assess the efficacy of treatment. The impact of treatment on the patient, as opposed to the disease, is crucial. Post-treatment progress should be monitored objectively and comparison of individual and group responses to different forms of treatment should be carried out using formally tested quality-of-life instruments.

Clark and Fallowfield's (1986) statement that 'Clinicians often forget that patients are frequently unwilling to accept the "life at any cost" philosophy of most doctors' still remains true today. For some patients the ability to lead what they consider a satisfying life may conflict with the clinician's perceived benefit from treatment. This is especially true in patients with trigeminal neuralgia. Some patients consider loss of facial sensation to be worse than intermittent trigeminal neuralgia. The discrepancy between patients' and clinicians' perceived treatment outcomes, as well as patients' need to feel in control of the treatment, is often the reason for non-compliance (Conrad, 1985). Our work in assessing outcome after different types of surgery for trigeminal neuralgia has shown discrepancies between clinicians' and patients' assessment of outcome. The questionnaire used, however, was self-constructed and not a well-validated instrument (Zakrzewska and Thomas, 1993). It does, however, highlight the crucial need for quality-of-life measures to be used in assessing outcome after different treatments. The choice of the correct instrument to assess outcome from the patient's perspective is not easy, but the same questions need to be asked as in any pain assessment questionnaire. These are summarized in Table 3.4. Textbooks such as *'Measuring Health: A Practical Approach'*, edited by G. T. Smith (1988), should be read by more clinicians.

When constraints are placed on the resources available for health-care, decisions have to be made about rationalization. Economists are looking at ways of making this simpler by developing health indicators. A health indicator has two components: a description of the outcome of a number of possible health interventions and a scale that expresses the relative value or importance of each so that outcome can be expressed numerically. The major ratings that have been used are the disability and distress matrix, as developed by Rosser and Kind (1978). Such indicators are needed if quality-adjusted life years (QALY) are to be used. 'The QALY is an index designed to take account of the quality as well as the duration of survival in assessing the outcome of health-care procedures or services' (Smith, 1987). The Kaplan–Meier life-time methodology (see Chapter 8), which is used to assess surgical outcome in patients with trigeminal neuralgia, forms the basis of the QALY. The index is particularly applicable in those conditions in which treatment results in increased quality of life.

However, it is extremely difficult to determine what the measures should be, as reaching a consensus on what constitutes an individual's quality of life is all but impossible (Smith, 1987).

The major health service reforms that are taking place in the UK will make these types of assessment crucial in the planning of future care for patients with trigeminal neuralgia.

HEALTH MEASURES

The Sickness Impact Profile (Bergner *et al.*, 1981) and its British adaptation—the Functional Limitations Profile (Patrick, 1981)—attempt to assess the impact of illness on those activities of interest to the patient.

The Nottingham Health Profile (Hunt *et al.*, 1986) is a short 38-item questionnaire used to assess outcome on the basis of physical mobility, pain, sleep, social isolation, emotional reactions and energy. It is fairly complex to score as it tries to weight replies. It has been used in a wide variety of conditions and is well validated and reliable, but has not been used in patients with trigeminal neuralgia.

CONCLUSION

Patients with trigeminal neuralgia should be assessed both on the basis of the pain history and also on a range of other factors known to influence the pain. To do this, an independent instrument is required. There are, unfortunately, no ideal measures for pain (in the broadest sense of the word) or quality of life, but some form of measurement will enable fuller pretreatment assessment of the patient (Table 3.5). This will then enable independent outcome assessments to be made, which may be 'crucial in the selection of alternative therapies when clinical outcomes are very similar or inconclusive' (Hunt, 1988).

It is vital that any instrument is used properly and taken seriously by clinicians, other health personnel and patients alike.

Table 3.5 Major instruments used for assessment of pain*

	Size or no. of questions	Pain	Psychology/ behaviour	Personality	Quality of life	Reported use in trigeminal neuralgia	Comment
VRS (Keele, 1948)	Short	✓	—	—	—	No	Very basic
VAS (Scott and Huskisson, 1976)	Short	✓	✓	—	✓	No	Descriptors allow flexibility
MPQ (Melzack, 1975)	Extensive	✓	✓	—	—	Yes	Shorter version
General Health Questionnaire (Goldberg, 1972)	60	—	✓	—	—	No	Shorter version
Beck Depression Inventory (Beck et al., 1961)	21	—	✓	—	—	No	Could be useful in trigeminal neuralgia
Hospital Anxiety and Depression Scale (Zigmond and Snaith, 1983)	14	—	✓	—	—	Yes	Very easy to use
State–Trait Anxiety Test (Speilberger et al., 1970)	—	—	✓	—	—	Yes	
Illness Behaviour Questionnaire (Pilowsky and Spence, 1975)	62	—	✓	—	—	Yes	
Eysenck Personality Inventory (Eysenck and Eysenck, 1969)	—	—	—	✓	—	Yes	
Minnesota Multiphasic Personality Inventory (Hathaway and McKinley, 1967)	566	—	✓	✓	—	No	Suitable only in the USA
Nottingham Health Profile (Hunt et al., 1986)	38	—	—	—	✓	No	

*The use of these instruments in patients with trigeminal neuralgia has been limited to a maximum of two reports.

4

Trigeminal Neuralgia: Do We Know the Cause?

INTRODUCTION

Numerous theories have been put forward to explain this rare condition, but none explains all the features. Work has been hampered by the lack of a suitable animal model (Fromm and Sessle, 1991; Rappaport and Devor, 1994).

ANATOMY

The trigeminal nerve provides sensation to the face and innervates the muscles of mastication, including the tensor muscles.

GROSS ANATOMY OF THE TRIGEMINAL NERVE

When performing any surgical treatment for trigeminal neuralgia the anatomy of the trigeminal nerve must be well known to obtain maximum pain relief with few complications.

The nerve roots emerge from the lateral aspect of the brainstem at the mid-pontine level and run to the gasserian ganglion. This ganglion contains the bi-polar sensory nuclei and lies on the apex of the petrous bone in the middle fossa. It is surrounded by a sac of arachnoid that is filled with cerebrospinal fluid and is termed the trigeminal cistern. Three divisions are then given off, each of which exits through its own foramen and supplies a specific area (Fig. 4.1).

The ophthalmic division passes through the superior orbital fissure and divides into branches within the orbit. It emerges from the supraorbital fora-men and its main branches are the supraorbital, supratrochlear and lacrimal nerves.

The maxillary division passes through the foramen rotundum into the ptery-gopalatine fossa and then through the infraorbital foramen, where it becomes

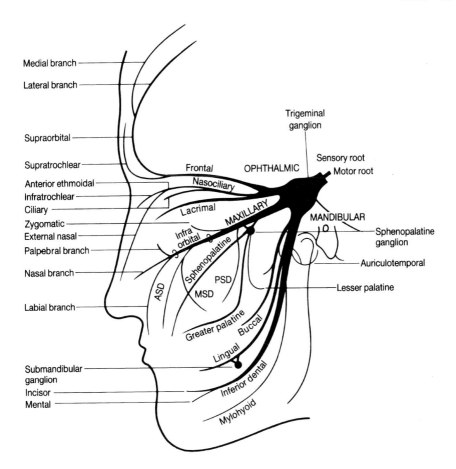

Figure 4.1 Main branches of the trigeminal nerve. ASD, MSD, PSD: anterior, middle and posterior superior dental nerves. (Modified from Mumford, 1976.)

the infraorbital nerve. Sensation to the gingiva and teeth is via the alveolar nerves.

The third division, the mandibular, leaves through the foramen ovale. The anterior trunk supplies sensation through the inferior alveolar nerve and carries the motor fibres for innervation of the masseters, pteryoids, temporals, and tensor tympani and tensor veli palatini.

The posterior trunk contains the lingual nerve, which supplies the anterior two-thirds of the tongue.

NEUROANATOMY

The trigeminal nerve is highly specialized to transmit cutaneous sensation. Pain sensation is carried by Aδ afferent fibres that are myelinated (Fields, 1990). The cornea and dental pulps have their own highly specialized sensory receptors.

The cell bodies of trigeminal primary afferent fibres lie in the gasserian ganglion. These are organized into three areas: the cell bodies of the ophthalmic division lie anteromedially, those of the mandibular region lie posterolaterally and those of the maxillary division lie between the two. The fibre bundles from the ganglion then enter the brainstem. The root divides into the portio major (sensory), minor (motor) and intermedia.

The portio major contains dorsal fibres from the ophthalmic division, ventral fibres from the mandibular division and the fibres in between are from the maxillary division. These fibres are arranged randomly, perhaps explaining why different sensory losses occur after seemingly the same operation. The root enters the lateral pons at the root-entry zone. The roots are covered by peripheral myelin derived from Schwann cells until the last centimetre, when the myelin sheath is formed by oligodendroglia. This sensory root contains around 125 000 fibres, of which half are unmyelinated. As the fibres descend down the spinal tract, they gradually lose their myelin.

The portio minor passes to the semilunar ganglion. Although it essentially innervates muscles it may contain some afferent fibres. This explains why some facial sensation may still be present after severing the portio major.

The portio intermedia enters the pons rostrally to the portio major, and probably carries different fibres.

In the lateral pons the trigeminal primary afferent fibres synapse with the brainstem nuclei. The mesencephalic nucleus has input from proprioceptive, large myelinated fibres mediating input from the muscle spindles and periodontal ligaments. Proprioceptive input also occurs into the subtrigeminal nucleus. The sensory nucleus receives input from light touch fibres and is thought to be divided into two parts: a ventral part receiving afferent fibres from the anterior part of the face and a rostrocaudal part with input from the posterior and peripheral parts of the face.

Pain sensation inputs into the spinal nucleus. This nucleus is divided into the oralis, interpolaris and caudalis nuclei. The caudalis nucleus appears to be homologous to the spinal dorsal horn and so has been called the medullary dorsal horn (Hu *et al.*, 1981). This nucleus has a laminar arrangement. Lamina 1 receives unmyelinated nociceptive C fibres, and laminae 2 and 3 (termed the substantive gelatinosa) is involved with integration. Laminae 4 and 5 (nucleus proprius) receive mechanoreceptors and wide dynamic-range neurons.

Thus, tactile and nociceptive input is received not only by the main sensory nucleus but also by all three divisions of the spinal nucleus. There are also numerous interconnections between the various parts of the trigeminal complex as well as periaqueductal or periventricular grey matter and nucleus raphe magnus, basal ganglia and cerebral cortex, and these can have inhibitory or excitory effects.

The brainstem nuclei project to the thalamus, superior colliculi, cerebellum and cranial nerve nuclei. Some neurons project to the contralateral side into the thalamic nucleus and end in the ventralis posteromedialis (VPM). The VPM nucleus projects to the sensory cortex where it is organized in a very complex manner (Fig. 4.2).

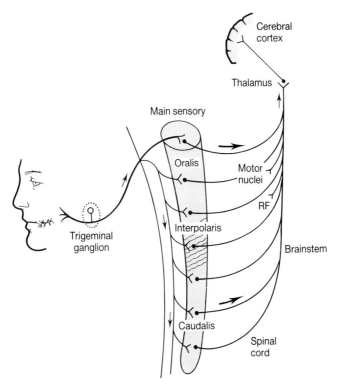

Figure 4.2 Major pathways transmitting sensory information from the mouth and face. Primary afferents project through the gasserian (trigeminal) ganglion to neurons in the trigeminal brainstem complex. These second-order neurons may project to neurons in higher levels of the central nervous system (e.g. thalmus) or in brainstem regions such as the cranial nerve motor nuclei or reticular formation (RF). (Modified from Sessle, 1986.)

Painful stimuli activate Aβ and C fibres and synapse with nociceptive neurons in the nucleus caudalis (Dubner and Bennett, 1983). However, pain can be modulated and elicited both by the nucleus caudalis and by the entire trigeminal complex due to the numerous interconnections. Yet trigeminal neuralgia appears to be set off not by Aδ and C fibres but by stimulation of Aβ fibres that normally transmit non-noxious mechanical stimuli.

PATHOGENESIS OF TRIGEMINAL NEURALGIA

Any hypothesis to explain trigeminal neuralgia needs to answer these questions:

1. Why is it of such severity?
2. Why is it short lasting?

3. Why is it paroxysmal with long remissions?
4. Why does it summate and then become refractory?
5. Why is it triggered by non-noxious stimuli?
6. Why is it unilateral and spread beyond the trigger area?
7. Why does it respond to some anticonvulsants and not to analgesics?
8. Why does it produce sensory loss in some patients?
9. Why are no other nerves affected?
10. Why does it occur mainly in the elderly?
11. Why do the various surgical techniques give pain relief?

There is no single hypothesis that fully explains all these features. There appears to be conflicting evidence from clinical and experimental data.

CLINICAL DATA

Clinically, most workers consider that compression of the trigeminal nerve results in aberrant conduction, but this is not a universally held view (Adams, 1989; Nurmikko, 1991). Compression occurs most commonly at the root-entry zone (Jannetta and Bennett, 1981; Richards *et al.*, 1983), but can occur at the level of the gasserian ganglion. Kerr (1963) suggested that, if the petrous bone is deficient, then pulsation of the carotid artery could affect the trigeminal nerve.

At the root-entry zone there is transition of peripheral and central myelin and it is postulated that a mismatch between differently myelinated axon segments may increase the potential for ectopic impulse generation (Loeser, 1977). However, others have suggested that this area is at the most 3 mm in length and therefore not visible to the naked eye (Adams, 1989).

Adams (1989) suggested that mere contact of a vessel with the nerve does not constitute compression and that a change in the position of the head does not alter this relationship. This is supported by the findings of Hardy and Rhoton (1978) that 60% of patients with non-trigeminal neuralgia had vascular contact with the trigeminal nerve.

Compression can be due to malignant or benign tumours, cysts and blood vessels, especially arteries and aneurysms (Fromm, 1987). Dental causes have also been implicated, including the formation of dental cysts (Ratner *et al.*, 1979). This is based on work showing that removal of tooth pulp can result in central degeneration (Black, 1974).

Multiple sclerosis has been associated with trigeminal neuralgia. It could result in ephaptic or non-synaptic transmission at the areas of demyelination. Calvin *et al.* (1977) and Burchiel (1980) have suggested that, within areas of focal demyelination, abnormal impulses may be generated. These demyelinated areas are the result of either multiple sclerosis or compression. Changes in evoked potential have been found in patients with multiple sclerosis, which would support this theory (Iragui *et al.*, 1986); it is thought that similar mechanisms are found in the peripheral nervous system. Hampf *et al.* (1990) postulated that nerve injury can occur as a result of cutaneous vasoconstriction, as thermal changes have been demonstrated in patients with trigeminal neuralgia. These areas of activity result in excessive central depolarization and reverberation, and lead to depolarization of small diameter nociceptive afferents and hence the perception of pain (Calvin *et al.*, 1977). It has been shown that up to 7% of damaged fibres in peripheral nerves show ephaptic transmission (Seltzer and Devor, 1979; Tomasulo, 1982). Studies with evoked potentials have tended to support these findings. Trigeminal evoked potentials show increased latency of the N_{20} potential peak and increased sensory threshold on the painful side; this is altered after surgery when the patient is pain-free (Bennet and Lunsford, 1984).

Other neurological diseases that may affect the trigeminal nerve, e.g. syringobulbia, rarely cause trigeminal neuralgia. All compressions would be present continuously, therefore not fully explaining the paroxysmal nature of the condition; so other factors must be looked for. If compression is the cause, microvascular decompression should result in a cure, and yet this does not happen in all patients and recurrences occur (Loeser, 1994). However, the long-term effects of microvascular decompression are better than those of any other procedure (Loeser, 1994). It has been postulated that compression results in dysfunction of the nerve that initially is reversible but later persists and so would account for recurrence (Bederson and Wilson, 1989).

EXPERIMENTAL DATA

It has been shown that peripheral nerve injury that results in damage to primary afferents and their cell bodies can lead to extensive repair and regeneration (Fromm and Sessle, 1991).

The major chemical mediators involved in nociceptive processes are amino acids, neuropeptides and monoamines. Injury results in release of neuropeptides such as substance P and calcitonin-gene-related peptide, as well as opioid peptides such as dynorphin. Dubner (1993) has proposed that the interaction of excitatory amino acids and opioid or non-opioid neuropeptides results in excessive excitation in the dorsal horn and possible excitotoxicity leading to loss of inhibitory mechanisms. Inhibitory amino acids, e.g. γ-aminobutyric acid (GABA), may also have an effect. The action of baclofen is mediated by GABA-B receptors and it has been postulated that they regulate the transmission of information from low-threshold mechanoreceptor afferents (Fromm *et al.*, 1992). Excitatory amino acids such as N-methyl-D-aspartate receptor antagonist (NMDA) primarily activate wide-dynamic range (WDR) neurons. WDR neurons are excited by non-noxious, e.g. tactile, stimuli as well as by noxious stimuli. As well as receiving C-fibre input, they may also receive input from large-diameter and small-diameter A fibres. Neuromodulatory chemicals similar to those found in the trigeminal brainstem complex have also been found in trigeminal afferents (Fromm and Sessle, 1991).

Dubner *et al.* (1987) and Fromm and Sessle (1991) proposed that trigeminal neuralgia has a peripheral aetiology and a central pathogenesis, and that the mechanisms suggested by Calvin *et al.* (1977) do not explain all the features of the condition. Segmental or afferent inhibition are central to this hypothesis.

Dubner *et al.* (1987) suggested that peripheral nerve damage results in alterations in the receptive field organization of WDR neurons in the dorsal horn. This results in altered processing, which includes anatomical as well as physiological and neurochemical changes. (The latter were discussed above.) Dubner and co-workers then suggest that there is an expansion of the touch receptive fields, which results in a greater overlap of receptive fields. A greater number of neurons are therefore activated by the stimulus, which previously would not have been activated. This would explain why the pain of trigeminal neuralgia radiates beyond the trigger area and yet is still perceived in the original site. The receptive fields of WDR neurons have extensive gradients of sensitivity. Dubner *et al.* (1987) postulated that the central zone responds differentially to touch, pressure and noxious stimuli and that the surrounding outer area is responsive only to more intense stimuli, such as pressure or pinch. Peripheral nerve damage leads to expansion of the low threshold portions of the receptive field owing to loss of surround inhibition. A touch stimulus will therefore result in activation of more low-threshold portions. Coupled with the greater overlap of the fields, this results in a punctate tactile stimulus being perceived as a sharp stimulus. Fromm (1991), however, suggested that as well as WDR neuron involvement there are also changes occurring to the low-threshold mechanoreceptors (LTMs) in the trigeminal nucleus oralis.

Fromm (1991) postulated that damage to the trigeminal nerve leads to focal demyelination. This results in both ectopic action potentials, as discussed above, and impaired segmental inhibition.

This afferent or segmental inhibition, which normally regulates the activity level of higher-order neurons in the trigeminal brainstem complex, is altered as a result of this increased activity. This in turn results in greater than usual excitability of the trigeminal brainstem complex neurons and results in a response that is more usual to noxious than to tactile stimuli. Fromm (1991) postulated that not only is there increased paroxysmal firing of the WDR relay neurons in the trigeminal nucleus caudalis, as suggested by Dubner *et al.* (1987), but that LTM interneurons are also unmasked before involvement of WDR neurons. They become hyperactive and begin to fire at frequencies normally elicited by noxious stimuli, and this results in the paroxysms of trigeminal neuralgia. This intermediate phase of hyperactivity of LTMs explains why attacks are set off by innocuous and not noxious stimuli.

Sessle (1993) suggested that LTMs are not required, as the spread of focus can occur just as well from WDR neurons to non-specific neurons. He also drew attention to the 'neuroplasticity' of WDR neurons (Sessle and Hu, 1991). Their properties can change depending on impairment of central inhibitory mechanisms. Previously inhibited tactile inputs can become unmarked and result in excitation of nociceptive neurons.

Fromm (1991) suggested that, although the nucleus caudalis may be involved in the pathogenesis of trigeminal neuralgia, the nucleus oralis may play an important role as it receives extensive tactile and some nociceptive input from the two branches most commonly affected by trigeminal neuralgia. Sessle (1993), however, does not consider this important, as WDR neurons are more important than LTM neurons and there may also be neurons in other parts of the central nervous system that are implicated. This hypothesis is supported by the finding that drugs that are effective in trigeminal neuralgia markedly facilitate segmental or afferent inhibition and depress excitatory transmission in the trigeminal nucleus (Fromm *et al.*, 1981). Anticonvulsant drugs result in sufficient inhibition to prevent the response normally seen to result in loss of sensation. Their physiological action closely correlates with their clinical activity in that carbamazepine is more effective than phenytoin. Carbamazepine has a much stronger depressive action on LTM neurons than phenytoin (Fromm *et al.*, 1981). Baclofen also both facilitates segmental inhibition and depresses excitatory impulses in LTM neurons (Fromm *et al.*, 1980). Amitriptyline also enhances segmental inhibition of WDR neurons, but it has less effect in nociceptor-specific neurons and does not depress excitatory transmission of LTM neurons (Fromm *et al.*, 1991). This would explain why amitriptyline is effective in some neuropathic pain conditions such as post-herpetic neuralgia but not in trigeminal neuralgia. None of the drugs used for neuropathic pain, however, is as effective as those for trigeminal neuralgia, suggesting that some other mechanism is involved (Burchiel, 1993).

Nurmikko (1991) suggested that expansion of receptive fields is clinically supported by the condition of pre-trigeminal neuralgia (see Chapter 5) and by the changes in cutaneous sensation that are found in some patients. He proposed that the degree of peripheral nerve injury in trigeminal neuralgia is much smaller than in post-herpetic neuralgia and therefore sensory changes are not as evident. This supports the findings of Hampf *et al.* (1990) of no quantitative sensory changes in 18 new patients with trigeminal neuralgia. However, this does not explain why relatively minor damage to the trigeminal nerve resulting from various surgical procedures does not lead to a worsening of the pain, but instead to temporary relief. In other forms of neuropathic pain, such ablative surgery may result in worsening of the pain. On this basis, Burchiel (1993) has argued that trigeminal neuralgia, although a neuropathic pain, has a different mechanism and so constitutes a distinctly different syndrome from other types of pain that are also described within the trigeminal sensory system, e.g. post-herpetic neuralgia, post-traumatic pain and anaesthesia dolorosa.

Recently Rappaport and Devor (1994) proposed the 'trigeminal ganglion (TRG) ignition hypothesis', which is based on experimental work of peripheral nerve pathophysiology. They postulated that a trigger stimulus sets off an autonomous self-sustaining neural process in the trigeminal ganglion as a result of damage to the ganglion or root. This can be of two types. One is based on the setting up of a 'circuit' between excitatory and inhibitory synapses that continues indefinitely (Fig. 4.3). The second type, called 'autorhythmic firing', is not based on synapses but on changes in transmembrane ion conductance, such as the sodium pump, that allow for continuous firing (Connor, 1985). This then

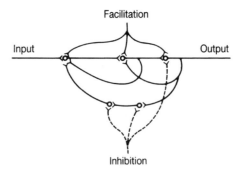

Figure 4.3   Reverberatory circuit.

spreads to other parts of the ganglion. Autorhythmic firing of these neurons continues until there is a change in ion concentrations, either because of depletion of stores or because other ions are brought in that act as suppressors. The whole cycle comes to an end as a result of hyperpolarization, and so produces a refractory period. This is based on the finding that ectopic discharges occur at the sites of nerve injury and there is increased mechano- and chemo-sensitivity, resulting in changes to local membrane potentials (Devor *et al.*, 1993). There is evidence that repetitive impulse activity in neurons can result in the depolarization of other neurons, causing them to fire. This is termed crossed afterdischarge (Mayer *et al.*, 1986). The rate at which this occurs would determine the rapidity of the attack. It would also explain why the pain extends beyond the trigger area. There may be various diffusion barriers within the ganglion that prevent the whole ganglion from being involved.

Rappaport and Devor (1994) hypothesized that remissions occur because of changes to the trigeminal ganglion ignition focus (a compact group of neighbouring trigeminal neurons), undergoing re-myelination or changes in the neurons themselves. The trigeminal ganglion could itself be damaged owing to a pathological process or other parts of the nerve, e.g. the root, could act as the focus. Impulses from these areas then travel to the trigeminal ganglion neurons and set off the whole activity. Cross-excitation appears to be triggered by low-threshold, fast-conducting myelinated fibres; for ganglia, light touch on the skin appears to be most effective. This would explain why trigeminal neuralgia is provoked by light touch. These changes are extreme and occur only in a small group of people.

All these hypotheses attempt to explain the occurrence of trigeminal neuralgia on purely anatomical, physiological and pharmacological bases. Pain, however, can be further modulated by higher centres, especially those concerned with psychological factors. It would seem likely that trigeminal neuralgia is also affected in the same way. Melzack and Wall's (1965) 'gate control' theory would explain the variability of the painful experience (Fig. 4.4).

An afferent impulse (thick myelinated fibres) arriving at the posterior horn has an inhibitory effect in the region of the substantia gelatinosa. Conversely,

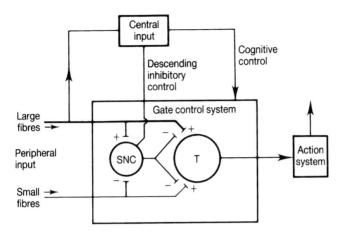

Figure 4.4 Cells of the subnucleus caudalis (SNC) exert an inhibitory effect on the afferent fibre input. These cells are themselves affected by the afferent fibres in such a way that their influence is increased by activity in the large fibres and decreased by activity in the small fibres (+ is excitatory; – is inhibitory). (Modified from Melzack and Wall, 1965.)

efferent impulses arriving in thin myelinated or unmyelinated fibres have an excitatory effect in the region of the substantia gelatinosa. The interaction between these inhibitory and excitatory fibres determines the activity of the second-order neurons of the spinothalamic pathway. As well as segmental influences, the higher centres also control the gate and form part of a feedback loop. The awareness of pain is brought about by projection from the thalamus to the cerebral cortex. This is greatly influenced by personality, mood and behaviour.

Although the aetiology of trigeminal neuralgia remains unknown, work in the field of neuropathic pain and on trigeminal neuralgia itself has increased our understanding of this complex disease. Not all the questions have been answered, but progress is being made.

5

Differential Diagnosis of Facial Pain

INTRODUCTION

'The patient with facial pain deserves a complete and careful study before the diagnosis of trigeminal neuralgia is made' (Walker, 1970). The commonest causes of facial pain are dental and oral problems, but not all facial pain should be labelled as such if the history and examination are unsupportive.

Facial pain that needs to be considered in the differential diagnosis of trigeminal neuralgia either shares the same characteristics, e.g. glossopharyngeal neuralgia, or occurs in the same site but originates from different structures. The differential diagnosis is shown in Table 5.1.

It is important to include neoplasia as a differential diagnosis for all facial pain: it should be considered especially if the pain is progressive and if sensory loss and other neurological features are noted. The neoplasm may be in the sinuses or other local structures but could also originate in the posterior fossa or medulla (Walker, 1970).

It is extremely important to ensure that facial pain is correctly diagnosed as treatments are so varied. In an attempt to address this problem diagnostic criteria have been put forward by the International Association for the Study of Pain (IASP, 1986, 1994) and the Headache Classification Committee of the International Headache Society (IHS, 1988), although others also exist (Maxwell, 1990).

IASP CLASSIFICATION

The IASP classification (1986) deals with pain affecting all parts of the body and is divided into primarily anatomical regions. The first group is made up of relatively generalized syndromes and subsequent groups are of relatively localized syndromes. The group entitled 'neuralgias of the head and face' (group II) includes trigeminal neuralgia, post-herpetic neuralgia and glossopharyngeal neuralgia. Temporomandibular joint pain is in a section called 'craniofacial pain of musculoskeletal origin' (group III), whereas dental and sinus pain are in

Table 5.1   Differential diagnosis of facial pain

Conditions affecting trigeminal nerve	Pre-trigeminal neuralgia Post-herpetic neuralgia Cluster headaches
Conditions not affecting trigeminal nerve	Hemifacial spasm Glossopharyngeal neuralgia
Dental conditions	Dentinal causes Pulpal causes Periodontal causes Cracked tooth Temporomandibular disorders Salivary gland diseases
Otolaryngological conditions	Maxillary sinusitis Frontal sinusitis Ethmoid sinusitis Sphenoid sinusitis
Eye conditions	Iritis Optic neuritis Glaucoma
Neoplasia	Sinuses Gasserian ganglion Posterior fossa
Vascular conditions	Migraine Giant cell arteritis
Idiopathic conditions	Atypical facial pain

a section called 'lesions of the ear, nose and oral cavity' (group IV). There is a separate group for primary headaches (group V), which includes migraine and cluster headache. There is also a section called 'pain of psychological origin in the head and face' (group VI). The term atypical facial pain is not used, but that of atypical odontalgia is used among the group IV lesions.

In every group each pain is described under the following headings: definition, site/system, main features, associated symptoms, signs and laboratory findings, usual course, complications, social and physical disability, pathology, summary of essential features and diagnostic criteria, and differential diagnosis. This classification was updated in 1994.

IHS CLASSIFICATION

The IHS classification deals exclusively with head and facial pain and is divided into 13 major groups. Trigeminal neuralgia belongs to group 12: cranial neuralgia, nerve trunk pain and de-afferentiation pains. Within this group are also included post-herpetic and glossopharyngeal neuralgia.

Cluster headache and migraine form groups on their own (1 and 3). Dental, temporomandibular joint and sinus pains belong to group 11 called 'headache or facial pain associated with disorders of cranium, neck, eyes, ears, nose, sinuses, teeth, mouth or other facial or cranial structures'. Atypical facial pain is considered a 'previously used term' and this classification calls them 'facial pains not fulfilling criteria in groups 11 and 12'.

The IHS classification gives three main diagnostic criteria:

A. clinical and/or laboratory evidence of disorder in a particular site;
B. headache located to affected facial or cranial structure with local or distant radiation;
C. pain disappears within 1 month of treatment or spontaneously remits. This last criterion is not met by all the disorders.

There is then a brief comment, but no attempt is made to summarize the major features of the disorder.

MAXWELL'S CLASSIFICATION

A simpler classification has been proposed by Maxwell (1990). The group of cranial neuralgias includes two major divisions: those involving the trigeminal nerve and those involving other cranial nerves. The non-neuralgic group includes pain due to ophthalmic, masticatory, sinus, neoplastic, vascular and idiopathic causes.

Maxwell (1990) lists over 30 different conditions, some of which are not included in either the IASP or IHS classification. Not all the conditions reviewed by Maxwell, however, are common enough to be considered in the differential diagnosis of trigeminal neuralgia.

PRE-TRIGEMINAL NEURALGIA

DEFINITION

This condition does not appear in any formal diagnostic classifications and yet may be an important condition to recognize. It is a prodromal dull aching pain preceding classical trigeminal neuralgia. It was first described by Symonds in 1949 as a dull continuous ache that later becomes classical trigeminal neuralgia.

It was called pre-trigeminal neuralgia by Mitchell (1980), and Fromm et al. (1990) have subsequently described more patients with this condition. It is, however, a diagnosis that is often made in retrospect, being treated initially as toothache or atypical odontalgia.

INCIDENCE

Incidence at present is impossible to estimate. It has been formally described in 62 patients (Mitchell, 1980; Fromm et al., 1990).

Age and sex
The mean age of onset is in the mid-fifties and there is a slight female predominance (Mitchell, 1980; Fromm *et al.*, 1990).

HISTORY (Table 5.2)

Character and severity
The pain is described as dull, aching, gnawing or burning. Patients compare it to toothache or sinusitis (Mitchell, 1980; Fromm *et al.*, 1990). The pain varies from mild to severe.

Table 5.2   Key diagnostic features: pre-trigeminal neuralgia

1. Moderately severe, dull, toothache-like pain
2. Unilateral, often one division of fifth cranial nerve
3. Paroxsysmal, short lasting
4. Provoked by light touch
5. Relieved by anticonvulsants
6. No signs
7. Progresses to trigeminal neuralgia

Site and radiation
Initially the unilateral pain is confined to one division, often a small specific part of a tooth-bearing area of the mouth, but when the trigeminal neuralgia develops it is often in more than one division (Mitchell, 1980). No one side predominates (Mitchell, 1980; Fromm *et al.*, 1992).

Periodicity and duration
The pain is sometimes intermittent and there may be, as with trigeminal neuralgia, periods of complete remission. In some patients the prodromal pain evolves directly into trigeminal neuralgia over a period of weeks or months (Mitchell, 1980; Fromm *et al.*, 1990). In other patients there will be periods of no pain and then trigeminal neuralgia may present 1–11 months later. The longest documented time before trigeminal neuralgia occurred was 12 years (Fromm *et al.*, 1990).

Each episode of pain may last for up to 3 hours and there may be one or two episodes a day (Mitchell, 1980). Sometimes the pain is continuous and lasts for weeks (Mitchell, 1980; Fromm *et al.*, 1990).

Provoking factors
In about one-third of patients the pain can be provoked by light touch, such as eating, brushing teeth, or by temperature variation (Mitchell, 1980; Fromm *et al.*, 1990).

Relieving factors
Dental causes are often looked for and dental treatment may give some

temporary relief. The pain may then return as classical trigeminal neuralgia (Mitchell, 1980). Anticonvulsant therapy is effective.

Associated factors
The dental status of the patient is often poor, with many people being edentulous.

EXAMINATION

This is unremarkable. No neurological signs are found.

MANAGEMENT

The most difficult aspect of this pain is the initial diagnosis, as it can easily be confused with atypical odontalgia. This diagnosis should be considered if there is persistent pain in the mouth for which there is no adequate dental explanation and which does not fit the criteria for atypical odontalgia (see below). Carbamazepine and/or baclofen are effective in most cases, the doses required often being low (Mitchell, 1980; Fromm *et al.*, 1990). Unfortunately, few clinicians recognize the disease entity and some patients undergo extensive dental therapy before it is diagnosed as an early sign of trigeminal neuralgia.

I have seen it in patients with trigeminal neuralgia, but have often made the diagnosis retrospectively when dental treatment and possibly tricyclic antidepressants have failed and anticonvulsants have been successful.

POST-HERPETIC NEURALGIA (TRIGEMINAL)

DEFINITION

Pain occurring in the distribution of the trigeminal nerve after an attack of acute herpes zoster.

FREQUENCY

The stage at which the pain becomes labelled as post-herpetic neuralgia, as opposed to the pain of acute herpes zoster, remains controversial.

The IHS classification (1988) specifies that the pain should have been present for 6 months, whereas the IASP classification (1986) does not specify a time. Watson *et al.* (1991), in their review of the literature, showed a wide variation, from 4 weeks to 6 months. They pointed out that the severity of pain also determines whether it is classified as post-herpetic neuralgia. The frequency may therefore range from 9 to 34% of all patients who had acute herpes zoster. It is therefore important to look at the diagnostic criteria used when evaluating drug trials, as some may be controlling pain of the acute attack rather than postherpetic neuralgia (Watson, 1989).

There is a rising prevalence of the condition in patients with increasing age: most patients are over 60 years of age. In their studies, Russell *et al.* (1986) and Watson *et al.* (1988b) found that 16% of patients were aged under 60 years and the remainder were over 60 years. Post-herpetic neuralgia is commoner in men. The condition resolves spontaneously within 3 months in 50% of patients but 22–50% will continue to experience problems for more than 2 years (Robertson and George 1990; Watson *et al.*, 1991). The longer the condition is present, the worse the prognosis (Watson *et al.*, 1991). Those patients with acute herpes zoster who ultimately develop post-herpetic neuralgia have been found to have had more severe pain, higher levels of anxiety and depression, decreased quality of life and a greater conviction of disease (Dworkin *et al.*, 1992).

HISTORY (Table 5.3)

Character and severity

The pain is described as a burning, itchy pain that can vary in intensity from moderate to severe. On the McGill Pain Questionnaire the ten most frequently used words are nagging, flickering, sharp, burning, gnawing, shooting, tiring, tender, itchy and stabbing (Watson *et al.*, 1988b). There are often three components to the pain: first, a constant nagging deep pain; second, a brief recurrent shooting tic-like pain; and third, allodynia—sharp unpleasant sensation evoked by light touch of the affected area. Often, one of these components predominates (Watson *et al.*, 1988; Rowbotham and Fields, 1989).

Table 5.3   Key diagnostic features: post-herpetic neuralgia

1. Severe burning pain with sharp excarberations
2. Unilateral, commonly ophthalmic division of fifth cranial nerve
3. Continuous
4. Provoked by light touch
5. No completely relieving factors
6. Associated with allodynia
7. Sensory disturbances common

Site and radiation

The pain is unilateral and in the distribution of the trigeminal nerve, just like trigeminal neuralgia, but the most commonly affected division is the ophthalmic (Watson *et al.*, 1988b), which is more frequently affected than in trigeminal neuralgia, in which it is rare.

Periodicity and duration

The pain begins at the time of the acute attack and persists from months to years. Very imperceptibly it gradually improves in many patients (Watson *et al.*, 1991). However, in some patients the pain may start several months later and become gradually more intractable (Watson *et al.*, 1991). It is a continuous pain and there are no periods of remission as with trigeminal neuralgia.

Provoking factors

Any non-noxious stimulus such as touching may exacerbate the pain (allody-nia) and, in a general series of patients with post-herpetic neuralgia, this trigger was found in as many as 50% (Watson *et al.*, 1988b). The pain thus elicited is sharp but not as fleeting as that of trigeminal neuralgia.

Relieving factors

Only some drugs will bring relief. Some patients avoid touching the face, as do those with trigeminal neuralgia.

Associated factors

Depression is often present but is severe in only a small proportion of patients (Watson *et al.*, 1988b). Sensory disturbance, ranging from hypoaesthesia (dimin-ished sensitivity to stimulation) to hyperaesthesia (increased sensitivity to nox-ious stimulation) and hypoalgesia (increased sensitivity to noxious stimuli), is often present in the pain area (Watson *et al.*, 1988b). This is markedly different from trigeminal neuralgia.

Examination

Examination may show cutaneous scarring and a range of sensory changes, e.g. decreased or absent response to pin-prick, touch, cold and light touch (Watson *et al.*, 1988b). Thermographic changes may be present in some patients (Row-botham and Fields, 1989).

Management

Attempts have been made to try to lower the incidence of post-herpetic neural-gia by vigorous treatment during the early acute phase. Evaluation of these studies are difficult as psychosocial factors can play an important role (Surman *et al.*, 1990; Dworkin *et al.*, 1992). There are poor control data but no one agent has been shown successfully to prevent development of the condition (Benoldi *et al.*, 1991). Acyclovir, corticosteroids, local anaesthesia, amantadine and levo-dopa have all been used prophylactically (Watson, 1989; Robertson and George, 1990).

Conventional analgesics are not effective for this neurogenic pain. Early treat-ment of post-herpetic neuralgias with amitriptyline is advocated, as Bowsher (1992) found a correlation between pain relief and time of commencement of treatment. Watson (1989) suggested doses of 10–70 mg daily in patients aged over 65 years and of 25–75 mg daily in younger patients. Desipramine, another tricyclic antidepressant, may be equally effective (Kishore–Kumar *et al.*, 1990). Mixed noradrenegic and serotonergic drugs may be useful (Watson *et al.*, 1992).

Topical medications have been in use for a number of years. Capsaicin (0.025%) used topically does cause some burning sensation but it appears to be effective in relieving pain (Watson *et al.*, 1988a; Peikert *et al.*, 1991). New topical analgesics such as lignocaine and prilocaine cream (EMLA) and benzydamine have been used, but the results must be interpreted with great care as these drugs have not been subjected to well-controlled randomized trials. (Stow *et al.*, 1989; McQuay *et al.*, 1990).

Other reported treatments have been with cutaneous argon laser with capsaicin (Bjerring *et al.*, 1990), opiates (Rowbotham *et al.*, 1991), trans-cutaneous electrical nerve stimulation (TENS) (Thompson and Bones, 1985; Watson, 1989) and acupuncture (Spoerel *et al.*, 1976). Somatic blockade with a local anaesthetic may decrease pain and allodynia (Nurmikko *et al.*, 1991). Anticonvulsant drugs are of no value in this condition (Watson *et al.*, 1988).

CLUSTER HEADACHE

Synonyms: migraneous neuralgia, Horton's syndrome, histamine cephalagia, sympathetic hemicrania.

DEFINITION

This pain is defined by the IASP (1986) as 'unilateral pain principally in the ocular, frontal and temporal areas recurring in severe bouts with daily attacks for several months and usually with rhinorrhoea and lacrimation'.

Cluster headaches are most often misdiagnosed as trigeminal neuralgia (Apfelbaum, 1988). Up to 42% of patients with cluster headache may also have unnecessary dental treatment (Bittar and Graff-Radford, 1992). If sharp shooting paroxysms in the distribution of the trigeminal nerve are reported, the condition can be classified as a cluster-tic syndrome (IASP, 1986).

PREVALENCE

This is a rare condition, found in less than 0.08% of the population and in about 10% of patients referred to a headache clinic (Krabbe, 1986).

Predisposing factors
It occurs mainly in men between the ages of 18 and 40 years. Smoking and high alcohol intake are predisposing factors. This may reflect more on personality characteristics as patients tend to be anxious, less sociable and more aggressive (Sjaastad, 1992; Levi *et al.*, 1992a).

HISTORY (Table 5.4)

Character and severity
The pain is described as stabbing, burning, intense pressure or throbbing. It can be extremely severe at the peak of the attack and will wake a patient from sleep (Sjaastad, 1992). In contrast to trigeminal neuralgia, it has more vascular-type characteristics with no shooting quality, but is equally severe.

Table 5.4   Key diagnostic features: cluster headache

1. Severe, stabbing, burning pain
2. Unilateral and often in distribution of fifth cranial nerve
3. Cyclic, predictable attacks, often nightly
4. Provoked by alcohol
5. Eye redness, nasal stuffiness and facial flushing
6. More prevalent in young men

Site and radiation

Characteristically the pain is unilateral and rarely changes side, a feature it shares in common with trigeminal neuralgia. The pain is commonly round the eye, zygoma, upper teeth and frontal area. It may radiate to the back of the head, down the neck and into the shoulders; if these features are present, the condition is easier to differentiate from trigeminal neuralgia.

Periodicity and duration

The most characteristic feature of this pain is its timing. The pain occurs in bouts and there are periods of remission as in trigeminal neuralgia. Each attack of pain lasts from 30 minutes to 2 hours and there may be one to three attacks per day, with one frequently occurring at night. The attacks have a much more regular pattern than those of trigeminal neuralgia, and some patients can predict the next attack. These attacks may then occur daily for 4–8 weeks. A pain-free interval then occurs which lasts for 6–18 months. In some cases the attacks persist for more than 6 months; these are called chronic cluster headaches (Krabbe, 1986; Sjaastad, 1992).

Although variations occur, this pattern of pain is more predictable than that of trigeminal neuralgia, and remissions are more frequent.

Provoking factors

Attacks may be precipitated by alcohol (Levi *et al.*, 1992b; Feinmann and Peatfield, 1993). Light touch does not act as a trigger as in trigeminal neuralgia.

Relieving factors

There is nothing the patient can do to prevent attacks or relieve them.

Associated factors

Ipsilateral lacrimation, ocular congestion and ptosis are very common. There may also be rhinorrhoea or nasal congestion, and rarely nausea. Another characteristic feature of this condition is that patients find it difficult to keep still and are very restless (Ekbom, 1970; Kudrow, 1980).

Blau (1993) studied behaviour patterns in 50 patients during an attack and found that walking and clutching the head or sitting and rocking backwards and forwards are the most common movements. Many used self-trauma as a distraction from the pain.

Unilateral forehead sweating may be noticed by the patient but can be sub-clinical (Sjaastad, 1992; Blau, 1993).

These factors are distinguishing features from trigeminal neuralgia.

EXAMINATION

Examination is unremarkable unless an attack is witnessed. There are no neuro-logical signs.

It is difficult to witness an attack and, in view of the lack of any clear diag-nostic test, various provocation tests have been introduced such as the admin-istration of histamine and nitroglycerin (Bogucki, 1990; Sjaastad, 1992). However, not all patients respond with an attack on being challenged. Nitroglycerin has been shown to affect the diameter of intracranial arteries, supporting the hypothesis that vasodilatation of intracranial arteries is respon-sible for the acute attack (Hannerz and Greitz, 1992).

MANAGEMENT

The drug of first choice is ergotamine given at the start of the attack in the form of inhalations, suppositories or orally. It is better as a prophylactic drug than when used during an acute established attack. Around 80% of patients respond (Kudrow, 1980). The smallest effective dose should be used and the drug should be stopped intermittently to ascertain whether remission has occurred (Sjaastad, 1992). Methysergide is used prophylactically, especially in young patients, but care must be taken as it causes retroperitoneal fibrosis (Sjaastad, 1992).

Systemic administration of prednisolone, 40–90 mg daily with a gradual tapering-off dose over 3–4 weeks, is useful in patients with a history of short but severe attacks (Krabbe, 1986; Sjaastad, 1992).

Lithium has been shown to be effective but its side-effects preclude regular use in all but the most difficult cases (Sjaastad, 1992). It has been compared with verapamil, which had a more rapid action but also more side-effects (Bussone *et al.*, 1990). Verapamil was used in an open study and improvement was found in 69% of patients (Gabai and Spierings, 1989). Another calcium channel blocker, sodium valproate, has also been shown in an open trial to be effective (Hering and Kuritzky, 1989).

Sumatriptan, an agonist of 5-hydroxytryptamine-like receptors, can be used subcutaneously or orally. It has been used in open trials (Hardebo, 1993) and double-blind placebo-controlled cross-over trials (Sumatriptan Cluster Headache Study Group, 1991), and was found to be effective for acute attacks and relatively free of side-effects.

In only the most intractable cases is surgery indicated. Retro-gasserian injec-tions of glycerol were used to control the pain in eight patients, with good results (Hassenbusch *et al.*, 1991). Other surgeons have performed partial sec-tioning of the main sensory root or nervus intermedius, with limited success (Morgenlander and Wilkins, 1990).

HEMIFACIAL SPASM (TIC CONVULSIF)

DEFINITION

This is a progressive condition, if not treated, that characteristically results in unilateral tonic contractions of the facial muscles. There may be mild ipsilateral facial weakness. In some cases, remission may occur.

HISTORY

The condition is painless in most patients, but Cushing (1920) and Harris and Wright (1932) described patients who had both trigeminal neuralgia and hemifacial spasm (Perkin and Illingworth, 1989).

The pain, if present, is ipsilateral and has all the features of trigeminal neuralgia. Most of these patients have compression or distortion of the relevant cranial nerve by tumours or abnormal blood vessels (Perkin and Illingworth, 1989).

MANAGEMENT

These patients are best treated by microvascular decompression.

GLOSSOPHARYNGEAL NEURALGIA

DEFINITION

Glossopharyngeal neuralgia is defined as a sudden severe stabbing recurrent pain in the distribution of the glossopharyngeal nerve (IASP, 1986).

INCIDENCE

This is a very rare disorder, with an incidence of 0.5 per 100 000 population per annum in the USA (IASP, 1986). Bruyn (1986), in a search of the literature, recorded 314 patients.

Sex and age
An analysis of all the reported cases shows no difference between the sexes, and the peak ages are between 40 and 60 years (Bruyn, 1986). Onset before 20 years is rare (Rushton *et al.*, 1981). The condition appears to be most common in left-handed people. There is no association with multiple sclerosis (Rushton *et al.*, 1981).

HISTORY (Table 5.5)

Character and severity
The sharp shooting bouts of severe pain are of the same quality as the pain of trigeminal neuralgia. Patients also report dull aching pains that persist for min-

Table 5.5 Key diagnostic features: glossopharyngeal neuralgia

1. Severe, sharp, shooting pain like trigeminal neuralgia
2. Unilateral in distribution of glossopharyngeal nerve
3. Paroxsysmal, cluster of attacks
4. Provoked by light touch
5. Relieved by anticonvulsants
6. No abnormal signs

utes to hours (Rushton *et al.*, 1981). The pain varies from mild to severe. There may also be a condition of pre-glossopharyngeal neuralgia (Rushton *et al.*, 1981).

Site and radiation
The only distinguishing feature from trigeminal neuralgia is that the pain is felt unilaterally in the tonsillar area and throat, and may radiate to the ear, eye, nose, maxilla and shoulder (Bruyn, 1986). Two forms may exist: one in which the pain is centred around the pharynx, and the other in which it is mainly auricular (Bruyn, 1986). Trigeminal neuralgia affecting the mandibular division, especially if the lingual nerve is involved, can make the diagnosis very difficult. Bilateral cases are rare (Rushton *et al.*, 1981).

Periodicity and duration
This is similar to that of trigeminal neuralgia: there are periods of pain attacks and then complete remission may occur. The attacks occur in clusters, which can last for weeks or months, mainly during the day but they may wake the patient at night.

Provoking factors
Mechanical stimulation of the fauces, especially during eating, talking and coughing, is the main trigger for the pain. Coughing can occur during an attack and intensifies the pain (Rushton *et al.*, 1981).

Relieving factors
As with trigeminal neuralgia, anticonvulsants provide the only relief.

Associated factors
Weight loss occurs as a result of the pain (Bruyn, 1986). Trigger points are less common than in trigeminal neuralgia (Rushton *et al.*, 1981). Cardiac arrhythmia and syncope during an attack have been described (Bruyn, 1986; IASP, 1986), and Bruyn (1986) described these attacks as the vagal variants.

If the pain radiates up to the eye it can cause lacrimation and redness of the eye, and so make the condition difficult to distinguish from cluster headache (Bruyn, 1986).

Both xerostomia and excessive salivation have been noted to occur in a few patients at the time of the pain (Rushton *et al.*, 1981; Bruyn, 1986).

The condition can coexist with trigeminal neuralgia, as well as being mis-diagnosed as trigeminal neuralgia (Rushton *et al.*, 1981; Bruyn, 1986). It is rare for both to occur simultaneously, and some patients develop trigeminal neuralgia first and glossopharyngeal neuralgia later, and vice versa (Rushton *et al.*, 1981).

EXAMINATION

Examination is unremarkable and there is neither sensory nor motor deficit.

INVESTIGATION

The only diagnostic test is the application of 10% cocaine to the trigger zone. It should, as in trigeminal neuralgia, result in pain relief for a short time (Bruyn, 1986).

MANAGEMENT

The same medical treatment is used as for trigeminal neuralgia. If cardiovascu-lar symptoms are present, atropine may be useful (Bruyn, 1986). Percutaneous radiofrequency thermocoagulation of Andersch's ganglion is not very effective as the vagus nerve is not treated (Langmayr and Russegger, 1992). A pharyn-geal approach to the glossopharyngeal nerve and upper vagal rootlets has been devised which allows for easier access (Mairs and Stewart, 1990). Otherwise, the treatment of choice is decompression of the ninth and tenth nerves in the posterior fossa, which is a major surgical procedure as used for trigeminal neur-algia (Fraioli *et al.*, 1989).

The approach is the same as for microvascular decompression for trigeminal neuralgia, but the ninth nerve is exposed so that the seventh and eighth cranial nerves are above and the ninth nerve is below (Apfelbaum, 1983).

OTHER NEURALGIAS

Sluder's or sphenopalatine neuralgia. This is extremely uncommon and thought to be due to an infection in the sphenopalatine ganglion. The pain occurs in and about the eye and in the roof of the nose, and can radiate backward to the ear and back of the neck. Nasal decongestants and topical cocaine may help.

Walker (1970), however, argues that this is a form of atypical facial pain, whereas McArdle (1970) suggests it is a mixture of syndromes, including clus-ter headache. This may explain why there are so few references to it in the present-day literature.

Geniculate ganglion neuralgia (Ramsay Hunt Syndrome). This type of neuralgia results in severe otalgia and has little radiation. This condition was first described by Ramsay Hunt in 1907 (Hunt, 1907); if it is secondary to a herpetic infection it is termed the Ramsay Hunt syndrome and is associated with a rash. The pain is paroxysmal with lancinating episodes located around the ear. There is also a dull constant background of pain. It may respond to carbamazepine (Maxwell, 1990).

DENTAL CAUSES OF FACIAL PAIN

If only a single nerve branch is affected by trigeminal neuralgia, it is common for patients to think they have toothache and seek dental treatment. However, the converse is also true, as Harris pointed out in 1926. It is important to check that there are no dental causes before making a firm diagnosis of trigeminal neuralgia. Both types of pain may be present simultaneously.

The signs and symptoms of dental pain are well established and can be found in most basic textbooks such as *Clinical Dentistry* edited by Rowe (1989), or Cawson's *Essentials of Dental Surgery and Pathology* (1991). They are summarized in Table 5.6. Pericoronitis (pain related to erupting teeth), dry sockets (pain after tooth extraction), acute necrotizing gingivitis and mucosal lesions all cause orofacial pain but they are not confused with trigeminal neuralgia as there are other highly specific signs and symptoms.

Treatment is varied and patients should be referred to their dental practitioner as most require surgical treatment, which is not discussed here. Some of the dental pains that may be confused with trigeminal neuralgia are discussed briefly.

DENTINAL PAIN

DEFINITION

This is most often due to caries or defective restoration, and results in short-lasting diffuse pain provoked by local stimuli. It is very common.

HISTORY AND EXAMINATION

Character and severity
The pain has a sharp quality and is of moderate intensity. Consequently it can mimic trigeminal neuralgia, especially when the latter is confined to a single peripheral branch.

Site and radiation
The pain is often poorly localized, and it can be difficult to differentiate between adjacent teeth and also upper and lower teeth. The pain does not cross the midline.

Table 5.6 Key diagnostic features: dental causes

Condition	Character	Severity	Ability to localize	Periodicity	Provoking factors	Relieving factors	Associated signs
Dentinal	Sharp	Moderate	Poor	Seconds	Hot, cold, sweet, sour	Removal of stimulant	Caries, defective restorations
Pulpal	Sharp, dull, throbbing	Severe	Poor	Intermittent then continuous	Thermal and pressure	Removal of stimulant	Deep caries, fractured tooth
Periodontal	Throbbing, sharp	Moderate	Good	Continuous	Percussion, palpitation of area	Drainage of pus	Periapical, lesion shows on radiograph; lateral or gingival pus and tooth extrusion
Cracked tooth	Sharp	Moderate	Good	Seconds	Biting	Removal of tooth	Fracture may be very fine

Duration
The pain is intermittent, lasting for a few seconds, rarely minutes, and so is similar to trigeminal neuralgia in its timing.

Provoking factors
Hot, cold, sweet and sour foods can all provoke an attack of pain. It is not related to the actual eating of the food. This is an important distinguishing factor from trigeminal neuralgia. Furthermore it is not provoked by light touch. It is, therefore, important specifically to ask whether different types of food provoke the pain as patients may not appreciate the difference.

Relieving factors
Removal of the stimulating factor results in immediate relief of pain, whereas with trigeminal neuralgia the pain may persist even though the trigger factor has gone.

PULPAL PAIN

DEFINITION

A sharp or dull pain related to pulpal inflammation that is often evoked by local stimuli. It is very common.

HISTORY AND EXAMINATION

Character and severity
The pain is sharp, dull or throbbing. Hall *et al.* (1986) found on the McGill Pain Questionnaire that it was described as throbbing, aching, annoying, radiating and nagging. These are very different descriptors from those used by patients with trigeminal neuralgia.

It is a severe pain, especially if irreversible pulpitis occurs, i.e. pulp dies and the tooth needs to be root-filled.

Site and radiation
It is difficult for the patient to localize the pain, which may radiate to both jaws but which does not cross the midline. The pain is more diffuse than that of trigeminal neuralgia.

Periodicity and timing
Initially the pain lasts only for as long as a stimulus is applied, but later it may last over 30 minutes. There may be a continuous aching pain that is exacerbated from time to time with sharp episodes. The pain often wakes a patient from sleep, in contrast to trigeminal neuralgia.

Provoking factors
Initially, thermal and pressure stimuli will initiate pain but later the pain persists and is continuous.

Relieving factors
At first, withdrawal of stimulus gives relief, but later this has no effect. Analgesics may help for a short time but ultimately only removal of the dead pulp tissue will lead to pain relief.

Associated factors
There is often a deep cavity (caries) or a new restoration in a large cavity that has resulted in exposure of the pulp. There may be a fractured tooth that has penetrated to the pulp. Careful examination and appropriate radiography often allows the correct diagnosis to be made.

PERIODONTAL PAIN

DEFINITION

This type of pain is easily localized by the patient; the affected teeth are often tender to percussion. These pains, therefore, are less likely to be mistaken for trigeminal neuralgia.

The pain can be due to involvement of the periodontium at the apex of the tooth (periapical), at the lateral borders of the tooth or at the gingival margin.

HISTORY AND EXAMINATION

Character and severity
The pain on the McGill Pain Questionnaire is described as throbbing, sharp, pressing, aching, tender, annoying, penetrating and nagging in type (Hall *et al.*, 1986). It is of moderate severity.

Site and radiation
Patients are able to localize the pain to the involved tooth. Radiation to the rest of the jaw may occur.

Periodicity and duration
The pain is continuous and tends to be worse at meal times owing to pressure on the teeth. Its continuous nature distinguishes it from trigeminal neuralgia.

Provoking factors
Initially nothing provokes the pain, but later biting on the tooth causes intense pain.

Relieving factors
An abscess forms and drainage of the pus is the most effective means of pain relief. Analgesics may help.

Associated factors
The affected teeth are mobile, tender to percussion and slightly extruded from the socket.

If a periapical abscess remains untreated it often results in gross facial swelling. A lateral periodontal abscess results in a more visible gingival lesion, and probing of the tooth will often result in the release of pus.

CRACKED TOOTH SYNDROME

DEFINITION

This diagnosis is often made in retrospect when the tooth finally fractures and results in a sharp transient pain. It is fairly common.

HISTORY AND EXAMINATION

Character and severity
The pain is described as sharp and of moderate to severe intensity; it is similar to trigeminal neuralgia.

Site and radiation
Although the pain is fairly well localized to the affected tooth, it is perceived in a tooth rather than over a nerve branch as in trigeminal neuralgia.

Duration
The pain lasts for a few seconds and so can be similar to that of trigeminal neuralgia.

Provoking factors
Biting or chewing on the affected tooth evokes pain.

Relieving factors
The only permanent relief of pain is restoration of the defective part of the tooth. Analgesics give no relief.

Associated factors
The cracked tooth can be difficult to diagnose as the fracture may be very fine and not evident without removal of part of the restoration. It is often tender to percussion.

The diagnosis is therefore often made in retrospect when the defective part fractures off.

TEMPOROMANDIBULAR DISORDERS

DEFINITION

Pain associated with the muscles, articulating structures of the joint, and soft tissue components of the joint including the disc are all included in the general term of temporomandibular disorders. The terminology that is used is extremely confusing and the following is a list of terms that describe either muscle pain, disc or joint problems, or any combination of these, and which are used in reports: myalgia, myofacial pain dysfunction, facial arthromyalgia, myositis, temporomandibular disorders, temporomandibular joint disorders, temporomandibular joint syndrome, temporomandibular pain dysfunction syndromes, oromandibular dysfunction, craniomandibular disorders, mandibular dysfunction disease, degenerative joint disease, Costen's syndrome.

Research diagnostic criteria for temporomandibular disorders have been proposed (Dworkin *et al.*, 1992), but these are very complex and simpler systems have been proposed for use in the clinical setting (Truelove *et al.*, 1992).

Diagnosis in patients who complain primarily of limitation of opening and clicking of the joint is not confused with trigeminal neuralgia. Absence of these symptoms and the presence of pain alone in the temporal area may cause confusion with trigeminal neuralgia.

INCIDENCE

Incidence is difficult to estimate owing to the variety of diagnostic criteria and the wide variability in assessing clinical signs with associated high inter-operator variability (Dworkin *et al.*, 1990b).

Population-based studies in America have shown that as many as 70% of those surveyed have one or more signs of a temporomandibular disorder, and about one-third of those with signs have one or more symptoms (Schiffman and Friction, 1988). However, several studies performed in a hospital setting have shown that less than 7% of clients seek or need therapy (Schiffman *et al.*, 1989; Dworkin *et al.*, 1990a).

Age and sex

Signs and symptoms of temporomandibular disorders first present in the mid-twenties and then become gradually more common in the fourth and fifth decades of life (Agerberg and Bergenholz, 1989; Salonen and Hellden, 1990). Although in population studies there is only a slightly higher proportion of females with signs and symptoms (3:1), a much higher proportion of them come forward for treatment—5:1 (Dworkin *et al.*, 1990a). Patients are likely to be low income earners and unemployed (Dworkin *et al.*, 1990a).

HISTORY (Table 5.7)

Character and severity

Temporomandibular joint pain is often described as a dull ache with a stiff tense sensation (Truelove *et al.*, 1992). The words chosen on the McGill Pain Questionnaire by patients with temporomandibular joint pain include throbbing, shooting, sharp, aching, tender and annoying (Hall *et al.*, 1986). The pain can vary from mild to severe.

Table 5.7   Key diagnostic features: temporomandibular disorders

1. Varying severity of dull, throbbing pain
2. Unilateral or bilateral in pre-auricular area
3. Intermittent pain for years
4. Provoked by jaw movement
5. Often settles after stress relief
6. May find tender spots

Site and radiation

The pain may be bilateral or unilateral, and diagnosis is confused with trigeminal neuralgia only in patients with unilateral symptoms. The pain is principally in the pre-auricular area, and radiates to all the associated musculature, sometimes including the top of the head and neck.

Periodicity and duration

The pain may last for minutes or hours. It may be present for many years before the patient comes forward for treatment, in contrast to the situation in most patients with trigeminal neuralgia.

Provoking factors

Use of the muscle often aggravates the symptoms (Truelove *et al.*, 1992). Pain is experienced not only during all jaw movements but also when palpating the joint or muscles (Dworkin *et al.*, 1990a). The most tender areas, however, do not correspond with nerve branches, which helps to distinguish temporomandibular disorders from trigeminal neuralgia.

Relieving factors

It is a self-limiting disease and many patients find that the pain subsides after resolution of stress factors.

Associated factors

Up to 84% of patients with a chronic temporomandibular disease have a psychological disorder, as diagnosed with the DSMIII (R) classification of the American Psychiatric Association (Kinney *et al.*, 1992). Depression, somatoform pain disorders, anxiety and personality disorders are most frequently encountered, as shown by a number of studies (Speculand *et al.*, 1983; McKinney *et al.*,

1990). However, the proportion of patients with psychological problems is lower than that in other patients with pain (Salter *et al.*, 1983).

Discrete clicking and popping sounds on joint movement are very frequent (Dworkin *et al.*, 1990a). The patients may also complain of tinnitus, vertigo, sensation of bite changes and deviation of the jaw (Truelove *et al.*, 1992). There is often a history of other facial pain (Feinmann *et al.*, 1984).

EXAMINATION

Examination may show some restriction in opening, deviation of the jaws, crepitus of the joint, and tenderness on palpation of the muscles of mastication. There are no neurological abnormalities.

MANAGEMENT

A vast array of treatments have been and are being used that have not been substantiated by well-designed clinical trials. These include simple physiotherapy, jaw rest and relaxation procedures, occlusal splints, occlusal adjustments and equilibration, non-steroidal anti-inflammatory drugs, analgesics, tranquillizers, muscle relaxants, surgery on the joint with open and arthroscopic treatment, and orthodontic and restorative treatments aimed at changing the position or occlusion of the teeth. If occlusal splints are to be used it is important to discontinue their use after 3 months (Harris *et al.*, 1993). If simple non-invasive techniques fail, then tricyclic antidepressants are used (Harris *et al.*, 1993).

Although temporomandibular disorder pain recurs for many years it is a self-limiting condition and there is little progression to physical changes (Dworkin *et al.*, 1990a). Those with abnormal illness behaviour (25%) benefit more from psychological therapy than conservative treatment (Speculand *et al.*, 1983).

ACUTE MAXILLARY SINUSITIS

DEFINITION

A throbbing pain over the cheeks resulting from an infection of one or both maxillary sinuses.

HISTORY (Table 5.8)

Character and severity
The patient complains of a heavy feeling of the face. The pain is described as aching or throbbing and may be severe. It is often more severe in the mornings and evenings.

Table 5.8 Key diagnostic features: sinusitis

1. Moderately severe, throbbing pain
2. Present over one or more sinuses
3. Continuous pain, acute or chronic
4. Worse with movement
5. Decompression gives relief
6. Often nasal discharge

Site and radiation
The pain is felt in the upper part of the cheek and may be unilateral or bilateral. It often radiates over the entire face and to the upper teeth. The unilateral cases may be more difficult to differentiate from trigeminal neuralgia.

Duration
The condition is acute and often follows a cold. It is a continuous pain. In some cases it is due to an oro-antral fistula in relation to dental problems, e.g. extractions. The condition resolves within 1 week if diagnosed correctly and antibiotics instituted.

Provoking factors
Lowering the head, as in bending down, worsens the pain. This is very characteristic and is an important distinguishing feature from trigeminal neuralgia.

Relieving factors
Only decompressing the sinuses by the use of decongestants, e.g. oxymetazoline, or surgery provides relief.

Associated factors
The patient often complains of a foul nasal discharge and a nasal stuffy feeling.

EXAMINATION

If an oro-antral fistula is present, an oral discharge will be found as well as a post-nasal drip. There is tenderness of the cheek and, in some cases, swelling and redness. Percussion of the upper teeth is often painful. The sinus transilluminates.

MANAGEMENT

Radiographs (15° occipital view) will show an opaque antrum or antra. Antibiotics and decongestants are used in the first instance. If a fistula is present it must first be enlarged to allow drainage and then closed once the infection has cleared.

ACUTE FRONTAL SINUSITIS

The history is the same as for maxillary sinusitis except for the location of the pain, which is directly over the sinus with radiation to the vertex or behind the eyes.

ACUTE ETHMOIDITIS

The pain is located between and behind the eyes, and may radiate to the temporal area. Otherwise it has the same characteristics as maxillary sinusitis. It could be confused with trigeminal neuralgia.

ACUTE SPHENOIDAL SINUSITIS

The boring pain is felt deep in the bridge of the nose and nasion, a location in which trigeminal neuralgia is rarely reported.

CHRONIC MAXILLARY SINUSITIS

This is a recurrent infection of the sinus. The symptoms and signs are similar to those of the acute form, but the pain is less severe. A prominent feature is the foul unilateral post-nasal discharge. The patient gives a history of recurrent pain attacks, and so the pain can initially be thought to be paroxysmal.

The condition is often due to dental infection, which must be eradicated to achieve resolution.

CARCINOMA

Very rarely, carcinoma of the maxillary antrum can present as chronic maxillary sinusitis and mimic trigeminal neuralgia. Tumours of the posterior fossa, gasserian ganglion or even other facial structures can present as trigeminal neuralgia. Most often the trigeminal neuralgia is progressive and other symptoms and signs can be found if looked for carefully.

CLASSICAL MIGRAINE

DEFINITIONS

The IASP classification (1986) divides migraine into classical, common and migraine variants. The IHS (1988) diagnostic criteria differentiate between migraine with or without aura, and then describe many variants.

Classical migraine is a unilateral head pain associated with nausea, vomiting and photophobia. The pain is preceded by an aura.

INCIDENCE

Migraine is a common condition: more than five million people suffer from it in the UK (Wilkinson, 1985).

Sex and age
Migraine is commoner in women than in men. The attacks begin in childhood but can start as late as 35 years of age.

HISTORY (Table 5.9)

Character and severity
The pain is described as throbbing or pulsating, never sharp or shooting in character. It gradually builds up into a severe pain and then reaches a plateau—a very different pattern to that of trigeminal neuralgia.

Table 5.9 Key diagnostic features: migraine

1. Severe, throbbing, pulsating pain
2. Unilateral but sides often change
3. Attacks of pain last several hours
4. Patients identify provoking factors
5. Self-limiting
6. Many accompanied by prodromal aura
7. Nausea, vomiting, photophobia

Site and radiation
The pain may be unilateral but is often described as a general head pain. Sides can change and this distinguishes it from trigeminal neuralgia, which changes to the opposite side in only a small proportion of patients.

Periodicity and duration
Each attack of pain lasts for several hours—up to 24 hours if untreated. Successive pain attacks may occur one to four times a month, but they may be more or less frequent. This periodicity is very distinct from trigeminal neuralgia, but the paroxysmal nature of the attacks is similar.

Provoking factors
Some patients have provoking factors such as stress, caffeine, certain foods and mood changes; other have none.

Relieving factors
The attack ends naturally after 4–10 hours in many patients, if they rest in a darkened room. Drugs, if used, may abort the attack.

Associated factors

Nausea, vomiting and photophobia are characteristic features. There is often a pro-dromal phase of mood change, which then leads on to the aura which passes from a blurring of vision and flickering changes in the visual field to scotoma. At this stage there still may be no pain. The pain commonly begins once the aura has finished.

EXAMINATION

During the aura a variety of disturbances may occur, ranging from dysaesthe-sia, aphasia and dysarthria.

COMMON MIGRAINE (MIGRAINE WITHOUT AURA)

DEFINITION

This type of migraine has all the characteristics of classical migraine but with-out the aura. The attacks tend to last longer and are more often bilateral.

MANAGEMENT

For many patients, rest and simple analgesics are enough. If nausea and vomit-ing are a major component, metoclopramide or domperidone should be given before analgesics. Suppositories or parenteral treatment may be necessary if vomiting is severe. Non-steroidal anti-inflammatory drugs can be more effec-tive than paracetamol (Pearce *et al.*, 1983; Johnson *et al.*, 1985).

Ergotamine has been used since the last century, but its side-effects have made it less popular, especially if used long-term. In patients who have frequent attacks that interfere with daily life some form of prophylaxis is indicated.

Propranolol 40 mg twice daily was the first drug used prophylactically and may be effective in 60–80% of patients (Peatfield *et al.*, 1986). Pizotifen, an antag-onist of 5-hydroxytryptamine, can be effective in 40–80% of patients and has the added advantage of being an antidepressant (Sjaastad and Stensrud, 1969). Methysergide is also very effective but, because of its ability to cause retroperi-toneal fibrosis, it should be used only in the short term—4 months (Lance *et al.*, 1963). Calcium channel blockers may be as effective as pizotifen (Olesen, 1986).

A variety of drugs may need to be tried, including aspirin 30 mg daily, until the most effective one for a particular patient has been found. Sumatriptan, both oral and subcutaneous, has also been shown to be effective, but it is short acting and the migraine tends to recur (Dechant and Clissold, 1992).

GIANT CELL ARTERITIS

Synonyms: temporal arteritis, cranial arteritis, polymyalgia rheumatica.

DEFINITION

This condition produces a diffuse aching pain related to the temporal arteries as a result of inflammatory lesions in blood vessels, especially branches of the external carotid artery. It may be a very localized disease, limited to the temporal arteries, or more generalized and associated with pain in the neck, hip or shoulder girdle, when it is more likely to be called polymyalgia rheumatica. It is very responsive to corticosteroids.

INCIDENCE, AGE AND SEX

The condition is unusual in people under 50 years of age and both sexes are affected.

HISTORY (Table 5.10)

Character and severity
The throbbing, aching, burning pain may be severe and intractable.

Table 5.10 Key diagnostic features: giant cell arteries

1. Severe, throbbing, aching pain
2. Unilateral or bilateral temporal areas
3. Intermittent or continuous
4. Worse on chewing
5. Relieved by steroids
6. Often tortuous, thickened arteries

Site and radiation
If the pain is limited to one temporal area, the condition can be confused with trigeminal neuralgia. In some patients pain may radiate to the whole of the head, and this will then be a distinguishing feature.

Duration and periodicity
The pain is intermittent or continuous and may, in some patients, be present for months because of an incorrect diagnosis.

Provoking factors
Chewing can make the pain worse as a result of intermittent claudication of the muscles of mastication.

Relieving factors
Only steroids provide relief.

Associated factors
Involvement of the ophthalmic artery can lead to sudden blindness, which may occur in up to 50% of patients. Other systemic manifestations include malaise, fear, weight loss and depression.

EXAMINATION

The temporal arteries may be thickened, tortuous and tender with loss of pulsation. The same changes may be found in facial and occipital arteries.

MANAGEMENT

Investigations usually show a marked erythrocyte sedimentation rate (ESR)—often over 100 mm h⁻¹—and a mild normochromic anaemia. Biopsy of the temporal arteries may be performed but, if the presentation is classical, it is more important to commence treatment. Patients respond dramatically to systemic steroids and may need treatment for 2 or more years (Schoenen and Maertens de Noordhout, 1994).

ATYPICAL FACIAL PAIN

Synonyms: atypical facial neuralgia, idiopathic facial pain, chronic facial pain.

DEFINITION

Persistent facial pain that does not have the characteristics of the cranial neuralgias and is not associated with physical signs or demonstrable organic cause is the definition put forward by the IHS (1988).

Throughout the literature on trigeminal neuralgia there are numerous references to patients with atypical trigeminal or facial neuralgia who may really have atypical facial pain—a condition in its own right. As early as 1924, Frazier and Russell identified this group of patients. Patients classified as having atypical trigeminal neuralgia do not do well after surgery and some may even complain of more pain afterwards, especially if part of the face has been rendered anaesthetic (Harris and Feinmann, 1990). Other patients develop atypical facial pain after classical trigeminal neuralgia has been treated surgically as a result of the de-afferentation (Loeser, 1984). It is, therefore, important to identify these patients before any surgical procedure is performed, as some will not be helped by surgery (Zakrzewska and Thomas, 1993). Unfortunately, the diagnosis is often used when the cause is unknown and all other terminology has been exhausted (Mock *et al.*, 1985). Atypical facial pain often coexists with facial arthromyalgia (temporomandibular joint dysfunction), atypical odontalgia and oral dysaesthesia (Harris *et al.*, 1993).

FREQUENCY

An estimated 5–7 million Americans suffer from chronic facial pain (Bonica, 1990). At some time in their lives, 25–45% of the population may be affected (Agerberg and Carlsson, 1972).

Age and sex
Atypical facial pain has a high female to male ratio in most series (Mock *et al.*, 1985; Pfaffenrath *et al.*, 1993). The mean age of onset is about 40 years, but the condition can occur in teenagers and the elderly (Feinmann and Harris, 1984; Mock *et al.*, 1985).

HISTORY (Table 5.11)

Character and severity
The character of the pain is extremely variable, ranging from a dull ache to a crushing, sharp, tearing pain (Solomon and Lipton, 1990; Pfaffenrath *et al.*, 1993).

Table 5.11 Key diagnostic features: atypical facial pain

1. Varying severity and character of pain
2. Varies from unilateral, localized to the whole face
3. Continuous with sharp excarberations
4. Provoked by stress
5. Relieved by appropriate treatment
6. Often associated with pain elsewhere in the body

The word most commonly chosen from the McGill Pain Questionnaire is nagging, as shown in an analysis of 195 patients with facial pain (J. Zakrzewska and C. Feinmann, unpublished data) (Fig. 5.1). Melzack *et al.* (1986) showed that the McGill Pain Questionnaire discriminates well between trigeminal neuralgia and atypical facial pain, although we have not found it so useful.

The pain can vary from mild to severe. There is often a marked discrepancy between the description of the severity of the pain and the behaviour of the patient (Solomon and Lipton, 1988; Feinmann and Peatfield, 1993). Patients say the pain is most severe and yet are capable of carrying on with the normal routine of life. I find this particularly noticeable in comparison with patients with trigeminal neuralgia who are having an acute exacerbation of the pain.

Site and radiation
The pain may be unilateral and fairly localized or more diffuse, affecting the non-muscular, non-joint areas of the face (Pfaffenrath *et al.*, 1993). The pain is deep-seated and does not follow any anatomical landmarks (Walker, 1970; Solomon and Lipton, 1990). It becomes bilateral in 20–35% of patients (Solomon and Lipton, 1990).

Frequency
Most patients have continuous pain, although it can have a fluctuating intensity and so mimic trigeminal neuralgia (Pfaffenrath *et al.*, 1993). Many patients give a long history of pain (Feinmann and Harris, 1984).

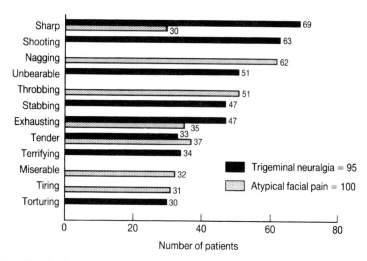

Figure 5.1   Words chosen from the McGill Pain Questionnaire by patients with trigeminal neuralgia or atypical facial pain.

Provoking factors

In many instances the pain occurs in response to stress and adverse life events (Feinmann and Peatfield, 1993). Some may be acute, e.g. bereavement, whereas others can be chronic.

Relieving factors

Many patients seek surgical remedies in the belief that there is a structural lesion; they obtain only temporary relief and the pain may worsen (Pfaffenrath *et al.*, 1993).

Associated factors

Many patients have pain in other parts of the body: headache, neckache, backache, irritable bowel pain and prurutis (Feinmann and Harris, 1984; Mock *et al.*, 1985; Feinmann and Peatfield, 1993).

Depression, anxiety and personality disorders may also be present (Weddington and Blazer, 1979; Mock *et al.*, 1985; Solomon and Lipton, 1990). Psychosocial problems are common, e.g. marital and financial problems or bereavement (Feinmann and Harris, 1984; Speculand *et al.*, 1983), and are often distinguishing features from trigeminal neuralgia (Weddington and Blazer, 1979). Despite the self-reported severity of pain, little life or work impairment occurs (Pfaffenrath *et al.*, 1993).

Up to 75% of patients may undergo unnecessary dental treatment on the assumption that the cause is dental (Mock *et al.*, 1985).

EXAMINATION

This is unremarkable and no neurological abnormalities are observed.

MANAGEMENT

Reassurance and careful explanation is crucial if treatment is to be effective. Patients need to be reassured that the pain is as real as any other type of pain and results from 'cramp' in muscles and blood vessels (Feinmann and Peatfield, 1993). This can be reinforced by an explanatory leaflet.

Up to half of patients may experience relief of symptoms with reassurance together with the administration of simple analgesics. If patients do not respond to this, antidepressants should be prescribed. However, it is essential that patients are first counselled in terms of stress and lifestyle (Feinmann and Peatfield, 1993).

Tricyclic antidepressants with low sedative qualities are preferred, and single nightly doses are used. Patients need treatment for several months and it is common for them to complain of unusual adverse reactions (Feinmann *et al.*, 1984). They must be counselled carefully regarding use of these drugs. Seventy per cent of patients will be pain-free 4 years later; those refractory to treatment will have a complex pain history and psychological problems (Feinmann, 1993).

Psychotherapy and cognitive behaviour therapy may be additional useful techniques, but have not yet been evaluated formally (Solomon and Lipton, 1988). Psychiatric referral, preferably within a pain clinic setting, may be necessary in some patients.

Surgical management is of no benefit and several surgeons have reported on the ineffectiveness of surgical treatments used for trigeminal neuralgia in these patients (Hakanson, 1981; Burchiel, 1988; Solomon and Lipton, 1988).

6

Medical Management

INTRODUCTION

Numerous preparations have been used for the treatment of trigeminal neuralgia. The earliest preparations contained poisons (e.g. hemlock, arsenic, venom of bee and cobra), metals (e.g. iron and copper), opioids, stilbamidine, ergotamine and numerous vitamins (Penman, 1968). However, the major treatments used between 1677 and 1940 were purgatives (1677), hemlock and quinine (1773), ferrous carbonate (1824), gelseminum powder (1874), galvanic therapy (1875), radiation and X-ray therapy (1847), trichloroethylene (1918) and thiamine hydrochloride (1940).

Perhaps the major advance in the management of trigeminal neuralgia occurred in 1876 with the use of the antiepileptic drug potassium bromide. The rationale for its use was based on the hypothesis that the paroxysmal nature of trigeminal neuralgia was probably due to abnormal conduction (Trousseau, 1853). Consequently, the disease was renamed 'neuralgia epileptiform'. However, the new era in the drug management of trigeminal neuralgia did not occur until 1942 when the antiepileptic drug phenytoin became available (Bergouignan, 1942). The next major advance occurred in 1962 when carbamazepine, another antiepileptic drug, was shown not only to be more effective than phenytoin but additionally was associated with fewer side-effects (Blom, 1962). The successful use of two further antiepileptic drugs, namely clonazepam (Caccia, 1975) and valproic acid (Peiris et al., 1980), and the drug baclofen (Fromm et al., 1980) have greatly enhanced the treatment options available for patients with trigeminal neuralgia. More recently, two new antiepileptic drugs, oxcarbazepine and lamotrigine, have shown encouraging antineuralgic properties (Farago, 1987; Zakrzewska and Patsalos, 1989; Remillard, 1994).

The most useful drugs for the management of trigeminal neuralgia at present are carbamazepine, phenytoin, valproic acid and baclofen, with carbamazepine being the drug of choice (Fromm and Terrence, 1987b; Zakrzewska, 1990; Zakrzewska and Patsalos, 1992). In this chapter seven drugs are reviewed in alphabetical order, namely baclofen, carbamazepine, clonazepam, lamotrigine, oxcarbazepine, phenytoin and valproic acid (Table 6.1). Table 6.2 shows the major antineuralgic drug formulations marketed in the UK. These formulations have been developed consequent to: (1) a better understanding of the phar-macokinetics and associated side-effects of the original formulation; (2) the

Table 6.1 Antineuralgic drugs available in the UK

Non-proprietary name	Trade name	Manufacturer	Year Introduced	First report
Phenytoin	Epanutin	Parke-Davis	1938	1942
Carbamazepine	Tegretol	Ciba Pharmaceuticals	1962	1963
Clonazepam	Rivotril	Roche	1974	1975
Sodium valproate (valproic acid)	Epilim	Sanofi–Winthrop	1974	1980
Baclofen	Lioresal	Ciba Pharmaceuticals	1972	1980
Lamotrigine	Lamictal	Wellcome	1991	*
Oxcarbazepine	Trileptal	Ciba Pharmaceuticals	†	1987

*Currently undergoing clinical evaluation; †available as a licensed drug in a number of countries (availability in UK within the next few years).

Table 6.2 Antineuralgic drug formulations available in the UK

Product	Formulation	Year introduced
Epanutin	Capsules	
	25 mg	1977
	50 mg	1975
	100 mg	1938
	300 mg	1992
	Infatab (chewable, spearmint flavoured)	1973
	Parenteral IV	1974
	Suspension	1954
Epilim	Plain tablets	1974*
	Syrup (cherry flavoured)	1976
	Enteric-coated tablets	
	500 mg	1977
	200 mg	1980
	Sugar-free liquid (cherry flavoured)	1983
	Crushable tablets	1983
	Liquid intravenous	1988
Lioresal	Tablets	1972
	Liquid	1986
Tegretol	Tablets	1963
	Liquid (caramel flavoured)	1974
	Chewtabs	1989
	Retard Divitabs	1989
Rivotril	Tablets	1974
Lamictal	Tablets	1991†

*Withdrawn 1983; †not licensed for use in trigeminal neuralgia.

therapeutic need to administer drugs parentally; and (3) patients' desires and needs. The drugs are reviewed in relation to their chemistry, pharmacokinetic characteristics including drug interactions and putative serum therapeutic (target) ranges, side-effects and antineuralgic efficacy. The pharmacokinetic characteristics of each drug are particularly emphasized since dosage regimens based on drug pharmacokinetics will often change a therapeutic failure into a success (Table 6.3). Finally, dosage recommendations are made based on available formulations for each drug.

BACLOFEN

Baclofen, which has been available since 1972, has been evaluated clinically in numerous neurological conditions and is now used effectively in the management of spasticity. Because baclofen resembles carbamazepine and phenytoin in depressing the response of spinal trigeminal neurons to maxillary nerve stimulation in cats, it was used in the management of trigeminal neuralgia; the first report of its use was in 1980 (Fromm *et al.*, 1980).

CHEMISTRY

Baclofen (molecular weight 231.67 Da) is a structural analogue of the naturally occurring brain inhibitory neurotransmitter γ-aminobutyric acid (Fig. 6.1a). It is available as Lioresal 10 mg tablets and as Lioresal Liquid (5 mg per 5 ml). Baclofen is also available generically as 10 mg tablets.

PHARMACOKINETICS

After oral ingestion the absorption of baclofen is rapid, with peak serum concentrations occurring within 3–8 hours. It is largely excreted unchanged by the kidney and has an elimination half-life in blood of 3–4 hours.

SIDE-EFFECTS

The most common side-effects of baclofen are shown in Table 6.4. Drug intolerance occurs in approximately 10% of patients and may be enhanced in those co-administered with carbamazepine.

DRUG INTERACTIONS

Pharmacokinetic drug interactions between baclofen and other drugs used in the treatment of trigeminal neuralgia are not expected (Tables 6.5 and 6.6).

ANTINEURALGIC EFFICACY

There have been three reports (a pilot study and two double-blind studies) on the use of baclofen in trigeminal neuralgia (Fromm *et al.*, 1980, 1984b; Fromm

Table 6.3 Pharmacokinetic characteristics of antineuralgic drugs

Drug	Nature (acid or base)	Bioavailability (%)	Distribution volume ($l\,kg^{-1}$)	Time to maximum concentration (h)	Bound to albumin (%)	Half-life (h)	Time to steady-state concentration (days)*	Therapeutic 'target' range ($\mu\,mol\,l^{-1}$)
Baclofen	Acid	—	—	3-8	—	3-4	1	—
Carbamazepine[†]	Neutral	>70	0.8-1.6	2-8	70-80	11-27	5[‡]	24-43
Clonazepam	Base	100	2.1-4.3	1-2	80-85	24-48	12	30-270
Lamotrigine	Acid	100	0.9-1.2	2-3	50-60	18-30	8	4-16
Oxcarbazepine	Neutral	100	0.3	1-2	40-45[§]	14-26[§]	7	35-110
Phenytoin	Acid	98	0.5-0.7	4-8	90-92	15-20[‖]	14	20-80
Valproic acid[†]	Acid	99	0.09-0.17	1-4	90-92	6-17	5	200-700

*Minimum elapsed time to achieve steady state after initiation of dosage regimen, change in dosage or as a result of a hepatic enzyme inhibitory interaction. Ideal sampling time for measurement of serum concentrations is immediately before ingestion of the next oral dose.

[†]Carbamazepine and valproic acid exhibit significant diurnal variation; sampling time in relation to dose is critical.

[‡]Twenty days if the drug has been introduced for the first time to allow complete autoinduction.

[§]Binding and half-life of the pharmacologically active metabolite 10,11-dihydroxycarbazepine.

[‖]Variability can be much greater due to saturation kinetics.

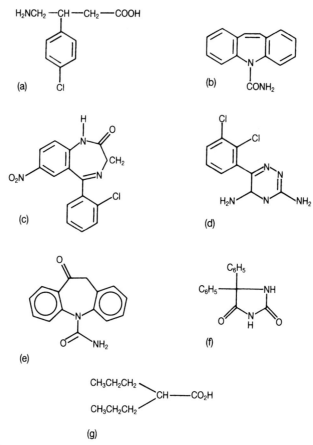

Figure 6.1 Structural representation of the different antineuralgic drugs: (a) baclofen; (b) carbamazepine; (c) clonazepam; (d) lamotrigine; (e) oxcarbazepine; (f) phenytoin; (g) valproic acid.

and Terrence, 1987a). In the pilot study of ten patients, paroxysms of trigeminal neuralgia were relieved with 60–80 mg baclofen per day (Fromm *et al.*, 1980). During 12 months of follow-up, seven patients had been pain-free or almost pain-free. Baclofen and carbamazepine were compared in ten patients with a double-blind protocol and in 50 with an open-label study design (Fromm *et al.*, 1984a). It was concluded that baclofen was not as effective as carbamazepine but that it was effective with phenytoin and was particularly effective in combination with carbamazepine, suggesting a synergistic effect. This synergism between carbamazepine and baclofen has also been reported by other authors (Herring *et al.*, 1982; Baker *et al.*, 1985). Two open studies of 16 and 20 patients with trigeminal neuralgia further confirmed the efficacy of baclofen (Steardo *et al.*, 1984; Parmer *et al.*, 1989). As baclofen is a racemic mixture, with L-baclofen as the active enantiomer (Olpe *et al.*, 1978) and as additionally the D-isomer

Table 6.4 Side-effects associated with antineuralgic therapy

Drug	Dose-related effects	Idiosyncratic effects	Chronic effects
Baclofen	Ataxia, lethargy, fatigue, nausea, vomiting		
Carbamazepine	Ataxia, dizziness, double vision, nausea, vomiting	Rash, reduced white blood cell count	Folate deficiency, hyponatraemia
Clonazepam	Lethargy, fatigue, dizziness	Rash, thrombocytopenia	
Lamotrigine	Ataxia, diplopia, dizziness, headache, irritability, somnolence	Rash	Not yet known
Oxcarbazepine	Ataxia, lethargy, diplopia, nausea, vomiting, hyponatraemia	Rash	Not yet known
Phenytoin	Ataxia, lethargy, nausea, headache, involuntary movements, behavioural change	Rash, pseudolymphoma, hepatitis	Gingival hypertrophy, dysarthria, hirsutism, coarsening of facial features, folate deficiency, intellectual blunting, mood and behavioural changes, cerebellar syndrome
Valproic acid	Irritability, restlessness, tremor, confusion, nausea, vomiting	Gastric irritation, rash	Alopecia, weight gain

antagonises the action of L-baclofen (Terrence *et al.*, 1983), a double-blind study was undertaken to compare L-baclofen and racemic baclofen in a cross-over design in 15 patients (Fromm and Terrence, 1987a). It was observed that L-baclofen was more effective than the racemic mixture in nine patients and that six of these continued to be pain-free 4–17 months (mean 10 months) later. Furthermore, as L-baclofen was better tolerated, it was concluded that L-baclofen represented a significant improvement over racemic baclofen in the management of trigeminal neuralgia.

CURRENT THERAPEUTIC STATUS

Baclofen can be used in patients hypersensitized to carbamazepine. Measurements of serum baclofen concentration are not generally available and individualizing optimum dosage requires careful titration. Treatment can be

Table 6.5 Expected changes in serum concentration when an antineuralgic drug is added to an existing antineuralgic drug regimen

Added drug	Existing drug						
	BCF	CBZ	CZP	LTG	OXC	PHT	VPA
BCF	NA	NA	NA	NA	NA	NA	NA
CBZ	NA	Auto-induction	CZP↓	LTG↓	10-OH-OXC↓	PHT↑↓	VPA↓
CZP	NA	NA	—	NA	NA	PHT↑↓	NA
LTG	NA	CBZ-E↑	NA	Auto-induction?	NA	NA	NA
OXC	NA	NA	NA	NA	—	NA	NA
PHT	NA	CBZ↓	CZP↓	LTG↓	OXC↓ 10-OH-OXC↓	—	VPA↓
VPA	NA	CBZ-E↑	NA	LTG↑	NA	PHT↓↑	—

Abbreviations: BCF, baclofen; CBZ, carbamazepine; CBZ-E, carbamazepine epoxide; CZP, clonazepam; LTG, lamotrigine; OXC, oxcarbazepine; 10-OH-OXC, 10-hydroxycarbazepine; PHT, phenytoin; VPA, valproic acid; NA, no change anticipated.
↑ = increase in serum concentration; ↓ = decrease in serum concentration

Table 6.6 Expected changes in serum concentration when an antineuralgic drug is withdrawn from an existing antineuralgic drug regimen

Withdrawn drug	Existing drug						
	BCF	CBZ	CZP	LTG	OXC	PHT	VPA
BCF	NA	NA	NA	NA	NA	NA	NA
CBZ	NA	Auto-induction	CPZ↑	LTG↑	10-OH-OXC↑	PHT↑↓	VPA↑
CZP	NA	NA	—	NA	NA	PHT↑↓	NA
LTG	NA	CBZ-E↓	NA	Auto-induction?	NA	NA	NA
OXC	NA	NA	NA	NA	—	NA	NA
PHT	NA	CBZ↑	CZP↑	LTG↑	OXC↑ 10-OH-OXC↑	—	VPA↑
VPA	NA	CBZ-E↓	NA	LTG↓	NA	PHT↓↑	—

Abbreviations: BCF, baclofen; CBZ, carbamazepine; CBZ-E, carbamazepine epoxide; CZP, clonazepam; LTG, lamotrigine; OXC, oxcarbazepine; 10-OH-OXC, 10-hydroxycarbazepine; PHT, phenytoin; VPA, valproic acid; NA, no change anticipated.
↑ = increase in serum concentration; ↓ = decrease in serum concentration.

initiated with a starting dose of 5–10 mg three times a day. The dose can then be increased by 10 mg every other day until pain relief is achieved or side-effects occur. The usual maintenance dose is 50–60 mg per day, but a maximum dose of 80 mg daily (20 mg four times a day) may be needed. If pain control is not achieved at this dose, carbamazepine (600 mg per day) or phenytoin (300 mg per day) should be considered in addition. If baclofen is no longer indicated, e.g. the patient is in remission, it should be withdrawn over a 3–4-week period as abrupt withdrawal may result in auditory and visual hallucinations, anxiety and tachycardia. Seizures may also be precipitated.

CARBAMAZEPINE

Carbamazepine, a tricyclic imipramine, was first described and synthesized in 1961 (Shindler, 1961). Its antineuralgic and antiepileptic properties were reported in the subsequent 2 years, and today carbamazepine is a major first-line antiepileptic drug, the drug of choice in the management of trigeminal neuralgia, and is also useful in the management of affective disorders (Blom, 1962; Theobald and Kunz, 1963; Elpick,1989).

CHEMISTRY

Carbamazepine, an iminostilbene derivative (molecular weight 236.26 Da), is a white crystalline compound that is virtually insoluble in water but highly soluble in ethanol, chloroform and other solvents (Fig. 6.1b). Carbamazepine is formulated as Tegretol to contain 100, 200 or 400 mg carbamazepine per tablet. Other Tegretol products include Liquid (100 mg per 5 ml), Chewtabs (100 and 200 mg) and Retard Divitabs (200 and 400 mg). Generic formulations of carbamazepine are also available.

PHARMACOKINETICS

Carbamazepine is slowly but almost completely absorbed from the gastrointestinal tract, with peak blood concentrations achieved within 2–8 hours. However, absorption rate can be erratic and unpredictable in chronic use (Morselli, 1989). As carbamazepine is poorly water-soluble, ingestion with food with concurrent release of gastic juices and bile can enhance absorption. Although no intravenous form of carbamazepine is available, the oral bioavailability of the capsule formulation has been estimated to exceed 70% (Bertilsson, 1978). Carbamazepine is approximately 80% bound to serum proteins, primarily albumin, and is distributed throughout the body.

Carbamazepine has some rather unique pharmacokinetic properties, which make its clinical use somewhat difficult:

1. A substantial intra- and inter-individual variation in serum concentrations occurs with the same dose in different patients (Elyas *et al.*, 1986; Macphee *et al.*, 1987).
2. It is extensively metabolized to carbamazepine-10,11-epoxide, which is present in blood and has been shown to have antineuralgic properties and to contribute to the side-effects associated with carbamazepine (Tomson and Bertilsson, 1984; Patsalos *et al.*, 1985; Bertilsson and Tomson, 1986; Gillham *et al.*, 1988).
3. Upon initiation of carbamazepine therapy, an elimination half-life of 20–40 hours can be expected. However, during chronic therapy, its half-life is decreased to 11–27 hours consequent to autoinduction (i.e. it induces its own hepatic metabolism). During combination therapy with

phenytoin, a carbamazepine half-life of 5–14 hours can expected (Eichelbaum *et al.*, 1975, 1979).

The extent of carbamazepine autoinduction of metabolizing enzymes, and possibly heteroinduction by other drugs (e.g. phenytoin), is considered to be responsible for the considerable diurnal variation in serum carbamazepine concentrations (Macphee *et al.*, 1987). Average variations of 80–90% are not uncommon and have been associated with intermittent neurotoxic side-effects (nausea, dizziness, diplopia and headache) coinciding with peak serum concentrations of the drug. By increasing the dosing frequency, these side-effects can be minimized, although often at the expense of patient compliance.

Pharmacokinetically, the new controlled-release formulation (Tegretol Retard Divitab) is very advantageous because the formulation was designed to reduce the significant diurnal variation in carbamazepine serum concentrations, to allow a reduction in dosing frequency to once or twice daily and also, since high serum peak concentrations are avoided, to enable the use of larger dosage regimens and thus achieve better pain control.

In a recent study comparing monotherapy Tegretol conventional versus Tegretol Retard, carbamazepine fluctuations decreased from 41 ± 3% to 28 ± 2% (McKee *et al.*, 1991). However, lower mean serum carbamazepine concentrations were observed with Tegretol Retard, suggesting that upon substitution a higher dose may be needed if pain control is to be maintained. Further, it should be emphasized that the different controlled-release formulations that are available (e.g. Timonil Retard, Neurotol Slow) should not be used interchangeably since significant differences in bioavailability have been observed (Jensen *et al.*, 1990; Reunanen *et al.*, 1992).

The chewable carbamazepine tablet (Tegretol Chewtabs), formulated for possible use by patients who have difficulty swallowing, is bioequivalent to the conventional formulation and thus can be used interchangeably (Patsalos, 1990; Patsalos *et al.*, 1990b).

Carbamazepine is also available in generic formulations of 100 and 200 mg tablets. However, caution needs to be practised when substituting one brand with another since biological equivalence may not occur (Hartley *et al.*, 1990; Welty *et al.*, 1992; Gilman *et al.*, 1993). Thus optimal pain control may be lost or toxicity may present after substitution.

SIDE-EFFECTS

Approximately 20% of patients treated with carbamazepine experience some side-effects; the most common are shown in Table 6.4 (Gram and Jensen, 1989). Haematological adverse reactions account for 6% of the total, and the incidence of symptoms is higher in the elderly and in those in whom the drug is introduced rapidly, or if the dose is increased rapidly.

These side-effects are usually mild and reversible. A 12–17% incidence of carbamazepine-associated folic acid deficiency and megaloblastic anaemia without associated peripheral neuropathy has been reported (Goggin *et al.*, 1987). Carbamazepine hypersensitivity takes the form of an allergic rash. This is seen in 5–10% of patients starting carbamazepine (Sillanpaa, 1981; Zakrzewska and Ivanyi, 1988). The rash usually develops within months of the initiation of therapy, is non-specific in type and resolves on discontinuation of treatment. More serious hypersensitivity reactions include the Stevens–Johnson syndrome, Lyell syndrome, dermatitis bullosa and an exfoliative dermatitis. Fortunately these are very rare indeed; however, if a patient develops oral ulceration in addition to a rash, this may herald the onset of a Stevens–Johnson reaction, and is an indication for immediate cessation of therapy and prescription of corticosteroids.

Carbamazepine at high concentrations has an antidiuretic hormone-stimulating effect that can produce fluid retention in patients with cardiac failure and in the elderly. Risk of hyponatraemia increases with age and higher carbamazepine serum concentrations (Lahr, 1985). Mild hyponatraemia is usually asymptomatic but if serum sodium falls below 120 mmol l^{-1} the patient may present with confusion and peripheral oedema.

DRUG INTERACTIONS

Carbamazepine is a potent hepatic enzyme inducer and also it indues its own metabolism (autoinduction), usually within 3–5 weeks. Carbamazepine metabolism is also highly inducible by other drugs. The metabolism of carbamazepine can also be inhibited, resulting in an increase in carbamazepine serum concentrations and greater risk of toxic effects. Thus drug interactions between carbamazepine and other antineuralgic drugs (Tables 6.5 and 6.6), and also with drugs used to treat other medical conditions, are common (Patsalos and Duncan, 1993; Patsalos, 1994).

Recently numerous drugs (e.g. lamotrigine, valproic acid and viloxazine) have been reported to inhibit selectively the metabolism of carbamazepine to its epoxide metabolite (carbamazepine-10,11-epoxide) or the subsequent metabolism of the epoxide (Pisani *et al.*, 1986; McKee *et al.*, 1992; Warner *et al.*, 1992). In the case of valproic acid, serum carbamazepine epoxide concentrations can be quadrupled in some patients (Rambeck *et al.*, 1990). These interactions may have considerable clincial significance, particularly since there is increasing evidence to suggest that the epoxide may contribute not only to the efficacy of carbamazepine but also to its toxicity (Patsalos *et al.*, 1985; Gillham *et al.*, 1988). Furthermore, these interactions may result in precipitation of neurological toxicity and may pass undetected since therapeutic drug monitoring of the epoxide is not commonly undertaken and carbamazepine concentrations are essentially unchanged.

The macrolide antibiotics, erythromycin, josamycin, triacelyloleandomycin, clarithromycin and ponsinomycin, have also been associated with carbamazepine toxicity. Erythromycin, in particular, strongly inhibits carbamazepine metabolism causing an up to threefold increase in serum concentration.

Toxicity (confusion, semnolence, ataxia, vertigo, nausea and vomiting) presents quickly after starting erythromycin therapy and is rapidly reversed upon withdrawal of the antibiotic. The severity of the interaction depends on the duration of antibiotic therapy. The monitoring of serum carbamazepine concentrations is advisable when macrolide therapy is contemplated.

Calcium channel blockers have variable effects on carbamazepine metabolism. Whilst nifedipine does not exhibit any significant interaction with carbamazepine, verapamil and diltiazem can almost double carbamazepine serum concentrations, resulting in toxic side-effects (Bahl *et al.*, 1991).

Cimetidine inhibits the metabolism of carbamazepine in a dose-dependent manner (Dalton *et al.*, 1986) and in clinical practice a 20–30% increase in serum carbamazepine concentrations can be expected during combination therapy. In some patients with peptic ulcers, the uptake of cimetidine may continue for a long time and thus the clinical significance of this interaction may increase with time as carbamazepine accumulates. For patients on carbamazepine, an alternative H_2-antagonist, such as ranitidine or famotidine, that is devoid of hepatic enzyme inhibitory effects, is indicated.

Isoniazid and nafimidone inhibit carbamazepine metabolism and increase serum carbamazepine concentrations by as much as twofold, with resultant signs of carbamazepine intoxication (Valsalan and Cooper, 1982). Carbamazepine metabolism is also inhibited by danazol, fluoxetine, fluvoxamine, propoxyphene and viloxazine (Patsalos and Duncan, 1993). As propoxyphene has only moderate efficacy as an analgesic, patients taking carbamazepine should avoid analgesic preparations containing propoxyphene and should use ibuprofen or codeine.

Carbamazepine increases the metabolism and lowers the serum concentration of a wide variety of concurrently administered drugs including the antiepileptic drugs phenytoin, primidone, valproic acid, clonazepam and ethosuximide. Drugs whose clinical effects may be significantly affected include oral anticoagulants, steroidal oral contraceptives, β-blockers, haloperidol, felodipine, and theophylline (Crawford *et al.*, 1990; Duncan *et al.*, 1991). The clinical significance of these interactions is variable and dosage adjustments may become necessary in some patients.

Finally, patients with highly induced hepatic enzymes may show a depressed response to the low-dose dexamethasone suppression test and to the oral metyrapone test even though adrenopituitary function is normal. This can be attributed to induction of steroid and metyrapone metabolism respectively.

ANTINEURALGIC EFFICACY

The pharmacological effect of carbamazepine is highly specific in that it relieves the pain only of trigeminal neuralgia. As other types of facial pain are unaffected by carbamazepine, it has been suggested that therapeutic benefit with this drug can be used as a diagnostic indicator (Illingworth, 1986; Killian and Fromm, 1968).

Early trials with carbamazepine are rather difficult to interpret since patients with atypical facial pain were included. Furthermore, the criteria for success (a difficulty in standardizing in any pain condition) were variable, with most results being classified as complete, partial or no relief of pain. Another difficulty is related to the fact that patient evaluation varied from 2 weeks to 5.5 years (Rockliff and Davis, 1966; Kiluk *et al.*, 1968; Sturman and O'Brien, 1969; Rasmussen and Rushede, 1970).

Approximately 70–80% of patients treated with carbamazepine respond well: 73–88% of these gain relief within 24 hours and 94% by 48 hours (Kiluk *et al.*, 1968; Rasmussen and Rushede, 1970; Sillanpaa, 1981; Tomsom and Ekbom, 1981). There is a significant lack of long-term studies of the efficacy of carbamazepine. In a series of 143 patients evaluated during a 16 year period, of the 69% who initially had therapeutic benefit from carbamezepine therapy, only 56% still had pain control 10 years later (Taylor *et al.*, 1981).

The interrelationship between carbamazepine dose and serum concentrations of carbamazepine and carbamazepine-epoxide and clinical efficacy was systematically investigated in a series of seven patients with trigeminal neuralgia (Tomson *et al.*, 1980). Carbamazepine serum concentrations and antineuralgic effect were significantly correlated in six patients and a serum therapeutic (target) range of 24–43 μmol l^{-1} was recommended. Side-effects were noted in two patients, both with carbamazepine serum concentrations in excess of 33 μmol l^{-1}. In a further study of six patients with trigeminal neuralgia, in which carbamazepine was substituted with carbamazepine epoxide, the two were comparable in efficacy (Tomson and Bertilsson, 1984). However, on a serum concentration basis, carbamazepine epoxide had a considerably higher pain-relieving potency than carbamazepine. Interestingly no side-effects were seen during carbamazepine epoxide therapy, suggesting that side-effects with the epoxide may in part be pharmacodynamic (acting at a common receptor) with carbamazepine. More recently a study was undertaken to investigate the efficacy of carbamazepine in neuralgic pain and to determine a therapeutic serum concentration range for carbamazepine (Moosa *et al.*, 1993). Of the 31 patients studied only 10 had trigeminal neuralgia (13 reflex sympathetic dystrophy, 4 post-hepatic neuralgia, 4 phantom limb). Significant correlation was observed between both carbamazepine and carbamazepine epoxide serum concentrations and pain control. The therapeutic serum concentration range for carbamazepine in this study of neuralgia, which was defined as the range of concentrations that would be expected to provide a 25–75% reduction in pain in 50% of patients, was 8–29 μmol l^{-1}.

CURRENT THERAPEUTIC STATUS

Carbamazepine is the drug of choice for the treatment of trigeminal neuralgia. The drug must be introduced at a low dose to offset the development of neurotoxicity, especially in elderly patients (e.g. 100 mg daily). If the pain is not too severe, a dose increase of 100 mg every 3 days should be made until pain control is achieved. Despite this careful approach, a few patients are unable to tolerate the central nervous system side-effects of the drug, with diplopia, dizziness and nausea being the most common complaints. Tolerance usually develops to these symptoms and the problem may be lessened by prescribing the controlled released formulation of carbamazepine.

Proportionately more of the daily drug dosage should be taken at night so that adequate serum concentrations are present in the early morning when most pain occurs. Provoking factors, e.g. shaving, brushing of teeth, face washing and eating tend to be prevalent in the morning. After approximately 20 days the dosage may have to be increased owing to the autoinduction characteristics of carbamazepine, which results in lower serum carbamazepine concentrations. Once complete pain control has been maintained for 1 month, the drug can be slowly withdrawn at a rate of 100 mg every 3–7 days. If pain returns, the dose should be increased again. The only way to determine whether there has been a remission is to withdraw the drug. It is therefore useful for patients to keep pain diaries.

As a result of the poor correlation between carbamazepine dose and serum carbamazepine concentrations, therapeutic drug monitoring is invaluable for optimizing and individualizing carbamazepine therapy. However, in most clinical settings, therapeutic drug monitoring is used only to check compliance or when the patient has unexpected side-effects. A therapeutic (target) range of 24–43 μmol l^{-1} should be targeted (Tomson *et al.*, 1980) and monitoring undertaken 5 days after a dose change, or serum concentration results will be underestimated. If a patient is exposed to carbamazepine for the first time, 20 days need to elapse (to allow autoinduction to complete) before therapeutic drug monitoring is undertaken. If autoinduction is not completed, serum concentration results will overestimate the efficacy of carbamazepine. If side-effects develop (e.g. ataxia or drowsiness) and if autoinduction has already occurred, the dose should be decreased by 100 mg. An average effective dose is 200 mg four times a day. Haematological and biochemical screens should be done before treatment and then 1 month after commencement of treatment, and thereafter perhaps at 6-monthly intervals, particularly if the patient continues on a high dose (more than 1000 mg per day) or is experiencing severe side-effects.

Finally, if adequate pain control is not achieved with carbamazepine, consideration should be given to duotherapy with phenytoin or baclofen. If phenytoin is added, treatment should be guided by monitoring serum concentration so that potentially toxic phenytoin concentrations are avoided (see section on phenytoin) and also to avoid problematic pharmacokinetic interactions (Tables 6.5 and 6.6).

CLONAZEPAM

Clonazepam has been used in the management of trigeminal neuralgia since 1975 (Caccia, 1975) and for the treatment of epilepsy and myoclonus since 1973 (Browne and Penry, 1973).

CHEMISTRY

Clonazepam (molecular weight 315.7 Da), a light yellow crystalline powder, is a chlorinated derivative of nitrazepam and is virtually undissociated throughout the physiological pH range (Fig. 6.1c; Kaplan *et al.*, 1974). Clonazepam is available as Rivotril (0.5 and 2.0 mg) tablets or liquid (1 mg ml^{-1}).

PHARMACOKINETICS

After oral ingestion, clonazepam is well absorbed with maximum blood concentrations being achieved within 1–2 hours. Clonazepam is approximately 80% bound to albumin. The blood half-life is 1–2 days and the relationship between dose and serum concentration is linear (Kaplan *et al.*, 1974).

SIDE-EFFECTS

Approximately 50% of patients taking clonazepam experience side-effects (drowsiness, fatigue, dizziness). However, during chronic use tolerance develops to these effects (Table 6.4).

DRUG INTERACTIONS

During co-medication with hepatic enzyme-inducing drugs such as carbamazepine or phenytoin, clonazepam concentrations can be expected to decrease; this may be associated with loss of pain control. Thus an increase in clonazepam dosage may be necessary.

ANTINEURALGIC EFFICACY

In the first report of the use of clonazepam in trigeminal neuralgia five of seven patients experienced significant benefit, but this was associated with marked drowsiness (Caccia, 1975). In a series of 19 patients studied over 18 months, 13 patients reported excellent or good response to clonazepam (0.1 mg per kg body-weight per day) and with no serious side-effects noted (Chandra, 1976). In a further series of 25 patients, 16 of whom were refractory to carbamazepine therapy, ten experienced complete pain control and six patients significant pain control (Court and Kase, 1976). However, the clonazepam dose used in this study (6–8 mg per day) was associated with drowsiness and ataxia in 85% of patients. Finally, in 21 patients with various neuralgias, of whom 14 were trigeminal neuralgia cases, doses of 1.5–6 mg per day clonazepam were used and were effective in 64% of patients. Side-effects were experienced only at daily doses of 6 mg, while none was reported at 3 mg (Smirne and Scarlato, 1977).

CURRENT THERAPEUTIC STATUS

Clonazepam is used only occasionally, usually when carbamazepine is contra-indicated, and is effective in only a small proportion of cases. The dose-dependent side-effects are reduced if two or three divided doses are taken daily. Dosage may be increased every 3–7 days by 0.5 mg per day. Doses of 4–8 mg daily have been found to be effective, but a dose of 1.5 mg per day is more commonly used. A putative therapeutic (target) range of 30–270 µmol l⁻¹ (based on studies of antiepileptic efficacy) is reasonable and serum monitoring should not be undertaken until 12 days after a dose change. During co-medication with carbamazepine, a higher dose may be necessary to compensate for the hepatic enzyme-inducing effects of carbamazepine.

LAMOTRIGINE

Lamotrigine became available in the UK for use in the management of epilepsy in 1991 and is currently licensed in numerous countries worldwide (Sander *et al.*, 1989; Loiseau *et al.*, 1990; Patsalos and Duncan, 1994; Patsalos and Sander, 1994). Its efficacy in trigeminal neuralgia is currently under clinical investigation.

CHEMISTRY

A white powder with low water-solubility, lamotrigine has a molecular weight of 256.09 Da and a pK_a of 5.5 (Fig. 6.1d). It is formulated as Lamictal 25, Lamictal 50 and Lamictal 100 containing 25, 50 and 100 mg lamotrigine respectively.

PHARMACOKINETICS

After oral ingestion, lamotrigine is rapidly and completely absorbed, with blood concentrations peaking 2–3 hours later (Posner *et al.*, 1991). It is approximately 60% bound to serum proteins and exhibits linear kinetics within the currently recommended therapeutic (target) range of 4–16 µmol l⁻¹ (Ramsey *et al.*, 1991). Lamotrigine is extensively metabolized by glucuronidation with 8% of the dose excreted unchanged in urine and 63% as a glucuronide. In healthy adult volunteers the mean elimination half-life of lamotrigine is approximately 24 (range 18–30) hours, whilst in the elderly it is 31 hours. The clinical relevance of a recent study in healthy volunteers suggesting that its metabolism may undergo autoinduction is uncertain (Yau *et al.*, 1992).

SIDE-EFFECTS

Side-effects commonly associated with lamotrigine therapy are primarily central nervous system related (Table 6.4). Overall, 8.6% of patients with epilepsy evaluated with lamotrigine have been withdrawn because of side-effects. These have included rash, dizziness, diplopia, somnolence, headache, ataxia, irritability and increases in seizure frequency (Betts *et al.*, 1991). The most common cause of withdrawal of lamotrigine therapy has been allergic cutaneous rash. Data from open studies demonstrate an overall rash rate of 10.8% (Yuen, 1992). The rash, which may be severe and is usually generalized maculopapular or erythema multiforme in nature, and has been described as Stevens–Johnson syndrome in two patients, resolves upon lamotrigine withdrawal (Betts *et al.*, 1991; Yuen, 1992). Alterations in biochemical and haematological parameters, including plasma and erythrocyte folate concentrations, have not been reported as clinically significant (Ramsey *et al.*, 1991; Sander and Patsalos, 1992).

DRUG INTERACTIONS

In patients with epilepsy already receiving enzyme-inducing antiepileptic drugs (e.g. phenobarbitone, carbamazepine, phenytoin, primidone) the half-life of lamotrigine is reduced from a mean of 24 to 15 (range 8–33) hours. In patients taking valproic acid only, the mean half-life of lamotrigine is increased to approximately 59 (range 31–89) hours. Finally, in patients on a combination of enzyme-inducing antiepileptic drugs and valproic acid, mean half-life values of approximately 24 hours have been reported (Jawad *et al.*, 1987). Thus, in prescribing lamotrigine, a different lamotrigine dosage strategy needs to be used depending on the patient's concomitant antineuralgic drug medication. Although lamotrigine does not affect the metabolism of commonly prescribed antineuralgic drugs, the possibility that it may inhibit the metabolism of carbamazepine epoxide, the pharmacologically active primary metabolite of carbamazepine, needs to be considered (Tables 6.5 and 6.6; Warner *et al.*, 1992)

ANTINEURALGIC EFFICACY

Anecdotal evidence suggests that lamotrigine may have antineuralgic properties. Clinical studies are presently underway to ascertain the efficacy characteristics of lamotrigine in trigeminal neuralgia.

CURRENT THERAPEUTIC STATUS

It is too early to ascertain the role of lamotrigine in the management of trigeminal neuralgia. The need to introduce lamotrigine slowly, so as to avoid induction of rash, may limit its use where acute intolerable pain needs to be resolved quickly.

OXCARBAZEPINE

Oxcarbazepine is a keto derivative of carbamazepine, and has been marketed in a number of countries since 1991. Current experience suggests that oxcarbazepine is equal and in some cases superior to carbamazepine in the treatment of those with epilepsy and in patients with trigeminal neuralgia (Farago, 1987; Dam *et al.*, 1989; Zakrzewska and Patsalos, 1989; Remillard, 1994).

CHEMISTRY

Oxcarbazepine is chemically related to carbamazepine (both consist of a dibenzapine nucleus) with a carboxamide group attached in the 5 position, but differs from carbamazepine by having a keto group in the 10 position instead of a double bond between positions 10 and 11. It is a neutral lipophilic compound with minimal aqueous solubility (Fig. 6.1e). Oxcarbazepine is formulated as Trileptal tablets containing 300 and 800 mg oxcarbazepine.

PHARMACOKINETICS

After oral ingestion the absorption of oxcarbazepine is rapid and essentially complete within 1–2 hours (Feldman *et al.*, 1981). Maximum blood concentrations of oxcarbazepine are achieved within 1 hour and by 3 hours the drug is not detectable in blood. Since oxcarbazepine is rapidly metabolized to a pharmacologically active metabolite, 10,11-dihydroxycarbazepine, it can be considered a pro-drug. 10,11-Dihydroxycarbazepine has a half-life of 14–26 hours in healthy volunteers (Theisohn and Heimann, 1982; Dickinson *et al.*, 1989). Approximately 70% and 40% of oxcarbazepine and 10,11-dihydroxycarbazepine respectively is bound to serum proteins (Patsalos *et al.*, 1990a). Oxcarbazepine is excreted via the kidney as 10,11-dihydroxycarbazepine, of which 50% is glucuronidated (Dickinson *et al.*, 1989). Its elimination has been described as biphasic since more rapid elimination occurs at lower serum concentrations of the drug (Theisohn and Heimann, 1982; van Heiningen *et al.*, 1991). The reason for this is not clear, but may be due to a minor pathway of elimination that is fast but saturable. However, as this non-linearnity occurs only at serum concentrations below the lower limit of the therapeutic (target) range, its clinical significance is minimal. Oxcarbazepine dose correlates significantly with both oxcarbazepine and 10,11-dihydroxycarbazepine serum concentrations (Zakrzewska and Patsalos, 1989; Patsalos *et al.*, 1990a).

SIDE-EFFECTS

Clinical interest in oxcarbazepine evolved because of its lack of hepatic enzyme induction and because it is not metabolized to an active epoxide metabolite, which has been attributed to carbamazepine-associated side-effects (Patsalos *et al.*, 1985; Gillham *et al.*, 1988). Clinical studies to date, primarily in patients with epilepsy, have suggested an improved tolerability with oxcarbazepine compared with carbamazepine (Houtkooper *et al.*, 1987; Reinikainen *et al.*, 1987; Dam *et al.*, 1989). While the incidence of allergic reaction is lower and psychomoter impairment is less during oxcarbazepine therapy, hyponatraemia may be as common with oxcarbazepine as with carbamazepine (Zakrzewska and Patsalos, 1989; Steinhoff *et al.*, 1992). Carbamazepine-associated skin rashes have been reported both to resolve (Jensen *et al.*, 1986; Houtkooper *et al.*, 1987; Zakrzewska and Patsalos, 1989) and to cross-react by approximately 25% (Jensen *et al.*, 1986; Beran, 1993) with oxcarbazepine.

DRUG INTERACTIONS

Unlike carbamazepine and phenytoin, which are metabolized by hepatic cytochrome P450-dependent enzymes, oxcarbazepine is metabolized by ketone reductase and glucuronyl-transferase enzymes (Faigle and Menge, 1990). These enzymes are less prone to induction and inhibitory effects, and consequently oxcarbazepine exhibits no or very weak enzyme induction (Dickinson *et al.*, 1989; Patsalos *et al.*, 1990c; Larkin *et al.*, 1991). Although clinically significant interactions with oxcarbazepine have not been reported to date, carbamazepine and phenytoin have recently been reported to induce the metabolism of 10,11-dihydroxycarbazepine (Tartara *et al.*, 1993; McKee *et al.*, 1994). The clinical significance of these interactions needs to be ascertained.

ANTINEURALGIC EFFICACY

Clinical experience of oxcarbazepine has primarily been in patients with epilepsy. Doses used ranged from 600 to 3600 mg per day and a substitution dose ratio of 3 oxcarbazepine for 2 carbamazepine was used. Only three studies have reported on the antineuralgic efficacy of oxcarbazepine (Farago, 1987; Zakrzewska and Patsalos, 1989; Remillard, 1994).

In the first report, 13 patients with trigeminal neuralgia were treated with oxcarbazepine over 1–43 (mean 11) months (Farago, 1987). Oxcarbazepine treatment resulted in either a reduction in pain or complete pain control in all patients. In six patients the onset of effect occurred within 24 hours, in four within 48 hours and in three within 72 hours. The effective dose in most patients was 10–20 mg per kg body-weight. Side-effects (sensation of heat in stomach) occurred in only one patient. In a subsequent study of six patients with trigeminal neuralgia intractable to carbamazepine, all experienced an excellent therapeutic response with onset of pain control within 24 hours (Zakrzewska and Patsalos, 1989). An overall serum therapeutic concentration range in the six patients of 50–110 μmol l⁻¹ of 10,11-dihydroxycarbazepine, corresponding to a daily effective dose range of 1200–2400 mg (14.6–35.6 mg per kg body-weight) oxcarbazepine, was observed. Oxcarbazepine was well tolerated and no significant side-effects were identified, although mild hyponatraemia was observed during high dosage (>28–35 mg kg⁻¹ day⁻¹).

More recently an open trial of 15 patients treated with oxcarbazepine over 20–44 months has been reported (Remillard, 1994). Patients were switched from carbamazepine to oxcarbazepine over a 7–10-day period. Thirteen of the 15 patients experienced pain reduction, with ten being pain-free at dosages of

900–1800 mg per day (one patient had intermittent dosage increases up to 2.4 g per day). Three patients experienced pain control with dosages over 2 g per day. Side-effects were not intolerable, were self-limiting, were often related to higher doses and comprised those indicated in Table 6.4.

CURRENT THERAPEUTIC STATUS

Double-blind studies and direct comparisons of oxcarbazepine and carbamazepine in patients with epilepsy suggest that the two drugs are of equal efficacy. However, oxcarbazepine has a much better tolerability profile and thus higher doses can be used. Although double-blind studies comparing oxcarbazepine with carbamazepine have not been undertaken in patients with trigeminal neuralgia, open studies indicate an impressive antineuralgic efficacy for oxcarbazepine. The dosing strategy is similar to that of carbamazepine except that 300 mg increments are used and a dose of 1200 mg per day is often effective. A therapeutic range for 10,11-dihydroxycarbazepine of 35–110 μmol l^{-1} should be targeted (Farago, 1987; Zakrzewska and Patsalos, 1989) and serum monitoring undertaken 7 days after a dose change if patient is on oxcarbazepine monotherapy.

Oxcarbazepine can also be effective when prescribed with phenytoin. Since the enzyme-inducing effect of oxcarbazepine is less than that of carbamazepine, on changing patient medication from carbamazepine to oxcarbazepine it may be necessary to reduce the dosage of concurrent medication. Finally, it is recommended that blood sodium concentration is monitored regularly during oxcarbazepine therapy.

PHENYTOIN

Phenytoin (diphenylhydantoin) was synthesized in 1908 (Biltz, 1908), first tested for possible hypnotic properties, and licensed for use in the management of epilepsy in 1938 (Meritt and Putnam, 1938). Phenytoin was first reported to be effective in the management of trigeminal neuralgia in 1942 (Bergouignan, 1942).

CHEMISTRY

Phenytoin, a white crystalline bitter-tasting powder, has a molecular weight of 252.28 Da and a pK$_a$ of 8.06 (Fig. 6.1f). It is soluble in aqueous bases and solvents (e.g. acetone, ethanol and chloroform) but only sparingly soluble in water and insoluble in acids.

Phenytoin first became available as a 100 mg Epanutin capsule (sodium phenytoin: equivalent to 92 mg phenytoin on a molecular weight basis). However, in the late 1960s and early 1970s, as serum concentration measurement techniques became widely available and it was observed that phenytoin undergoes dose-dependent or saturation elimination (Fig. 6.2 and see Pharmacokinetics below), it became apparent that individualizing drug therapy with only a 100 mg capsule formulation was clinically very difficult. Individualizing drug therapy with phenytoin became more feasible with the introduction of 25, 50 and 300 mg capsules (Table 6.2). These are formulated to contain 23, 46 and 276 mg phenytoin acid per capsule respectively. Other Epanutin products include chewable tablets (Infatabs) containing 50 mg phenytoin acid per tablet, a ready mixed suspension containing 30 mg phenytoin acid per 5 ml and a ready mixed parenteral solution containing 250 mg phenytoin sodium per 5 ml. Allowances should be made for differences in molecular weight between acid and sodium phenytoin when a patient's treatment is changed from one formulation to another. This principle was emphasized recently in a study of 20 adult volunteers in which Epanutin 25, 50 and 100 mg capsules, Epanutin Infatabs and suspension were compared (Sorayal *et al.*, 1991). While the three Epanutin capsule formulations were observed to be bioequivalent, and therefore could be used interchangeably during dosage titration, the Infatabs and suspension formulations were bioequivalent only when adjustments in dosage were made for phenytoin content.

Phenytoin is also available in various generic and brand name preparations and there are many reports of therapeutically inequivalent phenytoin products (Tyrer *et al.*, 1970; Melikian *et al.*, 1977; Sawchuk *et al.*, 1982; Mikati *et al.*, 1992). These products can differ significantly in both bioavailability and absorption (serum phenytoin concentrations can vary by as much as 20%) and thus patients should be treated with the drug product of a single manufacturer.

PHARMACOKINETICS

After oral ingestion phenytoin is rapidly absorbed with peak blood concentrations being achieved by 4–8 hours. However, peak concentrations may be achieved as early as 3 hours or as late as 12 hours, and the time to peak is independent of dose (Dill *et al.*, 1956; Sawchuk *et al.*, 1982). Its bioavailability is estimated to be 98% and phenytoin is primarily absorbed in the duodenum (Noach and van Rees, 1964). In the stomach, little absorption of phenytoin occurs because it is insoluble at the pH of gastric juice (about 2.0). Phenytoin is approximately 90% bound to serum proteins, primarily albumin (Hooper *et al.*, 1975). It exhibits an unusual pharmacokinetic property in that its metabolic elimination by the liver is zero-order at therapeutic doses (Remmer *et al.*, 1969; Bochner *et al.*, 1972; Richens and Dunlop, 1975). Thus, as the serum phenytoin concentration increases, the capacity of the hepatic mono-oxygenase enzyme system to metabolize the drug becomes saturated and a small increment in dose can produce an unexpectedly substantial rise in serum concentration (Fig. 6.2). Conversely, serum concentrations can decrease precipitously when the dose is modestly reduced.

Furthermore, this interrelationship between dose and serum concentration is substantially different in different patients, and therapeutic drug monitoring of

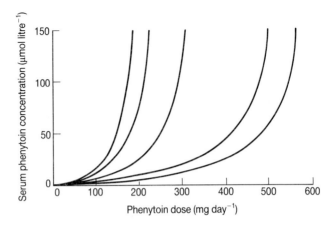

Figure 6.2   Phenytoin dose versus serum concentration for five patients. As a result of saturation kinetics, a small increase in dosage can result in a disproportionate increase in serum concentration. Wide interindividual variability is evident.

phenytoin is particularly invaluable in optimizing drug dosage to each patient's individual therapeutic requirement.

SIDE-EFFECTS

Phenytoin produces an array of side-effects, with cosmetic changes (acne, gum hyperplasia, hirsutism and facial coarsening) and psychosocial problems (aggression, depression, impaired memory, sedation) being the most problematic (Table 6.4). Accordingly, phenytoin should not be prescribed to younger women. Dose dependent and idiosyncratic side-effects can usually be made more acceptable by rational dosage adjustment based on therapeutic drug monitoring.

DRUG INTERACTIONS

Interactions with phenytoin are perhaps the most commonly observed, and this can be attributed in part to its frequency of use and the fact that it has been available for clinical use for a long time. Further, since phenytoin is extensively bound to serum proteins and also very loosely bound to hepatic cytochrome P450 enzymes, it is particularly susceptible to competitive displacement and metabolic inhibitory interactions (Patsalos and Lascelles, 1977a,b). Additionally, phenytoin is also a potent inducer of hepatic drug metabolizing enzymes and its metabolism is saturable at therapeutic concentrations (Bochner *et al.*, 1972; Patsalos *et al.*, 1988). Thus, inhibition of metabolism may produce a proportionately greater increase in circulating drug concentrations and enhance the risk of toxicity. Serum phenytoin concentrations should be monitored regularly when co-medication is introduced or withdrawn. Induction of phenytoin metabolism is often not clinically significant; nevertheless an important example is that with folic acid (MacCosbe and Toomey, 1983).

As alcohol is eliminated almost exclusively by the liver, an acute alcohol load reduces the liver's capacity to metabolize other drugs. However, long-term exposure to large amounts of alcohol results in hepatic enzyme induction so that the metabolism of other drugs can be enhanced.

The antacids aluminium hydroxide, magnesium hydroxide and calcium carbonate and the gastric protective agent sucralfate can reduce the bioavailability of phenytoin in some patients, resulting in lower phenytoin serum concentrations. Although small doses of antacids (<10 ml) generally have little effect, higher doses (15–45 ml) can reduce phenytoin absorption significantly (Carter *et al.*, 1981; Smart *et al.*, 1985). The variability of this interaction can be attributed to the complex effect of antacids in that they affect phenytoin dissolution, ionization, chelation and gastrointestinal tract mobility. Thus, ingestion of antacids and phenytoin should be separated by 1–2 hours to avoid interaction.

Cimetidine, a substituted imidazole compound and H_2-receptor antagonist, inhibits the metabolism of phenytoin dose dependently, causing toxicity within a few days in some patients (Levine *et al.*, 1985). Although the extent of this interaction is variable, 20–30% increases in steady-state phenytoin concentrations are likely and phenytoin dosage adjustments may be necessary.

The interaction between phenytoin and carbamazepine is controversial, with reports that serum phenytoin concentrations are both raised and reduced. These differences can be explained on the basis of carbamazepine acting both as an inhibitor and an inducer of phenytoin metabolism (Zielinski and Haidukewych, 1987). The mechanism that determines whether induction or inhibition prevails is not known, but probably relates to the relative dose and serum concentrations of the two drugs.

Patients on long-term phenytoin therapy who are administered isoniazid commonly experience drowsiness and intoxication. Intoxication occurs in approximately 10–15% of patients and can be attributed to inhibition of phenytoin metabolism by isoniazid (Miller *et al.*, 1979). Further, the risk is greater in individuals who are slow acetylators of isoniazid because they are more likely to achieve sufficiently high isoniazid serum concentrations to inhibit phenytoin metabolism. If the interaction is to occur it will present fairly rapidly (days) and the phenytoin dose should be adjusted accordingly, based on serum concentrations. In clinical practice, frequent monitoring of serum phenytoin concentrations after the introduction of isoniazid therapy is indicated.

Possibly the most clinically important interaction of phenytoin is with valproic acid. The dual nature of the interaction and its transient and unpredictable outcome make routine serum concentration monitoring potentially misleading. Valproic acid both displaces phenytoin from its binding sites and is also a weak inhibitor of phenytoin metabolism (Patsalos and Lascelles 1977a,b). These two effects can be opposite in nature. Thus, when valproic acid is introduced as a co-medicant, phenytoin is displaced from its serum protein binding sites and phenytoin free concentrations increase transiently, with rapid distribution throughout body tissues. Because phenytoin undergoes rate restrictive elimination (i.e. only unbound drug is cleared), a compensatory rise in metabolism occurs so that the free phenytoin concentration returns to that present before valproic acid was introduced. Although there is a fall in total phenytoin concentration, dosage should not be increased as the consequent pharmacological effect is minimal. This interaction profile occurs only in those patients in whom phenytoin metabolism is not saturated. However, in patients whose phenytoin metabolism is close to saturation, the displacement coupled with metabolic inhibition by valproic acid can result in a substantial increase in total phenytoin concentrations. In this situation neurological toxicity may occur and will require a reduction in phenytoin dosage.

Many other drugs have been reported to affect phenytoin serum concentrations and these are shown in Table 6.7. The clinical significance of the different interactions is variable but may be particularly important in patients already taking maximum tolerable phenytoin doses. The interaction with amiodarone justifies further comment since amiodarone can increase serum phenytoin concentrations by as much as 130–180% at 2–4 weeks after initiation of therapy (McGovern *et al.*, 1984). Further, in 4–9% of patients, amiodarone itself can cause similar central nervous system adverse effects to those observed with phenytoin. Thus, there is a need to be cautious about interpreting the clinical signs of apparent phenytoin toxicity.

Phenytoin effects on other drugs relate primarily to its potent hepatic

Table 6.7   Miscellaneous interactions affecting phenytoin

Drug	Phenytoin serum concentration	Mechanism
Allopurinol	↑	INH
Amiodarone	↑	INH
Cisplatin	↓	DA
Clobazam	↑	IHN
Chloramphenicol	↑	IHN
Cyclosporin	↑	INH
Disulfiram	↑	INH
Folic acid	↓	IND
Methotrexate	↓	DA
Miconazole	↑	?
Fluconazole	↑	INH
Nitrofurantoin	↓	?
Omeprazol	↑	INH
Oxacillin	↓	DA
Rifampicin	↓	IND
Sulphonamides (sulphaphenazole, sulphadiazine)	↑	INH
Theophylline	↓	DA
Vinblastine	↓	DA

Abbreviations: INH, hepatic inhibition; IND, hepatic induction; DA, decreased absorption.

enzyme-inducing properties (Patsalos *et al.*, 1988). Thus, essentially the same induction interactions as highlighted for carbamazepine occur with phenytoin and can be associated with serum concentrations decreasing by as much as 50% during phenytoin co-medication. Appropriate dosage adjustments need to be made and, if phenytoin is subsequently withdrawn, toxicity may result if re-adjustment of the dosage of the concomitant drug is not undertaken.

The possibility of a clinically significant age-dependent induction interaction between phenytoin and theophylline, a widely used bronchodilator with a narrow therapeutic index and requiring careful dose titration, needs to be considered. Particularly as phenytoin can increase theophylline clearance by as much as 35–75% and in contrast to other inducers in the elderly (e.g. rifampicin and dichlorphenazone), this induction effect by phenytoin is maintained in old age (Crowley *et al.*, 1987). Furthermore, the interaction can be further enhanced by cigarette smoking since smoking and phenytoin have an additive inducing effect on theophylline metabolism.

ANTINEURALGIC EFFICACY

The efficacy of phenytoin in the management of trigeminal neuralgia was first reported in 1942 in three patients (Bergouignan, 1942). Subsequently, a further five patients (four with trigeminal neuralgia and one with glossopharyngeal neuralgia) were reported to have benefited from phenytoin treatment (Iannone *et al.*, 1958). In two further studies of 20 and 6 patients, 19 experienced good pain control with phenytoin 100 mg three times a day (Braham and Saia, 1960; Chinitz *et al.*, 1966). All patients who benefited from phenytoin experienced an improvement within 24–48 hours and occasionally after the first dose. Data comparing phenytoin with carbamazepine are minimal and no double-blind comparison of the two drugs has been undertaken (Swedlow and Cundill, 1981; Zakrzewska, 1990)

CURRENT THERAPEUTIC STATUS

Phenytoin is currently used as an adjunct to carbamazepine or in patients hypersensitized to carbamazepine. Treatment should be instigated with a single dose of 200 mg per day. If pain persists, dosage should be increased, preferably with monitoring of serum concentrations, as needed for pain control or as limited by toxicity. A reasonable therapeutic range is 20–80 μmol l^{-1} (based on its antiepileptic properties) and serum monitoring undertaken 14 days after a dose change. In the absence of good pain control, and if the serum phenytoin concentration is less than 20 μmol l^{-1}, an increment of 100 mg is appropriate. If the concentration is 20–60 μmol l^{-1} an extra 50 mg can be prescribed, while with concentrations above 60 μmol l^{-1} the dose should be increased only by 25-mg increments. As there are significant differences in bioavailability between different phenytoin preparations, patients should be treated with the product of a single manufacturer.

VALPROIC ACID

Valproic acid, a short-chain branched fatty acid, was synthesized in 1882 but its antiepileptic activity was not realized until 1963 when it was used as a solvent in a drug screening programme (Burton, 1882). This fortuitous discovery culminated in the sodium salt of valproic acid being used clinically in the treatment of epilepsy in 1964 (Carraz *et al.*, 1964b) and in the treatment of trigeminal neuralgia in 1980 (Peiris *et al.*, 1980).

CHEMISTRY

Valproic acid (molecular weight 114.2 Da) is only slightly soluble in water and highly soluble in organic acids with a pK_a of 4.8 (Fig. 6.1g). The sodium salt, sodium valproate (molecular weight 166.19 Da), is highly soluble in water and is used to formulate Epilim as 200 and 500 mg tablets, the crushable tablet as 100 mg per tablet and the syrup as 200 mg per 5 ml. As gastrointestinal distress was the most common side-effect during initial therapy (Dreifuss and Langer, 1987), a 500 mg enteric-coated tablet was formulated and introduced in 1977. As enteric coating proved effective in minimizing gastrointestinal symptoms, a 200 mg tablet subsequently became available and the original plain tablets have now been withdrawn in the UK. In non-European countries valproate is marketed as the magnesium salt and these preparations can be used interchangeably since they are bioequivalent (Balbi *et al.*, 1991). Valproic acid is used to formulate Depakene capsules (250 mg per capsule) and the sodium salt is used to formulate Depakene syrup (250 mg per 5 ml). Also available are Depakote Sprinkle Capsules (125 mg) for sprinkling over soft food. Finally, valpromide, an amide derivative of valproic acid, has been available in Europe (Depamide in France, Vistora in Spain) for the past 30 years (Carraz *et al.*, 1964a; Musolino *et al.*, 1980; Lambert and Venaud, 1987). Although used interchangeably with valproic acid, caution needs to be exercised if patients are on carbamazepine co-therapy since up to eightfold increases in carbamazepine epoxide concentrations have been reported, leading to the development of clinical toxicity (Pisani *et al.*, 1988).

PHARMACOKINETICS

After oral ingestion, valproic acid is rapidly absorbed with peak blood concentrations achieved usually within 2 hours. However, if enteric-coated tablets are used peak serum concentrations may be achieved between 3 and 8 hours. The delay in absorption can be attributed to variable gastric emptying and dissolution rate of the enteric coating, which is pH dependent. Food ingestion delays absorption, but does not decrease bioavailability which is close to unity for all the currently available formulations. In adults, the half-life of valproic acid is

6–17 hours, with values being even shorter during duotherapy with enzyme-inducing drugs such as carbamazepine or phenytoin (Zaccara *et al.*, 1988).

Valproic acid is highly bound to albumin and binding is saturable so that the relationship between dose and serum concentration is not linear but convex. Valproic acid serum concentrations exhibit significant diurnal variability (up to 100%) and consequently intermitant side-effects can occur at peak concentrations (Pisani *et al.*, 1981). Elimination is via hepatic metabolism to numerous metabolites, some of which may be responsible for its pharmacological effects (Semmes and Shen, 1991). Valproic acid does not induce hepatic drug-metabolizing enzymes.

SIDE-EFFECTS

The most common side-effects associated with valproic acid therapy are tremor, weight gain, thining or loss of hair, and ankle swelling (Table 6.4). In patients who tolerate the drug, cognitive impairment is uncommon and stupor or encephalopathy, although potentially dangerous, are rare. Hepatotoxicity, which can be fatal, appears largely confined to children under 3 years of age (Dreifuss *et al.*, 1987). Chronic side-effects are reversible.

DRUG INTERACTIONS

Interactions affecting valproic acid are few and rarely of clinical significance. Perhaps the most important interactions relate to those with enzyme-inducing antineuralgic drugs (e.g. carbamazepine and phenytoin). Up to a 50% reduction in valproic acid serum concentrations as a result of hepatic enzyme induction and increased clearance has been reported during co-administration with these drugs (Duncan *et al.*, 1991). Chlorpromazine similarly interacts with valproic acid and the clinical consequence of these interactions can be a reduction in pain control necessitating an increase in valproic acid dosage.

Reduced valproic acid serum concentrations can also occur consequent to impaired absorption or a protein binding displacement interaction. Drugs that act in the former manner include antacids and the cytostatic drugs Adriamycin and cisplatin. Naproxen, phenylbutazone and salicylic acid displace valproic acid from serum albumin sites (Grimaldi *et al.*, 1984). The mechanism of the displacement interaction is similar to that between phenytoin and valproic acid discussed above. However, since valproic acid exhibits saturable binding, this interaction may on occasion be associated with an increase in serum total concentrations and with hyperactivity and acute toxic psychosis. Further, since salicylic acid also inhibits valproic acid metabolism, this interaction may not be consistently detected by monitoring total valproic acid serum concentrations (Goulden *et al.*, 1987).

Valproic acid is a potent inhibitor of both oxidative pathways and of glucuronide conjugation pathways. The inhibitory interactions with phenytoin, carbamazepine and lamotrigine are discussed elsewhere. Valproic acid also inhibits the metabolism of diazepam and nimodipine (Tartara *et al.*, 1991). As mean bioavailability of nimodipine can be increased by as much as 86%, this interaction may be particularly clinically significant.

ANTINEURALGIC EFFICACY

The first study on the use of sodium valproate in trigeminal neuralgia was a report on 258 patients over 10 years treated with different antiepileptic drugs (Savitskaya, 1980). In this series, of the 16 patients treated with sodium valproate, 14 benefited. Subsequently in an open study of 600–1200 mg per day sodium valproate in 20 patients, six were rendered pain free and three had a 50% reduction in pain (Peiris *et al.*, 1980). In four patients sodium valproate was effective only when used in combination with other drugs; however, the other drugs were not identified. One patient complained of nausea. Sodium valproate has also been shown to be effective in neuropathic pain (Swedlow, 1980). Of 70 patients evaluated, 34 responded successfully to sodium valproate (Swedlow, 1980). Unfortunately the study did not report on the doses used, although the effective therapeutic range was 190–550 μmol l^{-1} valproic acid (mean 386 μmol l^{-1}). Furthermore, no indication was given as to whether the reported serum concentrations were random, trough or peak.

CURRENT THERAPEUTIC STATUS

Valproic acid is only occasionally used in trigeminal neuralgia. The starting dose should be low, increasing in line with pain control and reported side-effects. Initially 600 mg per day is used and this can be increased by 100 mg per week (slower in the elderly). The dose should be divided so that ingestion is twice or three times a day. The maximum pharmacological effect of valproic acid may not occur for some weeks after steady-state serum concentrations have been achieved. A reasonable therapeutic range is 200–700 μmol l^{-1} (based on its antiepileptic efficacy) and therapeutic drug monitoring undertaken 5 days after a dose change.

OTHER TREATMENTS

In recent years numerous reports of a variety of medications for use in trigeminal neuralgia have been published. These include pimozide (Lechin *et al.*, 1989), tizanidine (Vilming *et al.*, 1986; Fromm *et al.*, 1993), tocainide (Lindstrom and Lindblom, 1987), chlormethiazole (Zurak *et al.*, 1989) and capsaicin (Fusco and Alessandri, 1992). The exact clinical role of these therapeutic agents in the management of trigeminal neuralgia will be clarified only when more clinical data become available.

CONCLUSION

During the past few years the drug treatment of trigeminal neuralgia has undergone considerable change owing to the introduction of many new anti-neuralgic drugs. Consequently the clinician has more choice but at the same time more decisions need to be taken. An understanding of the action, interaction and pharmacokinetics of the different drugs is crucial if medical management is to be optimized.

Today, many more patients can achieve better pain control with drugs then previously. Most patients should be prescribed carbamazepine in the first instance. If hypersensitivity, side-effects or poor pain control occur, a change in drug therapy is warranted. Baclofen or phenytoin may be added to the regimen or used on their own. If these are unsuccessful, then drugs such as valproic acid or clonazepam should be used. In those patients in whom the pain does not have all the features of trigeminal neuralgia, e.g. complex facial pain, the use of tricyclic antidepressants may be extremely beneficial and should be encouraged earlier rather than later. Two new promising antineuralgic drugs are oxcarbazepine and lamotrigine. Although oxcarbazepine is not licensed for use in the UK, it has been used successfully for a number of years and proven to be an excellent alternative to carbamazepine.

Although carbamazepine remains the gold standard at present, it may be superseded by newer drugs which have equally potent antineuralgic effects but with fewer side-effects.

7

Peripheral Surgery

INTRODUCTION

When medical treatment fails as a result of poor pain control or severe side-effects from drug therapy, surgical options need to be considered. The simplest procedures are those performed under local anaesthesia to the terminal branches of the trigeminal nerves, as summarized in Table 7.1.

All these procedures interrupt peripheral pathways as the nerves are temporarily or permanently destroyed by chemical, thermal or physical methods. The effects of these methods on nerve fibres have often been studied in animal models. Some of the procedures are selective in terms of type of nerve fibres affected, e.g. cryotherapy and radiofrequency affect mainly δ fibres. The effect of cryotherapy on nerve fibres has been shown to be reversible, although not all fibres recover at the same rate (Miles and Hribar, 1981).

When using these peripheral procedures it is essential to establish clinically which terminal branches are involved to ensure that treatment is successful. The trigger zone rather than the area of radiation is important. I use a local anaesthetic to confirm my clinical findings, as suggested by Mason (1972).

Table 7.1 Peripheral treatments used for the management of trigeminal neuralgia: first substantive reports

Procedure	Reference
Neurectomy	Horrax and Poppen (1935)
Alcohol injection	Grantham and Segerberg (1952)
Cryotherapy	Lloyd et al. (1976)
Jawbone cavity removal	Ratner et al. (1979)
Peripheral radiofrequency thermocoagulation	Gregg et al. (1978)
Adjustment of dental malocclusions	Blair and Gordon (1973)
Streptomycin and lignocaine injection	Sokolovic et al. (1986)
Glycerol injection	Stajcic (1989)
Acupuncture	Shuhan et al. (1991)

Complete abolition of pain after injection of a local anaesthetic into the trigger area indicates the nerve branch that requires treatment. Due to the localized nature of the treatment the pain-control periods are short. Even if the pain does not recur in the same branch, migration of the pain is common (Quinn, 1965; Barnard, 1989; Zakrzewska, 1991).

Peripheral treatments are easy to perform, repeatable, well tolerated even by patients unfit for general anaesthesia and result in no mortality and low morbidity (Mason, 1972). These factors are sometimes of more importance to the patient's quality of life than complete pain control (Zakrzewska and Thomas, 1993). However, peripheral procedures may delay more radical surgery to a time when the patient is older and less fit for surgery, and this needs to be taken into consideration (Henderson, 1967). These procedures are useful as temporary measures before more definitive surgery is performed, as they enable the patient to appreciate what loss of sensation really means.

It is difficult to compare results, especially in terms of pain relief, as very variable techniques of analysis are used and end-points are not clearly defined. Diagnostic criteria are not always specified. Often, the length of follow-up is not specified and there are few details of the statistical analysis. Complications after the procedures are reported more consistently, although usually only the major ones. Few prospective studies have been performed and relatively few reports have been made since the 1970s, probably due to improved techniques at the level of the gasserian ganglion.

NEURECTOMY

HISTORICAL BACKGROUND

Neurectomy is the oldest recorded surgical treatment for trigeminal neuralgia. André in 1756 attempted to destroy the infraorbital nerve by exposing it and applying caustic to it (Stookey and Ransohoff, 1959). This operation may, however, have been performed first by Schlichting in 1748 (Harris, 1926). Already in 1787 Pujol had suggested that several nerves may need to be cut to achieve pain relief (Sweet, 1985).

METHODS

Neurectomy can be carried out under general anaesthesia (Mason, 1972) or sedation and local analgesia with a short stay in hospital (Grantham and Segerberg, 1952; Quinn, 1965). Additional intraneural injections of local anaesthesia before avulsion are suggested by some clinicians to improve analgesia (Grantham and Segerberg, 1952; Quinn, 1965).

There are three stages in the performance of neurectomy:

1. Removal of an adequate length of nerve, leaving no small fibres.
2. Avulsion of the nerve including removal from the skin.

3.   Occlusion: blockage of the bony canal through which the nerve passes with non-resorbable material, e.g. bone, wax, silver plugs or polyethylene paint (Thoma, 1969).

The supraorbital nerve is approached through an incision in the eyebrow (Stookey and Ransohoff, 1959); the eyebrow does not need to be shaved. The infraorbital may be approached either extraorally through a skin crease (Hardman, 1967) or intraorally using the Caldwell–Luc incision (Grantham and Segerberg, 1952; Stookey and Ransohoff, 1959; Quinn, 1965; Mason, 1972).

The inferior alveolar nerve is normally approached intraorally (Quinn, 1965; Mason, 1972). The inferior alveolar nerve and vessels are traced to their foramen. The sphenomandibular ligament is cut at its attachment to the lingula to allow better visualization. The nerve can also be exposed in any other part of the inferior alveolar canal by cutting a window of bone (Thoma, 1969). Thoma (1969) advocated an extraoral approach in more difficult cases as it makes the field more aseptic and visualization is easier.

Both the lingual and inferior alveolar nerves can be exposed simultaneously (Ginwalla, 1961) and better results are reported using this technique (Khanna and Galinde, 1985). The lingual nerve can be exposed near the inner surface of the mandible in the third molar region.

Once exposed as far as possible, the nerve is removed. The relevant foramen is obliterated (Hardman, 1967; Thoma, 1969; Mason, 1972), or the nerve is cauterized electrosurgically (Grantham and Segerberg, 1952; Quinn, 1965). If the infraorbital foramen is roofless, care must be taken as orbital tissues can be injured (Mason, 1972). Ginwalla (1961) packed the mental foramen with bone chips after realigning the foramen with a drill. Dissection and excision of peripheral fibres may delay regeneration (Quinn, 1965).

Recurrences can be treated in the same way. If well done the first time, no nerve bundle will be visualized but some remnants may be found at re-exploration. Some neurosurgeons perform the procedure only once and then use other techniques (Grantham and Segerberg, 1952); others continue to do the procedure until it fails (Quinn, 1965). After the third procedure the foramen is usually completely filled in and so plugging the foramen is useless. However, new exploration may show the presence of nerve fibres in the surrounding fibrous tissue. These fibres can make contact with the periosteum and lead to recurrence of pain; they need to be avulsed (Quinn, 1965). Penicillin may be given for 72 hours as prophylaxis, as the periosteum is raised (Grantham and Segerberg, 1952). Re-exploration may show the presence of a neuroma, whose removal can lead to pain relief (Quinn, 1965).

RESULTS

Recurrence Rates
Although many texts describe the techniques, many either do not give results or describe them in broad terms such as 'all recurred within 3 years'. No random-

ized controlled trials have been performed and no recent reports have been made on the use of neurectomy, although the technique is still employed by maxillofacial surgeons (Zakrzewska, 1990).

Pain relief is not always immediate and pain may occur for another few days, but is of lesser severity (Quinn, 1965). There are a few patients in whom the procedure fails: up to 3% (Freemont and Millac, 1981). Quinn (1965) suggested that neurectomy performed within bone (mental and infraorbital) is less successful than that in soft tissue, whereas Mason (1972) had more success with infraorbital than inferior alveolar neurectomy. Mason (1972) postulated that regeneration is the reason for recurrence, as he found that operations involving avulsion alone were less successful than those including occlusion of the canal, as occurred when neurectomy was carried out on the infraorbital nerve. Regeneration results in hyperaesthesia, which often precedes recurrence of pain (Mason, 1972).

The pain-free period following a second neurectomy is usually shorter than after the first (Quinn, 1965). Quinn (1965) found it easier to perform repeat neurectomies on the third division, and could keep patients pain free for longer periods. A period of pain relief of 23–33 months is achieved in many patients. Other workers, by carrying out repeat neurectomies, find that they can achieve long-term pain relief in 75% of patients. Freemont and Millac (1981) were able to achieve pain relief in 20 of 26 patients for an average of 59 months, seven required serial neurectomies. Neurectomy needs to be performed on other nerve branches because of migration of the pain (Mason, 1972).

The main published results of neurectomy are presented in Table 7.2.

Table 7.2 Results of peripheral neurectomy

Reference	No. of patients	No. of nerves	Range of follow-up (years)	Average pain relief (months)	Success or failure rate
Grantham and Segerberg (1952)	55	55	0.5–8	33.2	—
Quinn (1965)	63	112	0–9	24–32	—
Ginwalla (1961)	15	—	1	—	100%
Mason (1972)	36	47	1–4	—	74% failed at 4 years
Freemont and Millac (1981)	26	43	—	23	—
Khanna and Galinde (1985)	118	145	1–5	—	75% success

Complications

Few authors have reported complications. Sensory loss in the area is inevitable but is not seen as a problem as the corneal reflex is kept intact (Mason, 1972). Grantham and Segerberg (1952) had one patient with postoperative infection, and Mason (1972) had one following obliteration of the canal by a wood paint.

ALCOHOL INJECTION

HISTORICAL BACKGROUND

Chloroform and osmic acid were the first substances to be injected into nerves (Stookey and Ransohoff, 1959). Alcohol injections were being performed by the beginning of this century, following some animal experiments carried out by Pitres and Vaillard (Stookey and Ransohoff, 1959). Schloesser injected alcohol (using an intraoral technique) through the foramen rotundum and ovale, as well as peripherally (Harris, 1926).

METHODS

Although essentially a simple technique, the alcohol must be injected very precisely as it is highly toxic; full patient cooperation is required. General anaesthesia is, therefore, not generally advocated. Local anaesthetics should be used to reduce the pain related to the injection of alcohol. A small amount of local anaesthetic can be given through the same needle without its withdrawal (Harris, 1926; Horrax and Poppen, 1935) or a different syringe can be used so that the alcohol is not diluted (Burchiel, 1987a; Fardy *et al.*, 1994).

Once anaesthesia of the correct branch has been achieved and pain relief obtained, the alcohol can be injected. The anaesthesia should not be too profound as it is then difficult to assess the effect of the alcohol (Grant, 1936). An external approach is favoured by most clinicians, although maxillofacial surgeons use intraoral techniques wherever possible. Harris (1926) and Stookey and Ransohoff (1959) gave precise details for a range of injections, including diagrams for those interested in the precise surgical details; a summary is found below.

The amount of alcohol injected should be between 0.5 and 1.5 ml, and 80–100% alcohol is used. Resistance to the injection indicates that the needle point has engaged the nerve (Grant, 1936; Harris, 1940). Care must be taken to avoid injecting into the companion artery as this can result in an area of necrosis. After injection of the alcohol, air can be injected to stop a sinus tract developing (Burchiel, 1987a).

First division
The injection is made directly into the supraorbital nerve, which has numerous branches. Care must be taken to prevent injection into the orbit.

Second division
The infraorbital foramen is easy to locate and inject. Horrax and Poppen (1935) and Harris (1926) also advocated the extraoral approach for the whole division, and precise instructions are given in their texts. Grant (1922) recommended the use of a 'zygometer' to calculate the angles accurately. It is important to move the tip of the needle around while injecting to ensure that any peripheral branches are also injected. Maxillofacial surgeons inject the alcohol peripherally into the infraorbital nerve through an intraoral injection given above the canine.

Third division
Horrax and Poppen (1935) describe in detail an extraoral subzygomatic approach which places the alcohol in the nerve trunk just below the foramen ovale. Radiographic checks on all needle positions should be carried out before injection (White and Sweet, 1969). Rotating the bevel upwards while injecting up to 3 ml alcohol may destroy a greater length of the nerve. Littler's technique (1984), using the standard intraoral approach for a dental inferior nerve block and checking its position by the use of radiographs, is much simpler. However, this technique affects only the inferior alveolar nerve.

Most descriptions of alcohol injection are found in the literature between 1930 and 1940. Extraoral approaches were used to inject the alcohol into the whole branch rather than just peripheral branches. The length of needles was carefully calculated and stops were put on them to prevent penetration into vital tissues. Alcohol injections are now given mainly by maxillofacial surgeons who inject peripherally into nerve branches using intraoral techniques (Fardy *et al.*, 1994). However, evaluation of outcome is poor.

RESULTS

Recurrence rates
Some patients obtain no relief from the injections: as many as 103 of 274 injections may be ineffective (Peet and Schneider, 1952; Stookey and Ransohoff, 1959). The average time for relief of pain varies from 6 to 30 months, as shown in Table 7.3. Stookey and Ransohoff (1959) combined several reports totalling 1500 patients and found the length of pain relief for each nerve to be as follows: supraorbital, 8.5 months; infraorbital and second division, 12 months; third division, 16 months; and ganglion injections, permanent. They postulated that the longer period of pain relief for the third division may be due to inadvertent injection into the ganglion.

Repeated injections are made more difficult due to fibrosis. No separate results are available for patients who have undergone subsequent injections, although these are usually less effective.

Complications
Complications are common with the more extensive injections but rare with peripheral injections. In a retrospective review of 413 peripheral alcohol injections, only three (0.7%) significant complications occurred (Fardy and Patton, 1994). Lateral rectus and facial palsies have been reported, some of which were only temporary (Grant, 1936; Peet and Schneider, 1952; Ruge *et al.*, 1958; Richardson and Straka, 1973).

Injection of the third division can lead to inadvertent injection of the gasserian ganglion (Grant, 1936; Stookey and Ransohoff, 1959) and to facial and orbital palsies (Richardson and Straka, 1973). Injection into the infraorbital nerve can produce loss of vision owing to spasm of the retinal artery (Markham, 1973) or temporary diplopia (Fardy and Patton, 1994). After injection into the supraorbital or infraorbital nerves, oedema and haematoma may result in

Table 7.3   Results of peripheral alcohol injection

Reference	No. of Patients	No. of injections	Nerve	Average pain relief (months)
Horrax and Poppen (1935)	Not specified	12	Supraorbital	6
		147	Infraorbital	12.4
		98	Maxillary	12.4
		345	Mandibular	14.3
Grant (1936)	185	255 (total)	Ophthalmic	18.0
			Maxillary	14.0
			Mandibular	16.0
Grantham and Segerberg (1952)	49	Not specified	All	15.5
Peet and Schneider (1952)	49	72	All	74% less than 2.0
Ruge *et al.* (1958)	298	821	All	7.23
Stookey and Ransohoff (1959)	274	Not specified	All	Less than 12
Henderson (1967)	165	208	Mandibular	12–4
	287	596	Infraorbital	6–24
White and Sweet (1969)	54		Maxillary	7
			Mandibular	30
Fardy *et al.* (1994)	68	68	Overall	13
		25	Infraorbital	13
		34	Inferior alveolar (median)	19

temporary inability to open the eye (Fardy and Patton, 1994). Alcohol causes local tissue necrosis and, if it occurs in mandibular muscle tissue, severe trismus can result (Phillips and Whitlock, 1976). On the skin, full-thickness

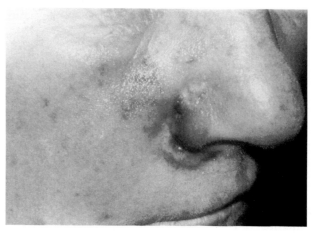

Figure 7.1   Skin necrosis as a result of alcohol injection into the infraorbital nerve using the external approach.

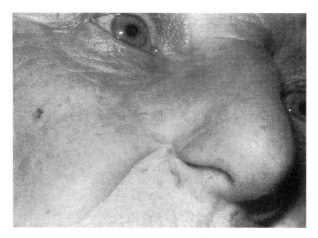

Figure 7.2 Healing of the necrotic area with no surgical intervention.

necrosis can occur (Fardy and Patton, 1994) (Figs 7.1 and 7.2). Intraorally this will result in mucosal ulceration, which gradually resolves (Fardy and Patton, 1994). Bony necrosis can lead to the formation of bony sequestra (Richardson and Straka, 1973; Fardy and Patton, 1994).

The procedure should be avoided in patients who have a skin infection at the site of injection (Horrax and Poppen, 1935). Herpes zoster of the ophthalmic division of the trigeminal nerve, with involvement of the trochlear nerve, has been reported after alcohol injection (Boucheret, 1971).

CRYOTHERAPY

INTRODUCTION

Cryotherapy is defined as the therapeutic use of cold in contrast to cryosurgery, which is the destruction of tissue by extreme cold (Dorland, 1974). Cryo-analgesia is a term introduced by Lloyd *et al.* (1976) to describe the use of cold to obtain pain relief. In this text, cryotherapy is used synonymously with cryoanalgesia.

HISTORICAL BACKGROUND

The use of cold for pain relief has been known since ancient times. The Egyptian papyri contain a reference to the pain-relieving properties of cold (Bracco, 1980; Whittaker, 1986) and Hippocrates also mentioned the use of cold in pain relief (Bracco, 1980; Hippocrates, 1978). References to the analgesic properties of cold are found in the Middle Ages in the writings of Bartholin; in 1661 he wrote the first book on the topic (Bracco, 1980). Napoleon's surgeon, Baron Von Larrey,

described painless amputations on soldiers trapped in the freezing temperatures of Moscow in 1812 (Larrey, 1829).

Further extensive uses of cold for therapeutic purposes were made by the
Arnott family, in particular by James Arnott (1797–1883). They used ice-cold
salt solutions and were able to achieve temperatures as low as –12°C. Among
other uses Arnott (1851) described its use in 'A mechanic suffering much for
seven days from tic douloureux in the face. One short application of the common frigorific mixture at once and permanently removed it'. In 1961 Cooper
and Lee developed the first cryoprobe and cryosurgery as such came into being.
The cryogenic system used by Cooper *et al.* (1962) employed liquid nitrogen as
the refrigerant and attained temperatures of –196°C. It was capable of maintaining temperatures from 37 to –160°C, but was a complex and expensive
machine. Amoils (1967) designed a small probe using carbon dioxide that was
capable of achieving temperatures of –50°C, and first used it in ophthalmic
surgery. It was later adapted for use with nitrous oxide, and temperatures of
–50 to –70°C were possible.

METHODS

To date, cryotherapy has been applied only to exposed peripheral nerve
branches and not to whole divisions, as with alcohol or neurectomy. Most
cryotherapy is carried out by oral and maxillofacial surgeons, who prefer an
intraoral to an extraoral approach. Clinicians usually perform the procedure
under local anaesthesia with or without sedation (Zakrzewska *et al.*, 1986).
General anaesthesia is used where the inferior alveolar nerve is to be exposed
(Barnard, 1989).

The individual nerves are exposed as detailed below.

First division
The supraorbital nerve is exposed by an incision in the eyebrow. Careful sutur-
ing should then leave no residual scarring (Barnard, 1986).

Second division
The infraorbital nerve is exposed using the Caldwell–Luc incision and dissect-
ing upwards towards the foramen (Barnard, 1986; Zakrzewska *et al.*, 1986)
(Fig. 7.3). The posterior and middle superior dental nerves are too fine to dissect
out, and a periosteal flap is raised in the area and the probe applied to the soft
tissues (Barnard, 1986).

Third division
The mental nerve is exposed by reflection of a mucoperiosteal flap in the pre-
molar region. The foramen is identified (Barnard, 1986; Zakrzewska *et al.*, 1986).
The long buccal nerve is exposed using the lateral incision line commonly
employed for the surgical removal of wisdom teeth (Barnard, 1986; Zakrzewska
et al., 1986). The anatomy of the long buccal nerve is variable and if difficulty is

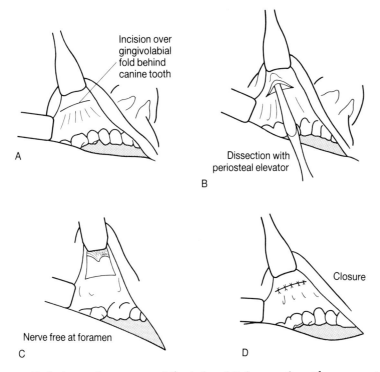

Figure 7.3 Technique of exposure of the infraorbital nerve for either neurectomy or cryotherapy. (Modified from Poppen, 1960.)

found in identifying it, the probe is simply placed in the assumed area of the nerve (Zakrzewska *et al.*, 1986; Politis *et al.*, 1988).

The inferior alveolar and lingual nerves are more difficult to expose. The standard incisions for the extraction of wisdom teeth are used, often necessitating general anaesthesia (Barnard, 1986). Politis *et al.* (1988) advocated a sub-periosteal rather than a supraperiosteal approach to avoid damage to the lingual nerve. To avoid the use of general anaesthesia in exposing the inferior dental nerve, Juniper (1991) used a C-arm image intensifier and a nerve stimulator. A slim Spembly–Floyd probe is then used for the cryotherapy. The lingual nerve is treated using the stimulator only.

Application of cryotherapy
Once the nerve or nerves have been exposed, cryotherapy is applied. The first descriptions of Lloyd *et al.* (1976) suggested two freeze–thaw cycles of 2 minutes each, using nitrous oxide to achieve a temperature of –60°C; this technique was also used by Barnard *et al.* (1981). Two freeze–thaw cycles of 90 seconds (Goss, 1984), or three cycles of 2 minutes each, can be used (Politis *et al.*, 1988). Liquid nitrogen capable of achieving temperatures of –120°C can be used in three 2-minute freeze–thaw cycles (Zakrzewska and Nally, 1988). It is impor-

tant to ensure as far as possible that the probe touches the nerve only and avoids the soft tissue as far as possible, especially the edges of the incision.

After cryotherapy the incision is sutured, and antibiotics and analgesics are given (Nally *et al.*, 1984; Politis *et al.*, 1988). Dexamethasone can also be given during operation to reduce swelling (Nally *et al.*, 1984).

RESULTS

Recurrence rates
Interestingly, Arnott in 1851, on the basis of a handful of patients, summarized the results of cryotherapy very accurately: 'one application of three minutes duration immediately terminated a state of torture ... in two others ... equally successful, though there was a necessity for repeating it several times. In a fifth ... relief is only of short continuance'.

In 1849 Arnott had already made the point that 'the assistance of quinine or other medicines ... will probably be necessary to prevent recurrence of paroxysms'. But he went on to write: 'but it is of great importance to have a means in our possession by which the agony of the patient may be instantly relieved on its recurrence while appropriate measures are being adopted for the removal of its persisting cause'.

Table 7.4 summarizes more recent results of peripheral cryotherapy. Several papers have been published from clinicians at the Eastman Dental Hospital in London, which involved the same patients. The latest paper is therefore used as it incorporates all the patients and used Kaplan–Meier analysis as described in Chapter 8. In Table 7.4 the overall mean pain control period is presented, although the median time to recurrence is a better reflection of the results. If individual nerves are assessed the median time to recurrence was 14 months for the infraorbital, 9 months for the mental and 11 months for the long buccal (Zakrzewska and Nally, 1988).

In some patients there is no relief of pain (Politis *et al.*, 1988; Zakrzewska, 1990). It would appear that results from liquid nitrogen therapy are better than those from nitrous oxide, but a more in-depth analysis of the liquid nitrogen group using Kaplan–Meier analysis gives comparable results (Zakrzewska, 1991). There appears to be no correlation between pain relief and the patient's age or sex, or duration of symptoms (Barnard, 1989; Zakrzewska, 1991). Cryotherapy performed on other peripheral nerves for the relief of other types of pain gives similar results: pain relief for 1–12 months (Wang, 1985); two 3-minute freeze–thaw cycles were used.

Cryotherapy can be used repeatedly, although it becomes technically more difficult (Barnard, 1989). Analysis of patients who have undergone cryotherapy for a second time shows that similar results are obtained (Zakrzewska, 1991), although in a smaller series Barnard (1989) obtained shorter pain relief times.

Many patients continue to take carbamazepine after treatment, although the doses required are lower. Although some patients use carbamazepine more as a placebo, in others it does act as adjuvant therapy (Barnard, 1989; Zakrzewska,

Table 7.4 Results of peripheral cryotherapy

Reference	No. of patients	No. of procedures	Range of follow-up (months)	Temperature (°C)	Time (s)	No freeze	Recurrence rate (months)	Loss of touch (months)
Barnard et al. (1978)	11	11	12 (mean)	−60	120	2	4 (median)	1.5
Barnard et al. (1981)	24	24	3–48	−60	60	2	6.1 (median)	2.1
Goss (1984)	11	11	0–36	—	90	2	15	2–3
Politis et al. (1988)	10	10	3–13	>0	120	3	2 recurred at 12	1.5–3
Zakrzewska and Nally (1988)	145	348	1–72	−140	120	3	Total: 10 (mean) 89 infraorbital: 20 85 mental: 17 66 long buccal: 13	2–3
Barnard (1989)	26	78	—	—	120	3	Total: 10 (mean) 41 infraorbital: 10 26 mental: 8.5 5 lingual: 17 6 inferior alveolar: 13	—

1991). In a postal survey on 102 patients who had cryotherapy, 71 were taking carbamazepine, compared with 45 of 180 following radiofrequency thermo-coagulation and two of 55 after microvascular decompression (Zakrzewska and Thomas, 1993).

Complications

Few complications have been reported, and there are no reports of neuroma formation, neuritis or anaesthesia dolorosa, as occurs after surgery on the gasserian ganglion (explained more fully in Chapter 8). Postoperative swelling and pain is common (Goss, 1984; Politis *et al.*, 1988). Up to 4% of patients may have postoperative infection (Zakrzewska and Nally, 1988). Although animal studies have indicated that nerve recovery is complete (Miles and Hribar, 1981), Zakrzewska and Thomas (1993) showed that 56% of patients complain of some loss of sensation beyond the expected time of 2–3 months (Barnard *et al.*, 1981; Goss, 1984). Sensory return does not signify the return of pain.

After operation patients may continue to complain of pain, but it has a different character and often responds well to a course of tricyclic antidepressants (Zakrzewska and Nally, 1988).

JAWBONE CAVITY REMOVAL

HISTORICAL BACKGROUND

In 1979 Ratner and colleagues proposed that the formation of jawbone cavities after tooth extraction was a major aetiological factor and that removal of these led to pain relief.

METHODS

A careful history is taken and examination performed to localize the possible areas of these cavities. Not all of them show up on radiographs; local anaesthesia is used to identify the areas and the methodology has been described in full by Ratner *et al.* (1979). Under local anaesthesia, a mucoperiosteal flap is raised and the area is very carefully curetted and then packed with gauze soaked in tetracycline. Penicillin is given a week before surgery and until all pain has ceased. If pain returns, the procedure is repeated (Ratner *et al.*, 1979; Roberts *et al.*, 1984).

RESULTS

The specimens show changes of chronic inflammation. In the series of Ratner *et al.* (1979) pain relief in 38 patients varied from 4 months to over 9 years. Roberts *et al.* (1984) reported on 131 patients with trigeminal neuralgia who had equally good results. Shaber and Krol (1980) operated on eight patients and only one failed to obtain complete pain relief; however, several procedures were necessary. Assessment of all the reported results (314 in total) by Roberts *et al.* (1984) gave a success rate of 70–90%. These authors reported on one patient who had been pain-free for 14 years. No complications, apart from mild temporary sensory loss and swelling, were reported (Roberts *et al.*, 1984). The results, however, have not been analysed using more sophisticated statistical methods, and few details have been given on the criteria used to assess outcome. Few centres have reported this technique.

RADIOFREQUENCY THERMOCOAGULATION OF PERIPHERAL BRANCHES

HISTORICAL BACKGROUND

Radiofrequency thermocoagulation of the gasserian ganglion showed that selective destruction of nerve fibres was possible (Sweet and Wepsic, 1974). Gregg *et al.* (1978) therefore investigated the use of this technique on peripheral nerves.

METHODS

Intravenous sedation and local anaesthesia are used. Full details of needle placement are given in the paper by Gregg and Small (1986). The first lesion is made at 60°C for 30 seconds and subsequent ones at 65–70°C. The placement of probes and the stimulation to elicit correct positioning can be painful.

RESULTS

Gregg and Small (1986) reported a 10-year follow-up of 71 patients who had had a total of 112 lesions. The mean length of pain control was 9.2 months; at 1 year the recurrence rate was 68%. As noted with other procedures, pain relief may not occur for 2–3 days (Gregg and Small, 1986). Sensory loss occurs but fine touch is often preserved, giving less profound anaesthesia than that following neurectomy or alcohol block. Apart from haematoma, there are few complications (Gregg and Small, 1986).

OTHER PERIPHERAL METHODS

DENTAL MALOCCLUSION

Blair and Gordon (1973) treated 39 patients by correction of a dental malocclusion. One of the seven dentate patients was rendered pain-free, whereas seven of the 32 edentulous patients had remissions for over 3 years. They postulated that malocclusion acts as a trigger for trigeminal neuralgia and hence its correction can be curative. However, there is no evidence to support the use of this technique.

PERIPHERAL INJECTION OF STREPTOMYCIN AND LIGNOCAINE

Sokolovic *et al.* (1986) reported on the use of streptomycin and lignocaine peripheral injections. Streptomycin (1 g) is dissolved in 2 ml 2% plain lignocaine, and this is then injected into the peripheral trigger nerve. Up to five injections may be required over a 5-week period. Sokolovic and co-workers (1986) treated 20 patients, and 16 were pain-free for periods up to 30 months.

A controlled trial was later performed, injecting lignocaine alone as a control. Although it appeared initially that those receiving streptomycin and lignocaine had better relief, this was not borne out in the long term (Stajcic *et al.*, 1990). A similar double-blind trial was performed by Bittar and Graff-Radford (1993), who also found that lignocaine alone had the same effect as streptomycin. No complications have been noted and there is no sensory loss (Stajcic *et al.*, 1990). I have found the injection to be as painful to administer as an alcohol injection, and much less successful in terms of pain relief.

PERIPHERAL INJECTION OF GLYCEROL

Just as Gregg and co-workers (1978) adapted the technique of radiofrequency thermocoagulation used on the gasserian ganglion, so Stajcic (1989) proposed the use of glycerol peripherally. After putting in a local anaesthetic of plain lignocaine, 1–2 ml sterile anhydrous glycerol is injected slowly into the infraorbital or mandibular foramen. If pain control is not achieved by 7 days, a further injection is given. The glycerol is very viscous and so difficult to inject but it is less painful than an alcohol injection.

Stajcic (1989) treated 17 nerves in 13 patients, and had no success in two cases. Pain relief varied from 3 to 24 months in the others; in six patients some sensory loss was noted.

We used glycerol in 22 of our patients, 17 of whom had undergone cryotherapy in the past. Five were failures, although one of these improved after a second injection. Pain recurred from 1 to 24 months later and the procedure was completely successful in only 11 patients. These patients had marked postoperative swelling and mild loss of touch sensation. No other complications were noted (Fardy *et al.*, 1994).

MISCELLANEOUS

Patients also seek alternative forms of medicine. Acupuncture has been used in patients with trigeminal neuralgia (Shuhan *et al.*, 1991; Beppu *et al.*, 1992). Shuhan and co-workers (1991) reported on the use of acupuncture in 1500 patients with trigeminal neuralgia; the full technique is described in their paper. They stress it is important to manipulate the needles to ensure that pain is elicited in the whole area. The course of treatment lasts 10 days (daily or alternate days), and may be repeated after 3–5 days if not successful. An average of 26 sessions is required.

Criteria for success are defined as short-term cure, markedly effective, improved and no effect. Patients are also classified as suffering from severe, moderate or minor attacks. Meridian acupuncture gave good results in five of ten patients (Beppu *et al.*, 1992).

The overall effectiveness was 99.2% of 539 patients followed for 1–6 years. A total of 237 patients (44.1%) had a recurrence but it was less severe. Patients who had had the disease for a shorter time had a higher success rate. There was no correlation with age, sex or nerve branch (Shuhan *et al.*, 1991). The only complication recorded was of nine patients who had transient difficulty in opening the mouth.

These results need to be evaluated further in controlled trials. Several of my patients have had acupuncture and I have had mixed reports about its effectiveness.

CURRENT STATUS

Peripheral techniques aim to cause selective trauma to a nerve in order to prevent the conduction of painful stimuli. They are relatively easy to perform and so can be done by a wide range of clinicians in both the outpatient clinic or in hospital. Except for radiofrequency thermocoagulation, the equipment is not expensive and is available in most settings. Peripheral techniques are now used mainly by oral and maxillofacial surgeons rather than neurosurgeons (Zakrzewska, 1990). The success of any technique is gauged on the recurrence rate, complication rate and patient satisfaction.

Recurrence rates for all techniques are similar: months rather than years. Neurectomy appears to give the best results in terms of pain relief, but these have not been subjected to rigorous statistical analysis.

Neurectomy, cryotherapy and removal of bone cysts all involve surgical procedures and may require intravenous sedation or general anaesthesia. Among oral and maxillofacial surgeons in the UK, cryotherapy has become the procedure of choice owing to its lack of complications. Jaw bone cyst removal is not carried out in the UK at present, but is widely practised by oral surgeons in the USA. The results of acupuncture appear very optimistic but there is only one substantive report.

The advantage of being able to administer a simple injection at the chairside at the time of acute pain has resulted in a search for the ideal solution to inject— hence the use of streptomycin, glycerol and alcohol.

Alcohol injections, especially when given into the division of the nerve, are difficult to administer and complications are not uncommon. The technique is performed blind, although recently radiographic localization has been possible. The injections are painful and patients are often unwilling to have them repeated. The formation of scar tissue also makes subsequent injections more difficult to administer. The sensory loss is often reversible but is more profound than after cryotherapy.

Streptomycin and glycerol have both been put forward as alternatives. I have been disappointed with both of these agents and find alcohol more predictable in its pain-relieving properties. With any injection one must be aware that its incorrect placement can have serious results. These can arise as a result of abnormal anatomy, overpenetration with the needle, too large a volume of solution or injection at too great a speed or force.

Just as glycerol given round the gasserian ganglion is highly successful as compared with its peripheral use, so radiofrequency thermocoagulation on peripheral nerve branches is a poor substitute for its use at the level of the gasserian ganglion. The outlay on special equipment is not justified if it is to be used only peripherally.

There is little to choose between the various methods. Complications are low with cryotherapy as the technique is performed with direct visualization of the nerve and sensory loss is low compared with other techniques. Although peripheral methods have a high recurrence rate, they remain valuable as a form of immediate pain relief in medically unfit patients and in those who refuse more extensive surgery. Complications are few and patients are satisfied with the treatment (Zakrzewska and Thomas, 1993). Patient preference must be taken into consideration, as I find that some patients prefer the immediacy of an injection rather than minor or major surgery. However, all the techniques should be evaluated using formal controlled trial techniques.

8

Surgery at the Level of the Gasserian Ganglion

INTRODUCTION

HISTORICAL

The earliest surgical treatments for trigeminal neuralgia were directed at peripheral nerve branches. It was soon realized that pain relief, if it did occur, was short lived. Treatment at the level of the gasserian ganglion seemed the next step. Techniques were developed to enter the foramen ovale and hence gain access to the gasserian ganglion without the need for an open procedure. It was not until radiological methods were used to guide the needle into position that all the techniques became safer and more precise (Penman, 1968). It is easier to enter the foramen, however, than to enter the ganglion and sensory root (Henderson, 1967). Techniques that have been used are summarized in Table 8.1.

A wide variety of substances were then injected into the gasserian ganglion, many of which are no longer in use. The first was osmic acid, described by Wright in 1907, who passed the needle under direct vision (Penman, 1968).

Table 8.1 Summary of main techniques used at the level of the gasserian ganglion

Technique	Reference
Osmic acid injection	Wright (1907)
Alcohol injection	Harris (1912)
Electrocoagulation	Kirschner (1931)
Phenol injection	Putman and Hampton (1936)
Compression	Taarnhoj (1952)
Boiling water injection	Jaeger (1957)
Phenol in glycerine injection	Jefferson (1963)
Radiofrequency thermocoagulation*	Sweet and Wepsic (1974)
Percutaneous retrogasserian glycerol rhizotomy*	Hakanson (1981)
Percutaneous microcompression*	Mullan and Lichtor (1983)

*Technique still in use

Harris' cadaver studies published in 1909 (Stookey and Ransohoff, 1959) showed that dyes injected into the foramen ovale resulted in staining of the gasserian ganglion, and this enabled Harris to give the first alcohol injections without doing an open procedure. Hartel (1912) described in detail the methodology of entering the foramen. If, however, the alcohol injections were incorrectly placed, multiple cranial nerve palsies occurred and so other agents were tried, e.g. hot water, phenol and glycerol.

Electrocoagulation was proposed by Kirschner in 1933 in lieu of destructive agents and led to the most commonly used procedure at present—radiofrequency thermocoagulation.

These procedures should not be used for other types of facial pain (Sweet, 1988). It has been shown by several workers that only the sharp shooting pain is relieved and that continuous pain remains (Hakanson, 1981).

EVALUATION OF RESULTS AND COMPLICATIONS

The reports on the various techniques vary so considerably that it is difficult to draw reliable conclusions. There is a dire lack of prospective controlled trials in which patients are randomly selected to alternative treatments (Loeser, 1993). I have listed some of these problems below.

Choice of patient
This has been remarked upon in discussions that attempt to evaluate different treatments (Burchiel, 1988). Some workers do not quote the criteria used for inclusion; others include other forms of facial pain and do not analyse them separately. In some series, patients who had previously undergone other procedures, ranging from peripheral neurectomy to microvascular decompression, have been analysed together, which no doubt influences the response to a particular procedure both in terms of recurrence rate and complications (Steiger, 1991).

Length of follow-up
Many series give no indication as to whether they are prospective or retrospective studies. Most, however, are retrospective. The length of follow-up is extremely variable with some series not even providing any details (see Tables 8.2 and 8.5). As the median recurrence rate for all procedures is around 24 months all series should have a minimum follow-up of at least 24 months. The range of follow-up is given most frequently but this provides no indication of how the patients are distributed within this range.

Classification of results
Results are often expressed as immediate failures, i.e. within 1 month, complete relief, good pain relief if adjuvant medication is required, or poor or no relief where other surgical procedures are required. Few workers have defined recurrence, and little mention is made of other forms of postoperative pain

(Zakrzewska and Thomas, 1993). It is also probably correct to assume that some who repeatedly report their results are using the same group of patients as previously and adding on further patients (Nugent and Berry, 1974; Nugent, 1982; Mittal and Thomas, 1986; Zakrzewska and Thomas, 1993). A recurrence in some patients is considered to have occurred only if a repeat operation is required (Nugent, 1982; Moraci *et al.*, 1992); in others, the taking of medication is classified as recurrence (Zakrzewska and Thomas, 1993).

Methods of analysis
Data analysis is variable and comparisons are therefore very difficult, not only between different procedures but also between the same ones. Life-table analysis of data is the only reliable method, but is used infrequently (Burchiel, 1988; North *et al.*, 1990; Steiger, 1991; Slettebo *et al.*, 1993; Zakrzewska and Thomas, 1993). Life-table analysis enables those patients who have died or been lost to follow-up to be included in the results (Peto *et al.*, 1977). These patients are 'censored,' but their inclusion prevents distortion of the data. The methodology assumes that some of those lost to follow-up are pain-free and that others are not. Patients who are pain-free are also classed as 'censored'. Fig. 8.1 is an example of the use of this method. It compares three different surgical techniques and shows the probability of having a recurrence at any one time. The statistical difference between the treatments can be calculated with a complex formula. If this method is not used, data are often rejected. This was seen very clearly in a series of 208 patients followed up for 5–8.5 years where only 135 patients were analysed because 23 had died and the rest failed follow-up

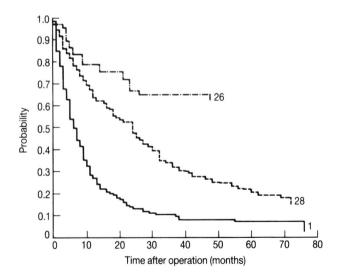

Figure 8.1 Kaplan–Meier plot of the probability of remaining pain-free. —·—·—, Microvascular decompression (*n* = 66); - - - - -, radiofrequency thermocoagulation (*n* = 273); ———, cryotherapy (*n* = 145).

appointments and were rejected from the analysis (Siegfried, 1981). These rejected data, however, may have had a considerable effect on the results and could have contributed significantly to the recurrence rate. Siegfried (1981) stated in the paper which patients were excluded, but other reports do not indicate how many were excluded from the analysis on the basis of having died or been lost to follow-up. One cannot assume that patients are pain-free if they do not return, as some will go to another centre.

RADIOFREQUENCY THERMOCOAGULATION OF THE GASSERIAN GANGLION

The use of heat for the production of a lesion in the gasserian ganglion was first used by Kirschner in 1933. The temperatures achieved were unpredictable and often too high. There were serious complications, including death, palsy of the sixth, fourth, eighth, and 12th cranial nerves and corneal ulcers, and the long-term recurrence rate was around 80% (Stookey and Ransohoff, 1959; Rovit, 1990). The problems were largely overcome by Sweet and Wepsic's (1974) procedure of controlled radiofrequency thermocoagulation of the gasserian ganglion. They modified the technique to allow for:

1. use of short-acting anaesthesia which allows patient to be woken during the procedure;
2. reliable radiofrequency current;
3. precise localization of the electrode within the gasserian ganglion by the use of electrical stimulation;
4. precise temperature monitoring.

Currently, radiofrequency thermocoagulation is the commonest surgical treatment for trigeminal neuralgia (Sweet and Wepsic, 1974). It is now called a variety of names, including radiofrequency heating, controlled thermocoagulation, percutaneous radiofrequency thermocoagulation/ablation or rhizotomy, percutaneous stereotactic thermocoagulation, percutaneous thermorhizotomy or simply percutaneous thermocoagulation.

MECHANISM

Sweet and Wepsic (1974), when first describing this procedure, called it 'controlled thermocoagulation of trigeminal ganglion and rootlets for differential destruction of pain fibres'. To achieve these aims a radiofrequency generator is needed with a precisely controlled heat source together with tiny thermistors to monitor the degree of heat developing. The placement of the electrode is crucial and several studies have been performed on cadaver skulls to establish the best position. (Henderson, 1967; Nugent and Berry, 1974; Sweet and Wepsic, 1974; Tew and Keller, 1977).

A lesion is produced by means of heat within the ganglion of the trigeminal nerve. It leads to differential destruction of pain fibres with the preservation of light touch and hence a reduction in the number of local complications such as complete sensory loss and corneal anaesthesia. Noxious stimuli are conducted in the smaller fibres of Aδ and C groups, whereas touch is transmitted by large A fibres. The former are thought to be more vulnerable to destruction by heat. In the trigeminal nerve this division is very distinct and so it is possible to be selective. The extent of the lesion depends on the length of uninsulated electrode protruding, the amperage of the current and the duration of lesion production time. Careful sensory testing immediately after production of the lesion shows loss of all modalities except cold. Six months later tactile and tragus pinch pain thresholds return to normal but those for warmth, hot pain and pinprick remain increased (Hampf *et al.*, 1990).

METHODS

Contraindications to radiofrequency thermocoagulation
This procedure cannot be performed in patients who do not want any sensory loss or in those with ophthalmic pain who would not be able to cope with corneal anaesthesia. Patients with bleeding tendencies that are not correctable cannot undergo the procedure as any intracranial penetration carries a risk of intracranial haemorrhage (Sweet, 1988).

Anaesthesia
For perioperative sensory testing to be carried out, the patient must be cooperative. Short-acting anaesthetic agents are therefore ideal for this procedure, as discussed in detail by Lowe *et al.* (1983).

Before operation diazepam or atropine may be given intravenously (Nugent and Berry, 1974; Sengupta and Stunden, 1977) or even droperidol (Rovit, 1990). During surgery most patients are given an injection of fentanyl and droperidol (Sweet and Wepsic, 1974; Sengupta and Stunden, 1977; Rovit, 1990), or fentanyl alone (Nugent and Berry, 1974; Lowe *et al.*, 1983). An injection of local anaesthetic xylocaine is given before insertion of the cannulae (Lowe *et al.*, 1983). At the moment of penetration of the foramen ovale, a short-acting anaesthetic such as methohexital, propofol (Kytta and Rosenberg, 1988) or althesin (Lowe *et al.*, 1983) is administered. The patient is thus able to respond when localization of the electrode is being achieved. During production of the lesion, further methohexital, thiopentone, althesin or etomidate can be given (Lowe *et al.*, 1983; Burchiel, 1987b; Meglio and Cioni, 1989), although the use of smaller insulated electrodes can obviate their use (Rovit, 1990).

A total of 150–300 mg methohexital, 5–10 mg droperidol and 0.05–0.1 mg fentanyl is used (Sweet and Wepsic, 1974; Sengupta and Stunden, 1977). The less methohexital is given the more changes in the conscious state can be picked up. In patients receiving methohexital anaesthesia, stimulation of the trigeminal ganglion can lead to marked arterial pressure rise, and it may be necessary to give vasodepressor agents (Kehler *et al.*, 1982). This is significant as many patients undergoing this procedure are elderly and have cardiovascular problems, especially hypertension which predisposes to intracranial haemorrhage owing to changes in blood pressure that occur during the procedure.

Naloxone 0.4 mg intravenously may be given at the end of the operation to ensure that no postoperative respiratory depression occurs (Sengupta and Stunden, 1977).

Patients are given intranasal oxygen (Lowe *et al.*, 1983; Rovit, 1990) and intravenous fluids if necessary. Vital signs are monitored throughout the 1–2-hour procedure (Rovit, 1990).

Technique

Most clinicians carry out the procedure in a radiography room, rather than an operating theatre, with the patient in the supine position. The anterior approach to the foramen ovale is used, as described by Hartel (1912). An 18-G spinal needle is placed in the scalp to act as the indifferent electrode (Onofrio, 1975; Sengupta and Stunden, 1977).

A hollow 19- or 20-G needle with a short bevel and sharp tip is used to make the lesion. The skin is penetrated at a point 2.5–3.0 cm lateral to the oral commissure. The position of the foramen ovale is estimated to be 3 cm anterior to the external auditory meatus and at the medial aspect of the pupil (Tew and Keller, 1977) (Fig. 8.2). This can be drawn out with a marking pen (Rovit 1990). The clinician places the index finger intraorally to touch the lateral wing of the pterygoid bone. This ensures that the buccal mucosa is not breached and infection avoided. The direction of the needle is crucial in determining its exact loca-

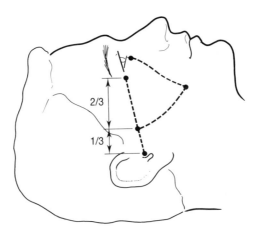

Figure 8.2 Guidelines for penetration of the foramen ovale. The needle enters the skin 2.5 cm lateral to the labial commissure for V2 and V3 trigeminal neuralgia pain. The direction of the needle is determined by two planes: a lateral plane directed at a point one-third of the distance from the external auditory meatus to the lateral canthus of the eye, and a medial plane directed from the puncture site to the medial aspect of the pupil. (Modified from Rovit, 1979.)

tion, and Sweet and Wepsic (1974) have described this in detail. Frequent radiographic verification (lateral and submento-occipital views) ensures that the needle enters the foramen ovale through the middle or medial third of it. If it is placed more posteriorly there is a possibility that the carotid artery may be pierced (Sweet and Wepsic, 1974). At the moment of entering the foramen a brief contraction of the masseteric muscles may be seen. As this is the most painful part of the procedure, it may lead to transient hypertension (Tew and Keller, 1977; Hitchcock *et al.*, 1983; Rovit, 1990).

The needle is advanced until the tip overlies the clivus. Fluoroscopy is used to check the position. Sweet and Wepsic (1974) performed very careful measures of the position of the tip in relation to sensory loss achieved and put forward their views on the best position. The technique has been well described by Rovit (1990) and by Sweet and Wepsic (1974).

The stylet is removed to ensure that cerebrospinal fluid (CSF) is obtained and not blood, although there may be some blood initially (Rovit, 1990). If the ganglion is penetrated there may be no CSF. The deeper the penetration the more likely it is that the first division will be penetrated, as shown in Fig. 8.3. It is not essential to obtain CSF before proceeding (Sweet and Wepsic, 1974).

Once the needle has been localized the stylet is removed and replaced by the radiofrequency electrode and monitor. Depending on the divisions to be treated, 5, 7 or 10 mm of the terminal portion of the electrode is left bare. The longest length is used for a lesion that involves all three divisions. A curved needle may be used as it is technically easier (Burchiel, 1987b; Tew and van Loveren, 1988). The curved needle is smaller and easier to manipulate accurately, and so reduces complications such as more extensive sensory loss, including corneal anaesthesia and masseteric weakness. Ideally the electrode should lie within the trigeminal rootlets rather than in the ganglion itself (Tobler *et al.*, 1983).

The final position of the needle tip is verified by electrical stimulation on the awake patient. A current is passed as an isolated square wave pulse of 1 ms duration, 100–400 mV and 50–75 Hz in order to stimulate pain or produce paraesthesia (see Fig. 8.2). If the correct area is not located the needle is advanced or withdrawn very slowly. During stimulation at 5 Hz it is essential

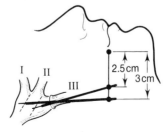

Figure 8.3 Guidelines for penetration of the gasserian ganglion. For VI trigeminal neuralgia, the puncture site is measured 3 cm lateral to the labial commissure and directed along the usual planes marked on the skin. (Modified from Rovit, 1979.)

to observe for any eye or masseteric movement. If either occurs, the needle must be repositioned.

McGlone and Wells (1991) have devised a bipolar electrode that obviates the need to wake up the patient. Electrical stimulation of the nerve results in an evoked potential that is interpreted by an averaging computer. The bipolar electrode has been tested in 12 patients: in eight it was successful. Being smaller, it producer a smaller lesion and this may lead to a higher recurrence rate.

Once all these checks have been carried out the lesion can be produced under light anaesthesia. The temperature at which the lesion is made is extremely variable, from 60 to 80°C (Table 8.2) (60°C: Sengupta and Stunden, 1977; 80°C: Siegfried, 1977; Onofrio, 1975). The temperature of the probe may also be affected by the amount of CSF, the position of the tip within the ganglion or rootlets, and by the consistency of the ganglion (Siegfried, 1981). Most clinicians make the first lesion for 60 seconds (Sweet and Wepsic, 1974; Burchiel, 1987; Tew and van Loveren, 1988), and then wake the patient to test for sensory loss. Further lesions can then be made and the temperature raised if necessary (Tew and Keller, 1977; Spincemaille *et al.*, 1985; Tew and van Loveren, 1988; Rovit, 1990). Timing ranges from 60 to 300 seconds (120 s: Sengupta and Stunden, 1977; 300 s: Zakrzewska and Thomas, 1993). Lower current settings are usually used for first division lesions (Nugent and Berry, 1974). Most clinicians make multiple small incremental lesions with intermittent sensory testing in order to ensure only pain loss and maximum preservation of touch. Most clinicians perform sensory testing with a sharp pin, and further lesions are halted once a pinprick is appreciated only as touch (Nugent and Berry, 1974; Rovit, 1990). Others may carry out fuller tests measuring touch appreciation in grams of pressure using calibrated touch (Tew and Keller, 1977) or use electrical stimulation (Hariz and Laitenen, 1986). Care must be taken when testing the corneal reflex as abrasions can be induced by the cotton wool. Rovit (1990) suggested the use of artificial tear drops instead of cotton wool to prevent this. Flushing of an area of the face during the procedure is considered useful, as it indicates the area being destroyed (Sweet and Wepsic, 1974; Onofrio, 1975). Flushing does not occur if the patient has previously had an injection or section (Onofrio, 1975). If

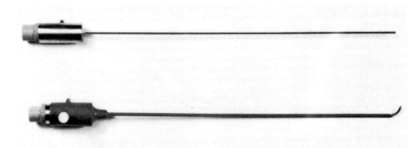

Figure 8.4   Electrodes from the Tew kit for lesion making. (Courtesy of Radionics Inc., USA.)

Table 8.2 Major results of radiofrequency thermocoagulation for trigeminal neuralgia, from the literature

Reference	No. of patients	Follow-up (months) Range	Follow-up (months) Mean	Temperature (°C)	Time (s)	No relief n	No relief %	Recurrence rate (%)	Comments
Nugent and Berry (1974)	65	1–41	13	—	30+	1	2	9	
Sweet and Wepsic (1974)	214	30–72	—	47–108	—	14	8	22	
Onofrio (1975)	135	—	—	80	30+	20	15	12	
Howe et al. (1976)	32	1–17	—	70–90	90			21	
Apfelbaum (1977)	48	0–36	—	—	—	6	12	13	
Hardy (1977)	53	0–36	—	65–70	—	3	6	—	
Rhoton et al. (1977)	149	1–53	—	80–85	30–60	3	2	19	
Sengupta and Stunden (1977)	39	2–20	—	60	120	3	8	8	
Siegfried (1977)	416	8–57	—	65	60	6	8	5	
Tew and Keller (1977)	400	12–84	48	60+	60+	4	2	14	
Silverberg and Britt (1978)	38	—	—	70–75	60–90	2	1	13	
Guidetti et al. (1979)	167	—	—	—	—	1	0.6	3	
Steude (1979)	104	10–48	24	70–85	—	—	—	11	Typical trigeminal neuralgia only 75% excellent
Burchiel et al. (1981)	78	—	33	—	—	15	19	23	
Ferguson et al. (1981)	55	2–52	30	—	—	2	4	42	Kaplan–Meier analysis (5 years)
Latchaw et al. (1981)	96	0–96	60	—	—	0	0	52	
Siegfried (1981)	135	66–96	—	60	60	—	—	21	
Choi et al. (1982)	72	1–36	—	—	—	—	—	13	
Nugent (1982)	800	—	55	—	—	—	—	23	
Schwarcz (1982)	400	—	72	—	—	7	17	9	
van Loveren et al. (1982)	700	—	72	—	—	7	1	20	14 others facial pain
Hitchcock et al. (1983)	33	—	14	—	—	1	3	8/33	
Kanpolat and Onol (1980)	256	0–96	—	—	—	16	6	17/256	
Frank et al. (1985)	930	6–60	—	—	—	1	13	21	
Spincemaille et al. (1985)	53	6–42	24	60–80	60	8	15	5	1 death
Mittal and Thomas (1986)	229	3–96	42	60	60	17	6	21	60% excellent, 27% good
Tew and van Loveren (1988)	950	1–204	96	60	30	22	2	14	
Sinduo (1987)	609	12–132	—	—	—	—	—	7	
Fraioli et al. (1989b)	474	2–132	78	—	—	4	1	11	
Meglio and Cioni (1989)	33	0–72	—	75–80	60–180	6	18	20/30	Mean time to recurrence 18.5 months
Broggi et al. (1990)	1000	60–188	111	65–70	60	52	5	18	
Rovit (1990)	550	0–240	—	—	—	25	5	19	
Choudhury et al. (1991)	40	—	—	—	—	5	3	15	
Moraci et al. (1992)	215	84–120	24	65	—	14	4	20	
	353	12–84	—	<65	—	—	—	26	
Sanders and Henny (1992)	240	12–96	50	65–70	60			28.3	
Broggi et al. (1993)	712	12–168	—	65–75	—	39	5	18	
Zakrzewska and Thomas (1993)	256	1–76	45	70–80	300	11	4	22	Kaplan–Meier median recurrence 24 months

the flushing spreads to the eyelids and forehead and first-division anaesthesia is not required, the procedure can be terminated at this point (Sweet and Wepsic, 1974). Ipsilateral lacrimation may occur. Careful sensory testing throughout the procedure reduces the incidence of corneal reflex loss and results in less deep anaesthesia and its consequences.

The patient should be kept on the radiography table for 15 minutes before being sent back to the ward. A careful check should be carried out to ensure that the correct degree of sensory loss has been achieved and the pain has gone. The sensory loss should be sufficient to cause a sharp prick to be appreciated as light touch, rather than not be felt at all (Tew and Keller, 1977; Burchiel, 1987b; Rovit, 1990).

The patient can be discharged the following day, or within 3 days. Medication is slowly tapered off. Antibiotics and ampicillin may be given for 5 days (Rovit, 1990). Patients must be given instructions about eye care, and warned of the effect of facial analgesia and possible masseteric weakness (Tew and Keller, 1977).

Further technical details are given by Rovit (1990).

RESULTS

Two large series have been reported from European centres but are not included in the tables as they have not been published in English and all the details are not known: 257 patients (Brandt and Wittkamp, 1983), 1357 patients (Siegfried, 1981). Siegfried has, however, published in English and probably used the same data (Siegfried, 1977, 1981). Brandt and Wittkamp (1983) followed 115 patients for 1–13 years and had excellent or good results in 71%.

Recurrence rate
No relief of symptoms occurred in 0–19% of cases, as shown in Table 8.2. Some of the failures are due to technical problems such as the inability to enter the foramen ovale (Sweet and Wepsic, 1974) or patient anxiety (Latchaw *et al.*, 1981).

Over 14 000 treatments have been reported, with variable follow-up (Table 8.2). The recurrence rate quoted ranges from 4% to 65%. The wide variation in recurrence rates in part depends on what constitutes a recurrence. In their series Tew and Keller (1977) quote a recurrence rate for those with pain severe enough to need surgery of 9% (37 patients), for those requiring medical treatment it was only 3% (13), and for those having no treatment 2% (six). Meglio and Cioni (1989) and Zakrzewska and Thomas (1993) had a high recurrence rate as any pain was classed as a recurrence; others class a recurrence to have occurred only if repeated surgery is required. Some clinicians expect higher recurrence rates owing to the use of lower temperatures but a decrease in the frequency of sensory loss (Tew and van Loveren, 1988). Recurrence rates and complications may be assessed together to give overall outcomes. Tew and van Loveren (1988) stated that, of their 950 procedures, 65% were excellent, 27% good, 5% fair and 1% poor. In the last three categories there was no trigeminal neuralgia pain but there were problems with dysaesthesia (to be discussed later). These results were based on patient questionnaires.

Life-table analysis of recurrence rates has been performed by some workers and indicates a sharp rise in recurrence in the first year and then a gradual tailing off (Burchiel *et al.*, 1981; Broggi *et al.*, 1990; Zakrzewska and Thomas, 1993). This was also found by Siegfried (1981) in a 12-year follow-up.

Factors affecting recurrence rates

Multiple sclerosis. Patients with multiple sclerosis appear to have a successful outcome (Guidetti *et al.*, 1979).

Previous surgery. Patients who have had previous peripheral surgery have the same recurrence rate, but those who have undergone craniotomy or some destructive procedure of the trigeminal roots such as alcohol injections have a higher rate (Hardy, 1977; Latchaw *et al.*, 1981). The recurrence rate after repeat radiofrequency thermocoagulation is the same as that after first surgery (Latchaw *et al.*, 1981).

Extent of sensory loss. There is some evidence to suggest that the more extensive the sensory loss the less likely a recurrence (Onofrio, 1975; Guidetti *et al.*, 1979; Latchaw *et al.*, 1981, Broggi *et al.*, 1990, Moraci *et al.*, 1992).

Broggi *et al.* (1990) showed a recurrence rate of 41% (71 patients) in 175 who had postoperative hypalgesia, whereas it was 13% (110 patients) in 825 with analgesia. Unfortunately the method of assessment of their results is not given. The extent of sensory loss must be assessed early in the postoperative period as there is gradual sensory return in most patients. Some clinicians report that no, or only short-lived, sensory loss after surgery normally results in immediate recurrence (Nugent and Berry, 1974; Sweet and Wepsic, 1974; Broggi *et al.*, 1990), but others have reported no statistically significant correlation between sensory loss and pain recurrence (Sengupta and Stunden, 1977; Meglio and Cioni, 1989; Zakrzewska and Thomas, 1993). Because of this some clinicians do not consider it necessary to test for sensory loss throughout the procedure (Zakrzewska and Thomas, 1993), although not all clinicians agree with this. Miserococchi and co-workers (1989) found that, when the area of sensory loss correlated exactly with the pain area, they had a recurrence rate of 15%, but when the sensory loss did not cover the whole pain area the rate was 39%.

Other factors. Age, number of divisions involved, length of time of disease and response to medication do not correlate with recurrence rate (Latchaw *et al.*, 1981; Siegfried, 1981). Patients classified as having 'non-classical trigeminal neuralgia' do less well than those with the classical condition (Latchaw *et al.*, 1981).

COMPLICATIONS

Sweet and Poletti (1988) reported on a postal survey carried out to elicit postoperative complications after radiofrequency thermocoagulation procedures.

They had reports from 140 neurosurgeons totalling around 8000 procedures. Some of the complications had not previously been reported and involved higher morbidity rates than is suggested in the literature; these have been detailed fully by Sweet and Poletti (1988). They suggested that the more skilled the neurosurgeon, the fewer complications are recorded. The major complications are summarized in Table 8.3.

Mortality and major morbidity
In over 14 000 reported cases, two deaths have been recorded. One was from intracerebral haemorrhage (Mittal and Thomas, 1986) and another from bilateral pneumonia after unsuccessful radiofrequency thermocoagulation (Nugent and Berry, 1974). However, Sweet and Poletti (1988), in their survey of neurosurgeons who had performed over 6000 operations, found that ten patients had suffered intracranial haemorrhage of whom five had died and one had permanent hemiplegia. Eight other deaths had been due to intracranial haemorrhage. In total, 13 deaths and four cases of major morbidity were reported. During radiofrequency thermocoagulation, temporary rises of blood pressure are common, and this, coupled with drugs causing prolonged bleeding, may account for the complications (Sweet *et al.*, 1985). Intracranial haemorrhage is the most serious complication and can be caused by puncture of a vessel by the electrode. However, in other cases the intracranial haematoma is in the opposite hemisphere. Sweet *et al.* (1985) suggested that these are due to the rise of blood pressure during the procedure. Monitoring of blood pressure during the procedure will enable vasodilators such as nitroprusside to be given when appropriate.

Peroperative complications
The most frequent complication is puncture of the carotid artery but this appears to have few sequelae (Sweet and Wepsic, 1974; Silverberg and Britt, 1978; Sweet, 1990). Minor carotid cavernous fistulae have been recorded in six patients of whom three needed surgical treatment (Sweet, 1986; Rovit, 1990). Other rare complications include an attack of angina (Sweet and Wepsic, 1974).

Other neurosurgical complications
These are rare and there have been only a handful of reports: aseptic meningitis (Sweet and Wepsic, 1974; Silverberg and Britt, 1978; Hitchcock *et al.*, 1983; Sweet and Poletti, 1988; Rovit, 1990), temporal lobe abscess (Sweet, 1986; Rovit, 1990) and bacterial meningitis (Silverberg and Britt, 1978; Sweet and Poletti, 1988). Other cranial nerve lesions have been reported: transient diplopia can occur in up to 2% of patients and is probably due to palsy of the sixth and fourth nerves (Siegfried, 1977; Tew and Keller, 1977; Broggi *et al.*, 1990) and oculomotor problems have also been reported (Siegfried, 1977; Sweet, 1986). Palsies of the sixth nerve have been described (Onofrio, 1975; Guidetti *et al.*, 1979) as well as one patient with seventh cranial nerve damage (Mittal and Thomas, 1986). Two peroperative seizures and one transient postoperative psychosis have also been noted (Sweet and Poletti, 1988).

Sweet (1990) reported on eight patients who became blind, mostly due to technical errors in the placement of the needle: one was due to subhyaloid haemorrhage, one to internal and external ophthalmoplegia, one to nerve paresis and a further two became blind for no known cause. Central retinal artery occlusion in a diabetic patient has also been recorded (Sweet and Poletti, 1988). It is essential that radiographs are taken after placement of the needle to avoid these types of complication (Sweet and Poletti, 1988).

Corneal reflex loss

One of the major complications of radiofrequency thermocoagulation is loss of the corneal reflex, either intentionally when there is pain in the first division or unintentionally, although this loss rarely causes problems (Cobb and Fung, 1983). Reporting is again very varied, with terms such as decreased or absent corneal reflex, corneal ulcers, scarring and neurolytic keratitis being used; up to 20% of patients may have some or all of these problems. The lower frequency of eye problems in the series of Moraci *et al.* (1992) may be due to the use of lower temperatures, 65°C or less (Table 8.3).

There is only one ophthalmological study that has attempted to assess the effect of corneal anaesthesia in 13 patients. Temperatures between 65 and 80°C were used for 30–90 seconds. The three patients who had neuralgia of the first division developed corneal anaesthesia; in the other ten patients, six had a reduction in corneal sensation and two had corneal anaesthesia. Of those with reduced corneal sensation, only one patient was aware of numbness. After 23 months of follow-up, no patient developed problems (Lewis *et al.*, 1982). This same group reviewed 16 other patients retrospectively who had corneal anaesthesia and found two with corneal scarring, one with a corneal ulcer treated unsuccessfully with tarsorrhaphy who later developed central corneal opacities and decreased visual acuity, and one with a corneal ulcer 3 years after operation treated with antibiotics who also developed opacities. The remaining 12 patients had no problems (Lewis *et al.*, 1982). However, two patients have been reported as going blind after radiofrequency thermocoagulation as a result of corneal anaesthesia (Sweet and Wepsic, 1974; Broggi *et al.*, 1990).

The cause of neuroparalytic keratitis remains unknown but, in some way, loss of corneal sensation affects normal corneal metabolism and function.

However, even patients with only decreased corneal sensation may develop blurred vision or keratitis (Tew and Keller, 1977), and it is important that all patients are given clear instructions on care of the eyes (see Chapter 10).

To avoid this complication, Rovit (1990) suggested combining radiofrequency thermocoagulation of the lower divisions with glycerol injection for the ophthalmic divisions in those who have pain in the first division, but no other surgeons have shown this to work.

Sensory loss

What exactly constitutes sensory loss is unclear in the literature but I define it as any decrease in sensation, be it to touch or pain. The procedure should produce

Table 8.3 Common complications after radiofrequency thermocoagulation for trigeminal neuralgia, from the literature

Reference	No. of patients	Disturbing sensory changes		Anaesthesia dolorosa	Motor paresis of masseter	Eye problems	Change in corneal reflex	Ocular palsy	Comments
		Mild	Severe						
Nugent and Berry (1974)	65	0 (0)	0 (0)	3 (5)	28 (43)	1 (1.5)	2 (3)	—	1 death
Sweet and Wepsic (1974)	214	6 (3)	2 (0.9)	0 (0)	119 (53)	1 (0.5)	45 (21)	1 (0.5)	1 blind
Onofrio (1975)	135	—	—	2 (1)	56 (40)	2 (1)	10 (7)	1 (0.7)	
Howe et al. (1976)	32	16 (50)	0 (0)	0 (0)	9 (12)	0 (0)	4 (5.2)	0 (0)	
Apfelbaum (1977)	48	Several	0 (0)	6 (13)	1 (2)	0 (0)	7 (14.5)	—	
Hardy (1977)	53	5 (9)		3 (5.6)	—	1 (1.8)	21 (39)	—	
Rhoton et al. (1977)	149	29 (19)	21 (14)	20 (13)	90 (60)	0 (0)	0 (0)	1 (0.7)	
Sengupta and Stunden (1977)	39	8 (21)		0 (0)	0 (0)	2 (5)	7 (18)	0 (0)	
Siegfried (1977)	416	9 (1.8)		4 (0.8)	126 (30)	8 (1)	—	6 (1.4)	
Tew and Keller (1977)	400	76 (19)		1 (0.3)	88 (22)	32 (8)	5 (13)	1 (0.7)	
Silverberg and Britt (1978)	38	—		1 (0.5)	2 (5)	0 (0)	7 (4)		
Guidetti et al. (1979)	167	10 (1)	1 (1)	1 (0.5)	6 (3)	0 (0)			
Steude (1979)	104	0 (0)		0 (0)	0 (0)	0 (0)			
Burchiel et al. (1981)	78	11 (15)		3 (4)	16 (28)	0 (0)	2 (3)		
Ferguson et al. (1981)	55	0 (0)	0 (0)	1 (2)	5 (5)	0 (0)	4 (7)		
Latchaw et al. (1981)	96	12 (13)	13 (13)	2 (2)	33 (24)	2 (3)	39 (40.6)		
Siegfried (1981)	135	32 (23)	0 (0)	5 (3.7)		8 (6)	6 (4.4)	5 (3.7)	
Choi et al. (1982)	72	12 (17)		1 (1)					
Nugent (1982)	800	70 (9)	41 (5)	6 (1)	198 (25)	—	90 (11)	—	
Schwarcz (1982)	400	211 (76)	0 (0)	1 (0.4)	Frequent	5 (2)			
van Loveren et al. (1982)	700	212 (33)	32 (5)	35 (5)	168 (24)	28 (4)		—	
Hitchcock et al. (1983)	47	4 (8)	0 (0)	1 (2)	4 (8)	1 (2)	2 (4.2)	4 (1)	
Kanpolat and Onol (1980)	370	—	—	6 (1.8)	9 (2.8)	1 (0.3)	24 (7.3)	—	
Frank et al. (1985)	930	—	109 (11)	6 (0.6)	9 (1)	—	10 (1)	—	
Spincemaille et al. (1985)	53	1 (2)	4 (8)	0 (0)	0 (0)	0 (0)	0 (0)	—	No patients with pain Va
Mittal and Thomas (1986)	229	15 (6)	—	22 (9)	2 (1)	10 (4)	34 (34)	2 (1)	
Tew and van Loveren (1988)	950	195 (20)	—	28 (3)	253 (27)	18 (3)	285 (30)	19 (0.2)	1 death
Sinduo et al. (1987)	609	90 (15)	—	30 (5)	154 (35)	25 (4)	140 (23)	25 (4)	
Fraioli et al. (1989b)	474	—	81 (15)	8 (1.5)	16 (3)	10 (1.9)	108 (20.3)	1 (0.2)	Only patients with typical trigeminal neuralgia
Meglio and Cioni (1989)	33	—	8 (24)	0 (0)	0 (0)	—	—	—	
Miserocochi et al. (1989)	111	38 (44)	9 (11)	1 (1)	—	2 (2)	—	—	
Broggi et al. (1990)	1000	37 (3.7)	52 (5)	15 (1.5)	105 (11)	5 (0.6)	197 (20)	5 (0.5)	1 eye loss
Rovit (1990)	550	254 (46)	—	1 (0.2)	35 (6)	—	23 (4)	—	
Choudhury et al. (1991)	40	2 (5)	—	—	4 (10)	1 (2.5)	—	—	
Moraci et al. (1992)	215	125 (20.6)	—	2 (0.3)	81 (13)	6 (0.9)	197 (20)	—	
Sanders and Henny (1992)	240	—	—	—	3 (1.2)	—	33 (13.7)	—	
Broggi et al. (1993)	712	—	130 (18)	0 (0)	73 (11)	4 (0.6)	142 (19.7)	—	
Zakrzewska and Thomas (1993)	256	28 (1.8)	0 (0)	14 (8)	—	26 (15)	—	—	Patient questionnaire

Values in parentheses are percentages.

sensory loss to pain, but light touch sensation should be preserved so resulting in hypalgesia (mild, moderate or severe) but not analgesia (Siegfried, 1981). Therefore, some sensory loss is inevitable if pain relief is to be obtained. However, loss of sensation to touch should be considered a complication as it does cause morbidity in many patients (Zakrzewska and Thomas, 1993). Preservation of touch sensation can only be done using lower coagulation temperatures. Temperatures between 60 and 65°C often result in only slight pinprick reduction whereas those above 76°C produce analgesia with resultant paraesthesia (Salar *et al.*, 1983). Differences in sensory loss may also be observed in patients treated at 65°C or less, but use of higher temperatures allows persistence for longer (Moraci *et al.*, 1992). However, Cobb and Fung (1983) found no clear relationship between lesion temperature and the likelihood of sensory change. They also found no relationship between the duration of electrode heating and sensory change, and this is reflected in the results from other workers, especially Zakrzewska and Thomas (1993) who lesioned for 300 seconds and yet did not have a grossly higher rate of sensory loss. Recovery of pinprick sensibility in the long term is more likely when lower temperatures are used (Salar *et al.*, 1983).

What may be more important is the threshold at which stimulation is perceived: 0.2 volts or less produces little change. This may be due to mechanical injury by the needle tip being very close to the rootlets rather than the stimulation.

The loss of light touch sensation can occur beyond the treatment area in as many as 46% of patients (Nugent and Berry, 1974; Onofrio, 1975; Latchaw *et al.*, 1981; Hitchcock *et al.*, 1983). The sensory loss is often less intense in these other areas (Cobb and Fung, 1983; Hitchcock *et al.*, 1983). This could be related to the placement of the needle primarily in CSF, as opposed to neuronal tissue. The CSF may diffuse heat away from the desired area into other areas (Tobler *et al.*, 1983). There is considerable variation in the reporting of sensory loss and its effects, and few define their terms. Dysaesthesia varies from a mild annoyance through to frank pain, and is classified by some as mild, moderate or severe. At the end of the spectrum is anaesthesia dolorosa. Some classify the severity of the dysaesthesia on the basis of drug use (Sweet, 1986; Broggi *et al.*, 1990). The risk of disturbing sensory changes can be as high as 21% and some suggest it is more common in the elderly (Tew and van Loveren, 1988). Anaesthesia dolorosa occurs in 1–5% of patients, but Apfelbaum (1977) reported a 13% frequency in an early series.

Loss of touch sensation can result in patients traumatizing the skin by scratching, which can result in excoriation of the skin (Tew and Keller, 1977). Loss of sensation intraorally is a particular problem in denture wearers. Not only do they have difficulty controlling their dentures, but they develop traumatic ulcers. This complication can be reduced with the use of a curved electrode (Tew and van Loveren, 1988).

Motor weakness: mastication and hearing

Weakness of the muscles of mastication has been reported in as many as 53% of patients (Table 8.3) but this improves over 3–6 months and is rarely permanent

(Nugent and Berry, 1974; Onofrio, 1975; Rovit, 1990; Moraci *et al.*, 1992). It is not always perceived by the patient. In an 8-year follow-up masseteric weakness was initially seen in 24% of patients but had dropped to only 1.5% at 5.5–8 years of follow-up (Siegfried, 1981). Weakness of the masseter, temporalis and pterygoids results in jaw deviation, but it is the loss of sensation that causes most problems with chewing (Tew and Keller, 1977).

As well as affecting the masticatory system, paralysis of the tensor veli palatini will result in failure of closure of the eustachian tube. This results in patients complaining of a feeling of fullness or even positional deafness (Onofrio, 1975; Sengupta and Stunden, 1977; Tew and Keller, 1977).

Other
It has been suggested that the use of a curved tip for making the lesion reduces masseteric weakness and depth of analgesia and, in a series of 150 patients followed for a maximum of 2 years, 7.3% had masseteric weakness, 9.3% minor paraesthesia, 2% keratitis and there were no patients with anaesthesia dolorosa (Tobler *et al.*, 1983). These results are better than those found in the series of van Loveren *et al.* (1982). Both clinicians used the same techniques and assessments.

CURRENT STATUS

Radiofrequency thermocoagulation of the gasserian ganglion is the commonest surgical method used for management of trigeminal neuralgia. It is a highly specific procedure. Its major advantages and disadvantages are listed in Table 8.4.

Considerable skill is required to carry out the procedure. If touch sensation is to be preserved but pain relief obtained, then multiple lesions must be produced, and careful sensory testing carried out during surgery. Relief of pain is immediate and lasts for 3–4 years. The procedure can easily be repeated.

However, patients must accept some loss of touch sensation. Controversy remains about the relationship between loss of touch sensation and recurrence rate. Loss occurs beyond the affected division but is often less severe; however,

Table 8.4 Advantages and disadvantages of radiofrequency thermocoagulation of the gasserian ganglion

Advantages	Disadvantages
Highly specific	Expensive equipment
Safe for older patients	Tedious skilled procedure
Immediate relief of pain	Must be able to wake the patient during the procedure
Relatively low recurrence rate	
Low mortality rate	Sensory loss beyond area affected
Few complications outside trigeminal area	Corneal anaesthesia
	Possible neuroparalytic keratitis
Can vary amount of sensory loss	Possible anaesthesia dolorsa

if it affects the first division the corneal reflex is lost. The less touch sensation has been preserved, the more likely it is for painful dysaesthesia to occur. Although rare, anaesthesia dolorosa is very debilitating and extremely difficult to manage. It can be a worse problem than the original trigeminal neuralgia because it is a continuous pain, unrelenting, untreatable and unresponsive to all analgesics (Rovit, 1990). Neuroparalytic keratitis is a relatively rare complication in comparison to the number of patients who have a reduction in corneal sensation.

This procedure remains the method of choice for most patients who are beyond medical management. It is the procedure most widely done, by both neurosurgeons and anaesthetists. Careful selection of patients is crucial as radiofrequency thermocoagulation may unmask other forms of facial pain that can become extremely difficult to manage (Zakrzewska and Thomas, 1993). In a 3-year follow-up (by regular questionnaire) of 56 patients who had radiofrequency thermocoagulation, those who did not have classical trigeminal neuralgia were found to have more postoperative pain, more complications and were more reluctant to undergo repeat surgery (Jassim, 1994). Sweet *et al.* (1981) have also commented that this group of patients has more complications. Depression, which is frequently present before operation, does lift after surgery in both groups of patients. Patients must be warned about loss of touch sensation and the area it will involve, as they are more willing to accept the loss if it has been explained to them beforehand (Tew and van Loveren, 1988). The procedure does provide a good period of pain relief, albeit not permanent.

PERCUTANEOUS RETROGASSERIAN GLYCEROL RHIZOTOMY

This technique was first described by Hakanson in 1978 as a result of a chance finding. Hakanson and Leksell planned to use stereotactically focused γ radiation to destroy the trigeminal ganglion. They first injected tantalum dust mixed in glycerol into the trigeminal cistern and noticed that glycerol relieved the pain. Until then, the injection of substances into the gasserian ganglion had been hampered by uncertainty of the precise position of the ganglion and the exact location of the needle. Contrast medium had been used previously but none had been effective until Hakanson (1978) suggested the use of metrizamide, a new water-soluble non-toxic medium.

Clinicians quickly took up the technique as it resulted in less loss of touch sensation than radiofrequency coagulation and yet resulted in pain relief. Since Hakanson's first evaluation (1981) in 75 patients, more than 20 papers involving over 1000 patients have been published.

MECHANISM

Glycerol is a simple three-carbon molecule used as a pure anhydrous sterile solution. Some workers have suggested that, although neurotoxicity occurs to both myelinated and unmyelinated nerve fibres, the latter are affected initially (Hakanson, 1981; Sweet, 1988). For this reason, it is postulated that pain relief can be obtained before loss of sensation. However, repeat procedures result in increasing neurotoxicity and hence gradual loss of touch sensation (Lunsford, 1990).

The glycerol is placed in varying amounts into the trigeminal cistern which surrounds the retrogasserian part of the trigeminal nerve within Meckel's cave. Rengachary *et al.* (1983) have shown in animals that glycerol is chemoneurotoxic in the same way as phenol and ethanol, and causes partial deafferentation with no selectivity for different fibres. Injected intraneuronal glycerol causes more extensive destruction than if applied to the surface of the nerve, where the fibres closest to the perineurium are destroyed first.

The high viscosity and poor miscibility of glycerol ensure that it diffuses out of the cistern very slowly and so has a slow neurolytic effect. This would account for its delay in action and also lack of complications in comparison with ethanol, which diffuses rapidly into the CSF. Stajcic (1990) also showed that destruction of rat nerve fibres was not selective.

METHODS

Anaesthesia

In the original descriptions all but one of the patients were operated on under local anaesthesia after premedication with oxycodone hydrochloride–scopalamine and droperidol or atropine (Hakanson, 1981; Lunsford and Bennett, 1984). Lignocaine (1%) is injected locally (Lunsford and Bennett, 1984) and in some patients postoperative intravenous analgesia is given (Young, 1988). Others insert an intravenous line and give continuous fentanyl throughout (Lunsford and Bennett, 1984; Waltz *et al.*, 1989). Methohexital can be given just before penetration of the foramen ovale (Lunsford, 1990).

Lunsford (1990) suggested that a general anaesthetic should be available. Careful cardiovascular monitoring is essential as changes in the cardiovascular system can occur in up to 20% of patients, with 15% having a vasovagal response (Lunsford, 1990).

Technique

The patient is in a seated or supine position (Lunsford, 1990). Entrance to the trigeminal cistern is the same as for radiofrequency thermocoagulation. Young (1988) has suggested that the foramen should be visualized radiographically before procedure is started. Fluoroscopic imaging has made the procedure easier.

A lumbar puncture needle, 20–22 G and 0.7 mm in length, is introduced under intermittent fluoroscopic control through the foramen ovale into the cistern until CSF just begins to flow spontaneously; the flow should not be rapid (van de Welde *et al.*, 1989). The flow is variable but cannot be used to confirm location of the retrogasserian cistern (Lunsford, 1990). The needle should be medial to the midpoint of the foramen, which is about 5–10 mm past the foramen ovale (Young, 1988).

Before the glycerol can be injected the precise location of the needle in the cistern and the size of the cistern need to be determined. To achieve this, metrizamide (contrast medium) is slowly injected until CSF drainage is achieved (Hakanson, 1978). Steiger (1991) uses iohexol, which leaves a permanent record.

As the medium is introduced (0.2–0.4 ml), it can be seen to be filling the cistern and then escaping posteriorly. Lateral and anteroposterior radiographs can then be taken to ensure the correct position (Hakanson, 1981). Young (1988) has argued that this is not an accurate method as some dye may not be visible on fluoroscopic examination, whereas Lunsford (1990) stated that as little as 0.01 ml medium will show up. If the position is incorrect, a second needle is introduced before the first is withdrawn. This may occur in up to 15% of patients (Hakanson 1981). Once visualization has occurred the contrast medium is drained, assisted by lying the patient down temporarily. It is important not to aspirate the contrast medium as this raises pressure. If the ophthalmic division is to be injected, some contrast medium can be left at the base, so preserving the mandibular branch (Lunsford and Bennett, 1984; Rappaport, 1986) (Fig. 8.5).

When cisternography is used, changes in the position of head are necessary and can result in the needle being dislodged. Others, therefore, do not perform cisternography and rely on sensory changes, the 'glycerol test' (Arias, 1986). A volume of 0.1–0.15 ml glycerol is first injected, which results in a change of sensation, e.g. warm, cold, numbness, pricking (Arias, 1986; Sweet and Poletti, 1988). After 3–5 minutes a further 0.05–0.1 ml glycerol can be injected, depending on the distribution of pain and area of altered sensation achieved (Saini, 1987; Young, 1988; Sweet and Poletti, 1988; Waltz *et al.*, 1989; North *et al.*, 1990). Lunsford and Bennett (1984) found this technique of no help. Whether cisternography alters the results is unknown. One worker found no differences in outcome (Arias, 1986).

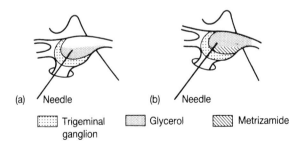

(a) Needle   (b) Needle

▒ Trigeminal ganglion   ▪ Glycerol   ░ Metrizamide

Figure 8.5 By adjusting the amount of the injected glycerol it is possible selectively to affect the different trigeminal divisions. Because of the density of glycerol it remains in the bottom of the cistern and therefore a small amount will affect only the third division (a). For the treatment of first and second division neuralgias, the rootlets of the third division may be spared by leaving a small amount of metrizamide in the bottom of the cistern (b).

Pure sterile 99.9% anhydrous glycerol is introduced very slowly via a 1-ml syringe (Fig. 8.6). The volume needed varies from 0.2 to 0.4 ml, depending on the results of cisternography. Some advocate filling the whole cistern regardless of the site of pain (Burchiel, 1987b), but others relate the volume injected to the number of branches involved (Hakanson, 1981) or suggest that it should be based on the degree of sensory loss required (Sweet, 1988). Lunsford and Bennett (1984) mix the glycerol with sterile tantalum dust to provide permanent visualization of the nerve and cistern.

The patient must be warned that facial pain may occur during the injection and last for a couple of hours (Burchiel, 1987b). Sophisticated intraoperative sensory testing is not required; however, some workers continue to test for sensory loss while injecting, arguing that it ensures the minimum volume of glycerol is used so that selective damage to the rootlets occurs (Arias, 1986; Sweet, 1988). The position of the head will also affect 'movement' of the glycerol (Sweet, 1988). Corneal sensory loss may also be reduced if the glycerol is not left in the cistern for more than 10 minutes when operating on the first division (Sweet, 1988).

After operation it is important to ensure that the patient sits up with the head flexed for 1–4 hours (Hakanson, 1981; Burchiel, 1987b; Lunsford, 1990; North *et al.*, 1990). To reduce sensory loss, Bergenheim *et al.* (1991) have proposed that different neck flexions be used, depending on the division in which pain occurs: 40° for the first division, 25° for the second division and upright for the third. Headache and facial pain after operation may be sufficient to cause hypotension, and opiates or atropine may be needed (Lunsford and Bennett, 1984; Burchiel, 1987b; Young, 1988). More pain and headache occurs in those having cisternography (Arias, 1986). Patients can be discharged on the same or the following day. Medication is steadily tapered off. In half the patients pain relief occurs within 24 hours but in others not for 6 weeks (Lunsford and Bennett, 1984; Rappaport, 1986; Burchiel, 1987b).

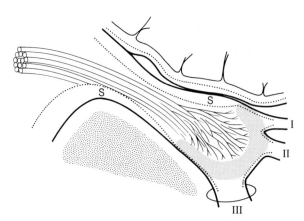

Figure 8.6 Schematic drawing of the dural and arachnoidal coverings of the trigeminal ganglion and roots. The arachnoid is drawn with a wavy line. S, subdural space within Meckel's cave. (Modified from Hakanson, 1981.)

If the procedure is to be successful, anatomical precision is essential. If the operation runs smoothly and there are no technical difficulties, the outcome is successful (Lunsford and Bennett, 1984). The complete procedure takes about 45 minutes. Repeat procedures are more difficult to perform (Slettebo *et al.*, 1993): the volume of the cistern is reduced, there is evidence of arachnoiditis, and it is more difficult to remove the metrizamide (Rappaport and Gomori, 1988).

RESULTS

Recurrence Rates
Pain relief may take 7–10 days to occur (Lunsford, 1990).

No relief of symptoms occurs in about 10% of patients, as shown in Table 8.5. Lack of response can also occur after a first successful procedure (Rappaport and Gomori, 1988). In some patients there are no identifiable causes for failure, but in others there are technical failures, e.g. abnormal anatomy, poor visualization, injection outside the cistern, insufficient glycerol, escape of glycerol from the cistern within 2 hours, or differences in the formulation of the glycerol (osmolarity or viscosity, addition of preservatives) (Hakanson, 1981; Lunsford and Bennett, 1984; Saini, 1987; Burchiel, 1988; Waltz *et al.*, 1989; Fujimaki *et al.*, 1990; Lunsford, 1990).

In some series patients were still included in the analysis if they had two different procedures (Steiger, 1991). There is a wide variability in recurrence rates (Table 8.5), due in part to different methods of analysis, as mentioned at the beginning of this chapter. Some workers excluded patients who died or were lost to follow-up (Saini, 1987; Fujimaki *et al.*, 1990) and yet this can affect the results considerably. Some used a disinterested party to interview patients after operation and so obtained more objective data (North *et al.*, 1990).

Recurrence rates vary from 10% to 72%, as seen in Table 8.5 (Arias, 1986; Fujimaki *et al.*, 1990).

In Saini's 1987 series of 469 patients followed up, only eight were pain-free at 6 years. This contrasts with Hakanson's short report (1984) on 100 patients with a mean follow-up of 4 years, where 78% were still pain-free after the first injection. Adherence to full details of the technique may also affect results (Sweet, 1988). North *et al.* (1990) quoted two different median times to recurrence. Three years is the mean time to recurrence, but at this stage patients may be on medication to which they are no longer refractory. However, at 2 years 50% of patients will have relapsed to their preoperative state and require surgery or medication.

Recurrence is most frequent within the first 6–12 months and the rate then gradually falls off, with a median recurrence time of under 3 years (Lunsford and Bennett, 1984; Rappaport, 1986; Burchiel, 1988; Young, 1988; Waltz *et al.*, 1989).

Factors affecting recurrence rates

Multiple sclerosis. Patients with multiple sclerosis are analysed separately; some authors have found that they have a higher recurrence rate (Beck *et al.*, 1986;

Table 8.5 Results following percutaneous retrogasserian glycerol rhizotomy for trigeminal neuralgia, from the literature

Reference	No. of patients	Cisternography	Follow-up (months) Range	Follow-up (months) Mean	No relief	Recurrence rate (%)	Mean/median recurrence (months)	5-year recurrence rate (%)	Comment
Hakanson (1981)	75	Yes, metrizamide	11–48	18	1 (1)	8	11		
Sweet et al. (1981)	27	Yes, metrizamide	0–30		3 (11)				High recurrence
Lunsford and Bennett (1984)	112	Yes, metrizamide	14–27		12 (11)	7			
Arias (1986)	100		6–36		5 (5)	10			
Beck et al. (1986)	58		2–40	18	10 (17)	11			
Rappaport (1986)	43	Yes, metrizamide	12–27	10	2 (5)	25	6		
Dieckmann et al. (1987)	51		12+		4 (8)	12			
Saini (1987)	469	No	12–72		0 (0)		24	82.6	
Apfelbaum (1988)	73		12–120		4 (6)	23			
Burchiel (1988)	60		3–44		12 (20)	47	18 mean	—	Kaplan–Meier analysis (46 typical trigeminal neuralgia)
Sweet (1988)	80		1.7 years	2.8 years		33			
Young (1988)	162	Not all, metrizamide	6–67		16 (10)	18.5			
Miserocchi et al. (1989)	111	No details	12–49			20			
Waltz et al. (1989)	200	Yes, non-ionic	24–63		36 (18)	24			
Campbell et al. (1990)	19		3–36						
De La Porte et al. (1990)	120	Yes, iohexol or amipaque	0–72						Analysed only 108, with good initial results
Fujimaki et al. (1990)	122	Yes, metrizamide	38–54		13 (11)	72	32 median	72	
Ischia et al. (1990)	112		1–66	42	10 (8)	20.5			
Lunsford (1990)	376	Yes, iohexol	6–90		51 (14)	40	36 median		Kaplan–Meier
North et al. (1990)	85	No	6–54	36			16 mean		Kaplan–Meier
Sahni et al. (1990)	58		6–51		9 (16)	29			Kaplan–Meier
Bergenheim et al. (1991)	106	Yes		3	4 (7)	12			
Steiger (1991)	122		1–96	24	20 (16)	23		41	Kaplan–Meier
Slettebo et al. (1993)	60	Yes	54–108	54 median	4 (7)		47 median	45	Kaplan–Meier

Values in parentheses are percentages.

Burchiel, 1988; Slettebo, 1993) whereas others have shown no difference (Lunsford and Bennett, 1984; Waltz *et al.*, 1989; North *et al.*, 1990).

Previous surgery. Recurrence tends to be more common in patients who have had previous surgery (Slettebo *et al.*, 1993). Previous surgery, such as radiofrequency thermocoagulation or alcohol injection, may affect results as it may have altered the anatomy of the cistern (Beck *et al.*, 1986; North *et al.*, 1990), although anatomical cisternal variation may also be present (Lunsford, 1990). In some of these patients repeated injections can be successful or radiofrequency thermocoagulation should be used (Steiger, 1991).

The time to recurrence after a second glycerol procedure is variable: it may be shorter (less than 1 year) (North *et al.*, 1990; Slettebo *et al.*, 1993) or no different (Rappaport and Gomori, 1988).

Extent of sensory loss. As with radiofrequency thermocoagulation, links with sensory loss and recurrence are looked for. Some workers have found that patients who had no postoperative loss of touch sensation remained pain-free for longer (Burchiel, 1988; Steiger, 1991), whereas others have observed a trend towards a higher recurrence rate in those with less loss (Lunsford, 1990; Slettebo *et al.*, 1993). Steiger (1991) reported that patients with intact sensation before operation had fewest recurrences and that the best prognostic factor for long-term pain relief was some transient or permanent sensory deficit.

Other factors. Patients with tumours in the posterior fossa do badly (Burchiel, 1988).

Predictors of good outcome include patients with classical trigeminal neuralgia, prior success with carbamazepine, and free flow of CSF at the time of needle placement, easy penetration of foramen ovale, normal appearance of the trigeminal cistern on cisternography, easy emptying and ipsilateral retroorbital ophthalmic pain at the time of injection (Lunsford, 1990; North *et al.*, 1990; Steiger, 1991). Age, sex and length of symptoms have not been found to be consistently good prognosticators (North *et al.*, 1990; Steiger, 1991; Slettebo *et al.*, 1993).

COMPLICATIONS

Mortality
Hakanson (1981) reported that one of his patients died from pulmonary embolism 1 week after operation, but no indication was given as to the possible cause. Another death occurred immediately after surgery from myocardial infarction (Lunsford, 1990). The major complications are shown in Table 8.6.

Perioperative complications
Vasovagal attacks are the main problem. Transient bleeding and haematoma formation at the needle site has been reported only by North *et al.* (1990).

Table 8.6 Complications after percutaneous retrogasserian glycerol rhizotomy for trigeminal neuralgia, from the literature

Reference	No. of patients	Loss of light touch sensation	Dysaesthesia	Anaesthesia dolorosa	Motor paresis of masseter	Eye problems	Change of corneal reflex	Comment
Hakanson (1981)	75	44 (60)	0 (0)	0 (0)	0 (0)	0 (0)	0 (0)	
Sweet et al. (1981)	31	20 (65)	4 (20)	0 (0)	—	0 (0)	5 (16)	
Lunsford and Bennett (1984)	112	31 (28)	9 (8)	0 (0)	0 (0)	0 (0)	2 (12)	
Arias (1986)	100	13 (13)	0 (0)	0 (0)	0 (0)	0 (0)	2 (2)	
Beck et al. (1986)	58	10 (17)	1 (2)	0 (0)	—	—	1 (2)	
Rappaport (1986)	24	9 (38)	3 (13)	0 (0)	2 (8)	0 (0)	0 (0)	
Dieckmann et al. (1987)	51	20 (40)	1 (2)	0 (0)	—	—	0 (0)	
Saini (1987)	466	—	61 (2)	26 (8)	16 (34)	—	23 (5)	Previous operations
Apfelbaum (1988)	73	—	4 (5)	—	—	—	3 (4)	
Burchiel (1988)	60	42 (72)	6 (10)	0 (0)	—	0 (0)	8 (23)	
Young (1988)	162	117 (72)	5 (3)	0 (0)	—	0 (0)	8 (5)	
Miserocchi et al. (1989)	111	9 (11)	1 (1)	0 (0)	—	2 (2)	—	
Waltz et al (1989)	200	13 (7)	—	0 (0)	20 (10)	0 (0)	18 (9)	
Campbell et al. (1990)	19	—	8 (50)	0 (0)	—	—	—	
De La Porte et al. (1990)	120	50 (41)	0 (0)	0 (0)	1 (1)	1 (1)	7 (6)	
Fujimaki et al. (1990)	135	20 (50)	23 (29)	3 (2)	—	—	1 (1)	
Ischia et al. (1990)	112	—	49 (44)	—	—	—	4 (3)	
Lunsford (1990)	376	110 (30)	0 (0)	0 (0)	0 (0)	0 (0)	4 (1)	
North et al. (1990)	85	3 (4)	3 (4)	0 (0)	0 (0)	0 (0)	5 (6)	
Sahni et al. (1990)	58	—	—	Some	0 (0)	0 (0)	—	
Bergenheim et al. (1991)	106	—	0 (0)	—	—	0 (0)	—	
Steiger (1991)	122	65 (53)	9 (13)	0 (0)	5 (7)	0 (0)	19 (16)	
Slettebo et al. (1993)	60	13 (76)	8 (38)	0 (0)	0 (0)	1 (2)	13 (22)	

Values in parentheses are percentages.

Headache occurs in 15% of patients for 2–6 hours and may be due to the iodine in the contrast medium, as fewer headaches occur in patients who have metrizamide (Lunsford, 1990).

Other neurological complications
Meningitis, both bacterial and aseptic, has been reported (Lunsford and Bennett, 1984; Beck *et al.*, 1986; Burchiel, 1988; Young, 1988; Waltz *et al.*, 1989; Lunsford, 1990; Slettebo *et al.*, 1993) and may be due to the irritant effect of the contrast medium (Sweet, 1990). Transient diplopia, Bell's palsy and masseteric weakness occur (Beck *et al.*, 1986; North *et al.*, 1990; Steiger, 1991).

Loss of corneal reflex
Corneal anaesthesia does occur and there may be slight or complete loss of the reflex (Lunsford and Bennett, 1984; Burchiel, 1988; Young, 1988; Sweet and Poletti, 1988). No ulceration has been reported, and only one case of corneal keratitis (Slettebo *et al.*, 1993). In evaluating this complication it is important to make baseline observations as up to 15% of patients may have preoperative loss of reflex (Slettebo *et al.*, 1993). Corneal sensory loss often occurs in those with no first-division pain (Burchiel, 1988; Lunsford, 1990; Bergenheim *et al.*, 1991).

Extracisternal or intraganglionic injection of glycerol does not appear to affect the presence or absence of the corneal reflex. Loss of corneal reflex appears to be totally unpredictable and may be due to anatomical variation of the ophthalmic division (Burchiel, 1988).

Loss of sensation
This is the most important complication. In assessing sensory loss, it is important to exclude patients who have had previous surgical procedures as these influence the effects. The timing of the evaluation is important, as numbness subsides with time (Arias, 1986; Waltz *et al.*, 1989) and it is also likely that an increase in sensory dysaesthesia occurs after a second procedure (Rappaport and Gomori, 1988). Loss of sensation may be related to intraganglionic injection or excessive amounts of glycerol (Arias, 1986). Fujimaki *et al.* (1990) have suggested that narrowing of the cisternal CSF space may in some way be related to the toxicity of the glycerol.

Patients complain of slight numbness of the face, but this is often not substantiated by careful sensory testing (Hakanson, 1981). A distinction must also be made between patients with mild loss of light touch (60%: Hakanson, 1981; 26%: Lunsford and Bennett, 1984; 71%: Young, 1988) and those who develop painful paraesthesia or dysaesthesia (2%: Lunsford and Bennett, 1984). The greatest area of sensory loss appears to occur after treatment of the third division, whereas patients treated for pain in the first division develop sensory loss only in that division (Bergenheim *et al.*, 1991). Sensory loss may be more substantial after previous procedures e.g. alcohol blocks or repeat glycerol injections (Fujimaki *et al.*, 1990; Lunsford and Bennett, 1984). After a second operation 50% of patients will have loss of light touch, and this proportion rises to 70% after the third procedure (Lunsford, 1990). Anaesthesia dolorosa has been reported in only two patients (Fujimaki *et al.*, 1990), but it may have occurred after other surgery. There have been other reports of anaesthesia dolorosa, but in patients who had undergone other ablative surgery resulting in sensory deficit before the glycerol treatment, which was later aggravated by the procedure (Slettebo *et al.*, 1993).

Other complications
As in many patients undergoing neurosurgery, a herpes simplex eruption may be found a few days after operation: 27–50% (Hakanson, 1981; Lunsford and Bennett, 1984; Arias, 1986; Beck *et al.*, 1986; Burchiel, 1988; Young, 1988; Steiger, 1991). In four patients it led to subsequent sensory loss (Lunsford and Bennett, 1984). Trigeminal motor weakness has been reported by a few workers (Saini, 1987; Steiger, 1991). Other minor complications include tinnitus (Burchiel, 1988), nasal congestion and rhinorrhoea (Burchiel, 1988); although transient and not serious, these do cause the patient discomfort.

CURRENT STATUS

The first reports on this technique appeared extremely encouraging and led to its adoption in many units, although some now perform the procedure less frequently than previously. It remains, as with other techniques, highly specific for trigeminal neuralgia (Rappaport, 1986; Lunsford, 1990). The advantages and disadvantages are shown in Table 8.7. It is a quick and easy procedure that can be carried out under general anaesthesia without intubation.

Cost is an important consideration in developing countries. If this procedure is done without cisternography, it is the cheapest method for control of trigem-

Table 8.7   Advantages and disadvantages of retrogasserian glycerol injections

Advantages	Disadvantages
Highly specific	Delayed relief of pain
Safe for older patients	Many initial failures
All ranges of anaesthesia possible; general anaesthetic not necessary	Correct needle placement essential
	High recurrence rate
Procedure less stressful and quicker to perform than radiofrequency thermocoagulation	Mild sensory loss in one-third of patients
Cheap equipment	
Few cases of anaesthesia dolorosa	
No complete sensory loss	
No keratitis	
Few complications beyond trigeminal area	
No mortality	
Repeatable	

inal neuralgia as long-term drug therapy is expensive, (Arias, 1986; Saini, 1987) and lesion-generating apparatus is not required.

Although loss of light touch occurs in up to one third of patients, it is not as profound as after radiofrequency thermocoagulation, and anaesthesia dolorosa is extremely rare. Bergenheim *et al.* (1991) suggested that the procedure is highly selective for pain of the first division but less so for other areas. However, it has a high initial failure rate, variable time of onset of pain relief, and a higher recurrence rate than radiofrequency thermocoagulation, causing some neurosurgeons to abandon it (Sweet, 1986).

Despite these disadvantages, I think the procedure has still an important role to play. It is more effective than peripheral techniques and yet does not lead to profound loss of sensation with anaesthesia dolorosa or keratitis. It is especially useful in patients with a trigger area in the first division (Sweet, 1988).

Those of my patients who are extremely reluctant to have surgery and yet cannot be controlled medically decide on this option. They are more willing to accept other surgical treatments in the future once they have seen the advantage of being off all medication yet pain-free. The procedure is extremely useful in the elderly, medically compromised, patient who may die from intercurrent disease before recurrence occurs.

OTHER INJECTIONS

ALCOHOL

The most frequently injected substance, after glycerol, is alcohol. Like glycerol, alcohol is neurotoxic but, in contrast to glycerol, it dissolves rapidly in the CSF and diffuses in the subarachnoid space, so producing more cranial nerve palsies than glycerol. Modern techniques involving fluoroscopic control allow more accurate placement and so reduce complications.

Burchiel (1987b) has described the procedure in detail. All clinicians stress the importance of injecting the alcohol slowly and only a small amount at any time.

Results

The technique was the most successful in Harris' series (1940): of 451 patients, 316 (70%) were pain-free for 3 years or more. Henderson (1967) reported on 217 procedures and, of 86 patients examined 1–17 years after injection, 65% were pain-free. Half of the recurrences were within the first year. Burchiel's (1987) analysis of the literature quoted 88% to be pain-free at 4 years.

Complications

Loss of corneal reflex. The most serious complication is that of keratitis which, even with very careful injection of small amounts of alcohol, cannot be avoided. Henderson (1967) reported that 19% (13 of 69) of patients in his series required tarsorrhaphy and one patient, in whom it was delayed, developed blindness.

White and Sweet (1969) in their review found 26 patients who became blind as a result of keratitis. Regular review of the eye and wearing of protective glasses can minimize keratitis, but its frequency is around 36%. An ophthalmological study, however, assessing 97 patients with corneal anaesthesia, showed that 75% of corneas were normal, 20% had some evidence of neurotrophic keratitis without decreased vision and 5% had permanent corneal changes with decreased visual acuity (Davies, 1970).

Sensory loss. All patients experience numbness, although Henderson (1967) reported that only 33% have total anaesthesia. Sensation returns most frequently to the mandibular division (Henderson, 1967). In some patients the numbness is associated with unpleasant paraesthesia and anaesthesia dolorosa.

The sensory loss can lead to persistent nasal ulceration and is observed in up to 18% of patients (Henderson, 1967).

Other complications. Damage to other cranial nerves (oculomotor, abducens and glossopharyngeal) can occur as a result of leakage into the subarachnoid space, although this may be transient (Henderson, 1967; White and Sweet, 1969). After operation herpes simplex may affect the lips (Harris, 1940).

White and Sweet (1969), in a review of the results of all the published data, suggested that, because of the high risk of corneal anaesthesia, the technique is rarely carried out in the USA.

OTHERS

Other techniques have been explored that injure rather than destroy the gasserian ganglion. Putman and Hampton (1936) injected phenol. Jaeger reported on the use of boiling water (80°C) in 1957 and 1959. He observed fewer complications and 96 of 100 patients had relief, but the recurrence rate was not established owing to the short follow-up (White and Sweet, 1969). No further reports of this technique have followed.

In 1963, Jefferson injected phenol in glycerine into the ganglion and reported his results in 50 patients in 1966. Thirty-six patients had relief but, of the ten in whom loss of touch was minimal, only five were pain-free for an average of 18 months. No corneal ulceration or anaesthesia dolorosa occurred.

OTHER TECHNIQUES

MICROCOMPRESSION

Taarnhoj (1952) first described a method of decompressing the ganglion through the middle cranial fossa, and around 1000 cases have since been reported (Stender and Grumme, 1969). Sheldon *et al.* (1955) then changed from decompression to compression, but the high relapse rate led to these procedures being abandoned. The procedure had a recurrence rate of 20% and so soon became less popular than radiofrequency thermocoagulation. However, the availability of newer technology led Mullan and Lichtor (1983) to develop a technique of percutaneous microcompression of the ganglion.

Methods

The technique has been described in detail by Mullan (1990) and Lobato *et al.* (1990). The procedure is performed under general anaesthesia and patients remain in hospital for 1–5 days. Short-acting barbiturate anaesthesia can be used, provided the patient has received premedication and then atropine, droperidol and fentanyl initially (Fraioli *et al.*, 1989b; Lobato *et al.*, 1990). Sodium thiopental or etomidate is administered at the time of skin puncture, entrance to the foramen ovale and ganglion compression. Oxygen is given through nasal prongs. Under fluoroscopic control a percutaneous needle or trocar (no. 14) is inserted into the foramen ovale, but not allowed to penetrate it, so decreasing the risk of haemorrhage. The catheter is then advanced into Meckel's cave. A Fogarty-type balloon with a capacity of 0.75 ml is filled with water-soluble contrast medium. A volume of 0.6–1 ml is required for adequate compression (Lobato *et al.*, 1990). It is marked on the external surface to ensure that it does not penetrate the posterior fossa. The balloon is then advanced into Meckel's cave and slowly inflated under fluoroscopic control until it assumes a pear shape. If it is in the incorrect position, it must be withdrawn together with the needle. A balloon pressure above 60 mmHg is required, with an average of 1200 mmHg (Lobato *et al.*, 1990). The compression is then maintained for 0.5–10 minutes. The longer the compression, the more likely it is for sensory loss to occur (Esposito *et al.*, 1985). Mullan (1990) and Lobato *et al.* (1990) now use 1 minute, provided the pressure is adequate. After aspiration of the contrast medium and withdrawal of the catheter, firm pressure is put on the cheek, as this helps to reduce haematoma formation. The whole procedure takes 15 minutes.

It is essential to monitor arterial blood pressure and heart rate throughout the procedure as significant falls have been recorded upon entry of the needle into the foramen ovale or upon balloon manipulation that causes compression of the ganglion or roots. Atropine must be at hand (Brown and Pruel, 1988). Lobato *et al.* (1990) advocated a bolus of sodium nitroprusside just before balloon distension.

Results

Lichtor and Mullan (1990) reviewed 100 patients followed up for 1–10 years, some of whom were part of the first report in 1983 (Mullan and Lichtor, 1983). Follow-up was by questionnaire and telephone; only three patients were lost to follow-up and eight died. At 5 years a recurrence rate of 20% (12 of 61) was found; of these, four had been controlled by carbamazepine, three had a repeat procedure and five (8%) went on to other neurosurgery. In this group there were also six patients with multiple sclerosis in whom less compression was used (Mullan, 1990). In the series of Lobato *et al.* (1990) of 164 procedures on 144 patients, the initial failure rate was 6% (nine patients); all failures were related to technical problems. Fourteen patients (10%) had pain recurrence 10–35 months after surgery. Fraioli *et al.* (1989b), in a series of 143 patients, had an initial failure rate of 10%; at a mean follow-up of 3.5 years 10% had had a recurrence. Another small group of 25 patients followed for a maximum of 7 years showed a 24% recurrence rate (Belber and Rak, 1987), whereas 50 other patients had a recurrence rate of 22% at 6 months (Esposito *et al.*, 1985).

It is estimated that at 10 years 70% of patients will still be pain-free, with an overall recurrence rate of 28%. Meglio and Cioni (1989), who have followed 74 patients for a maximum of 28 months, reported a mean recurrence time of 6.5 months. Recurrence rates were higher in those who had a shorter compression (1–3 minutes). About 5% will obtain no pain relief (Meglio and Cioni, 1989; Lichtor and Mullan, 1990), although up to 22% have been recorded as having no relief (Esposito *et al.*, 1985; Broggi *et al.*, 1990).

Complications

One death has been recorded from intracerebral haemorrhage due to penetration of the needle through the foramen ovale and the tip of the catheter entering the posterior fossa (Spaziante *et al.*, 1988).

Due to the severe brachycardia that can occur at the time of distension of the balloon, patients with cardiac problems may be excluded from having the operation (Mullan and Lichtor, 1983). Bleeding, venous or arterial, may occur in up to 13% of patients, but the procedure can still be performed (Lobato *et al.*, 1990). However, Meglio and Cioni (1989) reported that the procedure had to be stopped in three patients because of excessive bleeding, which may have been due to the large size of the cannula; arteriovenous communications can occur (Mullan, 1990).

There is always some loss of light touch sensation, the third division being most affected in half (Esposito *et al.*, 1985; Broggi *et al.*, 1990) to all patients (Lobato *et al.*, 1990). This gradually diminishes, but at 1 year 40% of patients may still have some areas of decreased sensation (Lobato *et al.*, 1990), and up to 10% of patients will have a distressing dysaesthesia (Broggi *et al.*, 1990).

The corneal reflex is maintained in most cases (Belber and Rak, 1987), although it is usually reduced initially (Lobato *et al.*, 1990).

Some masseteric weakness is present but rarely noticed by the patient (Mullan, 1990; Belber and Rak, 1987). The weakness is transient and generally lasts for only 3 months (Mullan, 1990; Belder and Rak, 1987), although it may persist in up to 12% of patients (Lobato *et al.*, 1990).

Dysaesthesia and hyperaesthesia occur, and may be related to the time of compression (Belber and Rak, 1987; Meglio and Cioni, 1989; Lichtor and Mullan, 1990; Lobato *et al.*, 1990). Disagreeable sensations may occur in 7–19% of patients, sometimes aggravated by stress (Fraioli *et al.*, 1989b; Lobato *et al.*, 1990). No keratitis or intracranial vascular injury has been recorded (Mullan,

1990), but one patient developed anaesthesia dolorosa (Fraioli *et al.*, 1989b). Transient diplopia may occur (Lobato *et al.*, 1990). Some impairment of mental function may occur (Meglio and Cioni, 1989). Herpes simplex occurs in up to 11% of patients.

Current status
I have no personal experience of this procedure and have not come across any patients who have had this type of treatment. From my reading of the literature there are certain advantages and disadvantages of the technique that are summarized in Table 8.8.

Table 8.8   Advantages and disadvantages of percutaneous microcompression

Advantages	Disadvantages
Highly specific	Recurrence rates not yet adequately assessed; may be 25% at 5 years
Safe for all patients	
General anaesthesia used, so pain-free	Relatively few reports
Technically easy with short operation	Mild sensory loss
Low mortality rate	Bradycardia and hypotension occur peroperatively; not suitable for some patients with cardiac disease
Few complications beyond trigeminal area	
No reports of anaesthesia dolorosa	Requires general anaesthesia with intubation
No loss of corneal reflex	

RETROGASSERIAN RHIZOTOMY

This open procedure, in which all or parts of the sensory root are cut, was first described by Frazier. However, few series have been repeated since closed techniques have been used. Petri (1970) reported on 308 patients and, more recently, Guidetti *et al.* (1979) reported on 170.

The recurrence rate is around 7–10% of patients who have been followed up for an average of 10 years (Petri, 1970; Guidetti *et al.*, 1979). Three deaths (two from anaesthetic problems and one from stroke) have been reported (Petri, 1970).

Anaesthesia dolorosa occurs in 1–3% of patients, and 8% have unpleasant dysaesthesia (Petri, 1970; Guidetti *et al.*, 1979). Keratitis may occur in up to 6% of patients (Petri, 1970), although this rate was much lower in other series: one patient with neuroparalytic keratitis and eight with loss of corneal anaesthesia (Guidetti *et al.*, 1979).

A complication not often encountered with other procedures is the development of transient seventh nerve palsies; this been reported in 17 patients (Petri, 1970; Guidetti *et al.*, 1979).

CONCLUSIONS

At present, procedures at the level of the gasserian ganglion are the most popular worldwide treatments for patients with trigeminal neuralgia.

Most procedures can be performed on all patients, whatever their age or past medical history. It has to be accepted, however, that these procedures are not curative and that recurrence often occurs within 3–4 years. The major complication is sensory loss, including loss of corneal reflex.

More objective, prospective, evaluation of the different techniques is required if comparison is to be made between different treatments.

9

Posterior Fossa Surgery

HISTORY

Cushing, in 1920, first hypothesized that trigeminal neuralgia could be caused by the pressure of a tumour on the posterior trigeminal root, but it was Dandy in 1925 who first performed partial sections of the sensory root in the posterior fossa (Taarnhoj, 1982). Dandy (1934) observed that blood vessels, and occasionally tumours, compressed the trigeminal nerve but he excised only the tumour. Few neurosurgeons, however, followed his lead as the operation was considered dangerous; only recently has it been advocated by a group who performed the procedure on 20 patients with good results (Gelber et al., 1989). Gardner and Miklos (1959) dissected off an artery compressing the trigeminal nerve using the posterior fossa approach. Gardner (1962) then reported on 18 patients on whom he had performed posterior fossa surgery, but in six he found no compression or tumour and was at a loss to explain the cause of the symptoms. It was Jannetta (1967) who refined the technique of decompression with the use of the operating microscope. His technique, microvascular decompression, has become popular.

MICROVASCULAR DECOMPRESSION

This procedure is based on the concept that compression of the trigeminal nerve causes trigeminal neuralgia. Jannetta (1967) postulated that, with increased age and development of arteriosclerosis, arteries in particular come into contact with the root entry zone of the trigeminal nerve and cause demyelination leading to abnormal electrical impulses. The root entry zone is defined as 'a junctional area between central and peripheral myelin and measures 0.5 to 1 cm in length'. These concepts are discussed in greater detail in Chapter 4. Pain does recur and is postulated to be due to an intrinsic lesion of the nerve, which therefore cannot be relieved by decompression (Bederson and Wilson, 1989). Some

157

neurosurgeons also consider that patients should be offered this procedure early in the condition when irreversible intrinsic lesions of the nerve are less likely to have occurred (Lunsford and Apfelbaum, 1985; Bederson and Wilson, 1989).

METHODS

Microvascular decompression is a major neurological procedure and patients must be carefully assessed medically before operation. Those who are medically unfit are not eligible, e.g. bleeding diathesis, poorly controlled hypertension or coronary artery disease (Lunsford and Apfelbaum, 1985).

Some neurosurgeons will not operate on patients with multiple sclerosis (Illingworth, 1986; Pollack *et al.*, 1988; Wilkins, 1988). Age is often a determining factor. Some neurosurgeons will operate only on patients aged under 70 years (Apfelbaum, 1984; Steiger, 1991), others will operate on older patients if medically fit. The oldest patients operated on have been in their nineties (Breeze and Ignelzi, 1982).

As well as radiological examination, some neurosurgeons perform audiometry to assess hearing function as this can be impaired by the procedure and it is important that the patient has adequate hearing on the contralateral side (Piatt and Wilkins, 1984).

Anaesthesia
A full general anaesthetic with endotracheal intubation is given and patients are hyperventilated (Zorman and Wilson, 1984; Bederson and Wilson, 1989). The patient is positioned either in a semi-sitting position (Jannetta, 1976; Burchiel *et al.*, 1981; Apfelbaum, 1984; Piatt and Wilkins, 1984) or lateral recumbent position (Jannetta, 1976; Piatt and Wilkins, 1984; Shapiro *et al.*, 1988). The latter position is used more frequently as it is safer: there is less risk of perioperative air emboli and hypotension (Pollack *et al.*, 1988). Chest Doppler ultrasonography and right atrial catheter are used for the detection of air emboli by most surgeons if the modified sitting position is used. Doppler monitoring may indicate air embolism in about 25% of patients, but this is clinically significant only in about 2% of patients (Jannetta, 1990). The Doppler monitoring will also alert the surgeon to bradycardia, which can occur during manipulation of the trigeminal nerve (Jannetta, 1976; Burchiel, 1987). Auditory evoked potentials may also be monitored during operation to avoid hearing loss (Hanakita and Kondo, 1988; Wilkins, 1988). Lumbar puncture is performed and a catheter is placed to aid exposure by draining cerebrospinal fluid (CSF). Antibiotics are given during operation (Zorman and Wilson, 1984; Bederson and Wilson, 1989), but not by all (Burchiel *et al.*, 1981), as well as dexamethasone (Bederson and Wilson, 1989). Mannitol may be given to decrease intracranial pressure and aid exposure, as an alternative to CSF drainage (Jannetta, 1976; Zhang *et al.*, 1990; Bederson and Wilson, 1989).

Surgical procedure

This has been described in detail by Jannetta (1976, 1981, 1990), and few changes have been made since. A summary is provided here. Two different sites on the ipsilateral side of the pain are used for the initial incision. The landmarks for one of the incisions is an imaginary line drawn between the tip of the mastoid and a point two-thirds of the way from the inion. A 10-cm vertical incision is made halfway above and halfway below a line that joins these landmarks (Jannetta, 1976; Burchiel, 1987a). Others make a C-shaped incision on the right and a reverse C incision on the left side, behind the hairline slightly above the mastoid (Adams *et al.*, 1982; Zhang *et al.*, 1990). This approach avoids encroachment on the mastoid cells (Fig. 9.1).

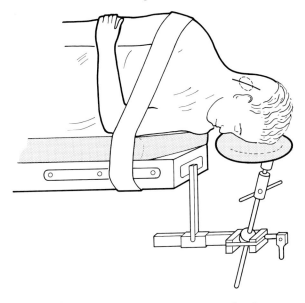

Figure 9.1   Position of the patient for microvascular decompression.

Craniectomy is then carried out to expose the lateral sinus superiorly and the sigmoid sinus laterally (5 cm in diameter) (Jannetta, 1976). The dura is opened in a cruciate form and sutured out of the way to reduce the amount of retraction that needs to be done. A self-retaining retractor is used to retract the cerebellum and vision is helped by aspirating CSF. The CSF must be removed very slowly as rapid withdrawal can lead to laceration of veins and hence haematoma (Hanakita and Kondo, 1988). Suction should be used minimally (Jannetta, 1976; Hanakita and Kondo, 1988). It is important to keep retraction to a minimum, and some neurosurgeons avoid exposure of the internal meatus and seventh and eighth cranial nerves (Fritz *et al.*, 1988). Any small veins are divided and coagulated.

Further surgery is now carried out with the operating microscope (magnification ×10 and ×16) (Richards *et al.*, 1983). The petrosal vein may need to be coagulated and divided to obtain good visualization of the trigeminal nerve area (Burchiel, 1987a; Adams *et al.*, 1982).

The arachnoid investment is carefully removed from the nerve to visualize it fully, especially at the junction of the nerve with the brainstem at the root entry zone. Sources of compression are then looked for carefully (Fig. 9.2).

The definition of compression remains controversial. Adams *et al.* (1982) have stressed that in a large proportion of patients vascular structures are seen close to the nerve but, to be classified as a compression, the nerve should be indented, grooved or distorted. Jannetta (1990), on the other hand, has argued that experienced surgeons find more compression than more junior ones if they look for it. For this reason some clinicians classify three categories of compression: (1) close contact but compression difficult to verify; (2) cross-compression with or without displacement; and (3) cross-compression causing distortion or grooving (Piatt and Wilkins, 1984; Szapiro *et al.*, 1985).

The frequency of compression reported in 2548 patients is very variable, as indicated in Table 9.1. The artery most commonly involved is the superior cere-bellar (80%); others are the anterior inferior cerebellar and the basilar (Apfelbaum, 1984). Goya *et al.* (1990) suggested that there is a correlation between the distribution of pain and the type of compression encountered. Negative findings have been reported in around 8% of patients (Table 9.1). The lowest compression rate was reported by Adams *et al.* (1982). Tumours, aneurysms, bony compression and even inflammation of the arachnoid have been reported, but these involve less than 2% of all patients (Table 9.1).

If no compression is found, or if plaques of multiple sclerosis are identified, most surgeons perform partial rhizotomy (Jannetta, 1976; Piatt and Wilkins, 1984; Adams *et al.*, 1982; Burchiel *et al.*, 1988), although Adams *et al.* (1982) and Bederson and Wilson (1989) have also combined partial sectioning with microvascular decompression in cases where vascular contact was found with no deformity.

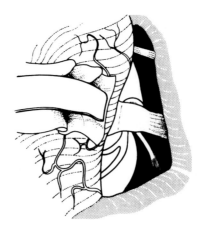

Figure 9.2 Compression of the trigeminal nerve by the superior cerebellar artery. The spatula is retracting the cerebellum. Redrawn from Illingworth (1989), with permission.

Table 9.1 Operative findings during microvascular surgery

Reference	No. of patients	Arterial Alone	Arterial Other vessels or aneurysms	Venous	Tumour/ cholesteatoma	Negative findings	Comment
Jannetta (1976)	100	86 (86)	8	2	4	0	Acoustic neuroma, meningioma, glioma
Lazar (1978)	14	6 (42)	7	1	1	1	
Ferguson et al. (1981)	24	12 (50)	5	5	1	1	Cholesteatoma
Burchiel et al. (1981)	42	26 (62)		10	15	1	
Jannetta (1981)	411	242 (59)	98	57	1	1	Cholesteatoma
Breeze and Ignelzi (1982)	52	40 (77)	2	7		8	
Swanson and Farhar (1982)	14	11 (79)	1	2	1		
Taarnhoj (1982)	86	44 (50)		15	1		
van Loveren et al. (1982)	50	14 (28)	24	4		4	
Richards et al. (1983)	52	37 (71)	2	4	3	10	
Apfelbaum (1984)	289	151 (52)	98	43	10	1	2% thick arachnoid
Kolluri and Heros (1984)	72	42 (58)	23	7		24	
Piatt and Wilkins (1984)	104	74 (70)	—	7		26	
Zorman and Wilson (1984)	125	75 (60)	2	15	5	12	Schwannoma, epidermoid, meningioma
Szapiro et al. (1985)	68	46 (67)	7	5		10	
Apfelbaum (1988)	300	235 (78)		45	5	5	
Burchiel et al. (1988)	45	26 (72)		10		0	Acoustic neuroma, more than one vessel
Shapiro et al. (1988)	36	40 (88)	1	16	1	30	56 contact with artery, 2 meningiomas, 3 epidermoids, 2 schwannomas
Bederson and Wilson (1989)	252	166 (65)	4	15	7	1	2 adhesions
Dahle et al. (1989)	57	28 (49)	16	10		0	
Goya et al. (1990)	36	34 (94)		4		0	
Zhang et al. (1990)	200	186 (93)	2	12			
Adams et al. (1982)	55	5 (11)	1		4	10	
Zakrzewska and Thomas (1993)	64	44 (69)		6			
Total	2548	1670 (66)	301 (12)	302 (12)	57 (2)	144 (6)	

Values in parentheses are percentages.

Three cases of arteries transfixing the nerve have been reported which made decompression impossible and rhizotomy had to be performed (Tashiro *et al.*, 1991). Veins can be coagulated and divided where they are thought to be indenting or deviating the nerve.

Any lesion lying on the nerve is removed for histological diagnosis.

Arteries are mobilized and a small piece of inert material may be interposed to prevent compression. It is important that the implant does not touch the nerve or it may cause compression (Goya *et al.*, 1990). Others secure the prosthesis with cyanoacryate cement to the pons or nerve (Zorman and Wilson, 1984; Bederson and Wilson, 1989). Teflon (Burchiel, 1987), sponge (Apfelbaum, 1984), gauze (Richards *et al.*, 1983), muscle (Kolluri and Heros, 1984; Zhang *et al.*, 1990) and periosteum (Szapiro *et al.*, 1985) have all been used. Periosteum is less effective than Dacron (Szapiro *et al.*, 1985). Slippage or even compression by these materials can be the cause of recurrence, so they must be positioned very carefully (Goya *et al.*, 1990) (Fig. 9.3).

Haemostasis must be carried out carefully and all the layers closed meticulously. Mastoid air cells, if exposed, are filled with bone chips or wax, which is very important to prevent middle-ear effusions (Jannetta 1976; Fritz *et al.*, 1988; Zhang *et al.*, 1990). After surgery patients are nursed with the head of the bed elevated about 10° (Jannetta, 1976).

Medication is continued for several days and then gradually tapered off as pain may not disappear immediately (Jannetta, 1976). Patients can be discharged 5–10 days after surgery, but should not return to active work for several weeks.

The procedure can be repeated if recurrence occurs (Burchiel *et al.*, 1988; Pollack *et al.*, 1988) and some find no further compression (Piatt and Wilkins, 1984) whereas others have reported slippage of the inert implant (Goya *et al.*, 1990) or fibrotic adhesions (Yamaki *et al.*, 1992). Some neurosurgeons perform

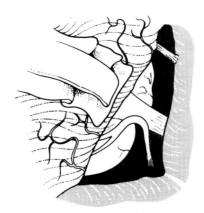

Figure 9.3 The superior cerebellar artery has been elevated away from the nerve. An inert material may now be interposed between the nerve and artery. Redrawn from Illingworth (1989), with permission.

microvascular decompression; others do a partial rhizotomy (Piatt and Wilkins, 1984; Pollack *et al.*, 1988).

The operation requires skill in microsurgical techniques and meticulous attention to detail as mortality and morbidity rates are higher for less experienced surgeons (Sweet, 1986). Apfelbaum (1988) has described it as 'an unforgiving operation in which there is little room for error in either judgement or technique'.

RESULTS

Recurrence rates
As with all other surgical evaluations, recurrence rates are extremely difficult to compare owing to the varied methodology as detailed in Chapter 8. Many report their findings in three groups: (1) excellent results; (2) minor recurrences that are often transient and require only medication; and (3) major recurrence requiring surgical intervention (Piatt and Wilkins, 1984; Burchiel *et al.*, 1988; Zakrzewska and Thomas, 1993). Others quote recurrence rates in relation to the degree of compression (Dahle *et al.*, 1989). The length of follow-up is crucial and in only one series has the mean follow-up been over 5 years (Burchiel *et al.*, 1988).

The results after a mean follow-up of 8.5 years show that, overall, 70% have a good result but only 58% are completely free of pain, 12% have minor recurrences and 30% major recurrences (Burchiel *et al.*, 1988). Using Kaplan–Meier analysis it is postulated that the half-life for a pain-free state is 10 years; for a good result it is 14 years (Burchiel *et al.*, 1988). Unfortunately, Jannetta, who has operated on the largest number of patients with the longest follow-up, has not published all his results and so progression of recurrence over time is impossible to predict. The results of various workers are shown in Table 9.2.

Initial reports suggested that most recurrences occur within 2 years (Burchiel *et al.*, 1981; Apfelbaum, 1984; Kolluri and Heros, 1984) but the long-term series of Burchiel *et al.* (1988) and Bederson and Wilson (1989) show that recurrences at a rate of 2–3.5% annually continue to occur, although the rate falls over the years.

Factors affecting recurrence rates
Numerous prognostic factors have been looked at to see whether outcome can be predicted.

Age, sex or duration of condition. The age of the patient was found not to play a role by Kolluri and Heros (1984) and Steiger (1991), but Bederson and Wilson (1989) reported that patients with an excellent outcome were older at the onset of symptoms. One group found a higher recurrence rate among women (Kolluri and Heros, 1984) but this has not been substantiated by other workers (Steiger, 1991).

The duration of symptoms does not appear to affect outcome (Kolluri and

Table 9.2 Results of microvascular decompression

Reference	No. of patients	Follow-up (months) Range	Mean	No relief	Major recurrence	Minor recurrence	Recurrence rate (%)	Kaplan–Meier 5-year survival rate (%)	Mortality	Eighth nerve injury	Comment
Jannetta (1976)	100	2–94	—	2 (2)	0 (0)	2 (2)	—	—	1 (1)	—	
Apfelbaum (1977)	55	1–14	6	3 (4)	5 (9)	8 (14)	—	—	0 (0)	2 (4)	
Lazar (1978)	15	3–24	—	0 (0)	0 (0)	0 (0)	0	—	0 (0)	0 (0)	
Weidmann (1979)	10	6–18	—	0 (0)	0 (0)	0 (0)	—	—	0 (0)	1 (10)	
Ferguson et al. (1981)	24	5–44	28	3 (12)	—	4 (17)	29	—	0 (0)	3 (12)	
Burchiel et al. (1981)	36	1–40	25	3 (7)	—	—	17	—	1 (2)	0 (0)	
Jannetta (1981)	411	—	—	—	—	—	—	—	4 (1)	20 (5)	
Breeze and Ignelzi (1982)	52	1–53	23	8 (15)	22 (5)	40 (10)	13	—	0 (0)	11 (21)	40% no complications
Taarnhoj (1982)	120	1–348	11.5	6 (5)	6 (11)	5 (10)	—	—	1 (1)	5 (4)	
van Loveren et al. (1982)	50	3–36	36	2 (4)	25 (20)	—	12	—	0 (0)	9 (12)	14% dysaesthesia
Richards et al. (1983)	52	6–60	30	1 (2)	6 (12)	—	0	—	0 (0)	1 (2)	
Apfelbaum (1984)	289	—	55	5 (2)	28 (11)	0 (0)	36	—	3 (1)	9 (3)	
Kolluri and Heros (1984)	72	36–84	60	3 (4)	14 (19)	2 (3)	18	—	0 (0)	14 (19)	
Piatt and Wilkins (1984)	104	—	48	3 (4)	24 (23)	—	—	71	1 (1)	15 (14)	30% cranial nerve complications, 15% minor complications
Zorman and Wilson (1984)	92	6–156	26	6 (5)	8 (9)	6 (7)	16	—	0 (0)	4 (3)	
Szapiro et al. (1985)	68	12–60	—	3 (4)	2 (3)	—	12	—	—	2 (3)	82% excellent results
Apfelbaum (1988)	300	12–120	63	0 (6)	—	—	—	—	—	—	
Burchiel et al. (1988)	36	1–120	102	—	11 (33)	6 (17)	—	70	0 (0)	—	
Shapiro et al. (1988)	45	6–108	51	0 (0)	2 (4)	—	4	—	0 (0)	1 (2)	
Bederson and Wilson (1989)	252	6–192	61	13 (5)	14 (5)	19 (8)	12	82	0 (0)	1 (1)	Includes rhizotomy 3.6% major morbidity: recurrence rate related to compression
Dahle et al. (1989)	54	36–84	37	11 (20)	—	—	40	—	0 (0)	—	
Goya et al. (1990)	35	6–72	—	1 (6)	2 (12)	—	6	—	0 (0)	3 (18)	
Zhang et al. (1990)	200	3–34	—	0 (0)	3 (1)	—	1	—	0 (0)	0 (0)	
Steiger (1991)	22	1–96	24	0 (0)	4 (18)	2 (9)	—	68	0 (0)	1 (4)	
Klun (1992)	178	—	62	0 (0)	—	—	6	—	0 (0)	1 (1)	
Sinduo and Martens (1993)	410	1–120	—	16 (4)	24 (6)	—	—	—	2 (0.5)	2 (0.5)	
Zakrzewska and Thomas (1993)	65	1–120	45	0 (0)	7 (9)	8 (12)	—	78	0 (0)	6 (11)	

Values in parentheses are percentages.

Heros, 1984; Piatt and Wilkins, 1984; Steiger, 1991), although Bederson and Wilson (1989) reported improved results in patients with a shorter duration of symptoms (less than 8 years) and nerve compression.

Previous surgery. Some have found previous surgery makes no difference to outcome (Piatt and Wilkins, 1984), whereas others have reported a higher recurrence rate in those who had undergone surgery, especially if at the gasserian ganglion (Barba and Alksne, 1984; Szapiro *et al.*, 1985; Bederson and Wilson, 1989). Burchiel *et al.* (1988) reported excellent results in this group of patients, but with an increased incidence of minor recurrences.

Sensory loss. Preoperative loss of light touch, either found incidentally or surgically induced, leads to worse results (Szapiro *et al.*, 1985), especially initially (Steiger, 1991). Sensory loss after microvascular decompression does occur, and Steiger (1991) found it to be related to lower a recurrence rate, although Burchiel *et al.* (1988) found no correlation.

Degree of compression. This factor has been analysed most closely. Bearing in mind the varying definition of compressions, as explained above, most neurosurgeons consider that arterial compression is related to lower recurrence rates, whereas venous compression does not affect the results (Kolluri and Heros, 1984; Piatt and Wilkins, 1984; Szapiro *et al.*, 1985; Burchiel *et al.*, 1988; Wilkins, 1988; Dahle *et al.*, 1989). However, Apfelbaum (1988), in a large series, found no difference with the source of compression. Arterial cross-compression is inversely related to the risk of major recurrence but is not related to the risk of minor recurrence (Burchiel *et al.*, 1988). Using Kaplan–Meier analysis, Piatt and Wilkins (1984) predicted that 73% of patients would be pain-free if arterial contact were established, but only 51% if no contact were found. The more significant the distortion, the lower the recurrence rate (Piatt and Wilkins, 1984). All agree that if there is doubtful compression, the recurrence rate is higher. Neither age at onset, age at operation nor duration of symptoms appears to relate to the type of nerve/blood vessel contact, although fewer women have been found to have arterial distortion (Steiger, 1991). Szapiro *et al.* (1985) found that the use of periosteum to relieve the compression was less successful than Dacron. Trauma to the nerve does not result in a higher frequency of recurrence, and this is borne out by the good results obtained after partial sensory rhizotomy (Burchiel *et al.*, 1988).

Other factors. The only other clinical feature considered as an important prognosticator is the type of pain and its distribution. Szapiro *et al.* (1985) showed that patients with pain that was only paroxysmal and who had no background, continuous dull to sharp pain had a much lower recurrence rate. This may be because the background pain is not true trigeminal neuralgia but atypical facial pain, which is unmasked by surgery (Zakrzewska and Thomas, 1993).

The fewer divisions involved the better the outcome (Szapiro *et al.*, 1985), although Bederson and Wilson (1989) did not find this to be a factor.

Recurrence rates after repeated microvascular decompression are difficult to establish as few cases are reported, but not all obtain relief (Yamaki *et al.*, 1992). In many patients rhizotomy is performed, and appears to lead to better outcome (Bederson and Wilson, 1989).

COMPLICATIONS

Mortality

Deaths, although few in number, do occur, especially among less experienced surgeons (Jannetta, 1981; Wilkins, 1988). They are due to cerebellar haemorrhage or cerebellar infarction, and involve 0–1% of patients, as shown in Table 9.2. Two of the deaths were in patients with tumours (Jannetta, 1981). In 24 units, 29 patients died or suffered permanently disabling sequelae after microvascular decompression. In two of these units over 100 procedures have been performed, whereas in the others fewer than 50 patients had been operated on. Four of the deaths occurred in patients who appeared to be fit and well (Sweet and Poletti, 1988). The average postoperative mortality rate in units in which over 100 patients had been treated was around 1% (Sweet, 1990).

Peroperative complications

Major complications that occur during operation are air embolism (Breeze and Ignelzi, 1982; Kolluri and Heros, 1984; Piatt and Wilkins, 1988), haematoma (Ferguson *et al.*, 1981; Jannetta, 1981; Piatt and Wilkins, 1984), CSF leaks (Jannetta, 1981; Breeze and Ignelzi, 1982; Zorman and Wilson, 1984; Shapiro *et al.*, 1988; Bederson and Wilson, 1989; Goya *et al.*, 1990) and supratentorial or cerebellar infarction leading to hemiparesis or cerebellar dysfunction (Apfelbaum, 1988).

In the immediate postoperative period nausea, cerebellar nystagmus, confusion and ataxia are common (Jannetta, 1976; Breeze and Ignelzi, 1982; Kolluri and Heros, 1984; Shapiro *et al.*, 1988; Bederson and Wilson, 1989). CSF leaks may occur from the mastoid air cells (Zorman and Wilson, 1984). Headaches can become very severe, and removal of CSF appears to relieve them (Kolluri and Heros, 1984).

Major morbidity

Overall, the immediate morbidity rate may be as high as 60% (Breeze and Ignelzi, 1982) but persisting morbidity is around 10–30% after 3 months (Breeze and Ignelzi, 1982): 3% major, 15% minor (Piatt and Wilkins, 1984). Intracranial haemorrhage was recorded in 19 patients who underwent microvascular decompression: ten died, five had major residual sequelae, three suffered transient hemiplegia and one recovered (Sweet and Poletti, 1988).

Aseptic meningitis (Jannetta, 1981; Breeze and Ignelzi, 1982; Zorman and Wilson, 1984; Shapiro *et al.*, 1988; Bederson and Wilson, 1989; Dahle *et al.*, 1989) as well as pulmonary embolism, cerebellar oedema, bacterial meningitis and chronic subdural haematoma (Piatt and Wilkins, 1984) occur, but are rare

(Jannetta, 1981; Sweet and Poletti, 1988; Bederson and Wilson, 1989). Ataxia may become permanent in some cases (Jannetta, 1976; Kolluri and Heros, 1984).

Other neurological complications
Occipital neuralgia has been noted by some (Breeze and Ignelzi, 1982; Szapiro *et al.*, 1985; Shapiro *et al.*, 1988) and in one case was severe enough to require a neurectomy (Shapiro *et al.*, 1988). Other minor complications include herpes infection (Breeze and Ignelzi, 1982; Kolluri and Heros, 1984; Bederson and Wilson, 1989; Zhang *et al.*, 1990), as well as middle-ear effusions (Fritz *et al.*, 1988) and wound infections (Apfelbaum, 1977). Impairment of function of the fourth, sixth and seventh cranial nerves has also been recorded by a variety of workers (Apfelbaum, 1977; Ferguson *et al.*, 1981; Breeze and Ignelzi, 1982; Kolluri and Heros, 1984; Piatt and Wilkins, 1984; Zorman and Wilson, 1984). Some of these injuries are associated with the removal of tumours (Apfelbaum 1983; Kolluri and Heros, 1984).

Hearing loss
Cranial nerve problems are more likely to occur in patients who have tumours removed (Kolluri and Heros, 1984). The most significant complication is hearing loss. In a carefully controlled study on 21 patients using audiometry before and after operation, five (24%) were found to have hearing impairment, which was transient in three. Hearing loss may be transient in up to 21% of patients (Breeze and Ignelzi, 1982) but is permanent in 3–8% (van Loveren *et al.*, 1982; Kolluri and Heros, 1984; Piatt and Wilkins, 1984; Bederson and Wilson, 1989). Some patients may experience only partial hearing loss (Kolluri and Heros, 1984; Zorman and Wilson, 1984). Middle-ear effusions clear up within 1 month, but positional vertigo may last for up to 3 months (Fritz *et al.*, 1988).

Sensory loss/corneal reflex
Although microvascular decompression should not in theory cause sensory loss, this complication is found in 5–31% of all patients (Szapiro *et al.*, 1985; Burchiel *et al.*, 1988; Shapiro *et al.*, 1988; Dahle *et al.*, 1989; Steiger, 1991). All reports stress that loss of touch is minor and has not caused unpleasant dysaesthesia or anaesthesia dolorosa. Sensory loss may occur in patients who had less compression (Szapiro *et al.*, 1985). The corneal reflex may be lost (Shapiro *et al.*, 1988). It must, however, be remembered that many of these patients will have had previous surgery that left them with loss of touch but which was not recorded preoperatively.

BILATERAL MICROVASCULAR DECOMPRESSION

Only one paper has been devoted to the management of bilateral trigeminal neuralgia. Pollack *et al.* (1988) reported 35 patients with bilateral trigeminal neuralgia: 25 had unilateral microvascular decompression and ten bilateral procedures (in total 45 operations). At operation, multiple compressions were seen.

At 5 years 66% still had good or excellent results; six had a recurrence between 1 and 5 years, the rest occurring within the first year. Six had further surgery. On average this group had few complications except for hearing loss (two minor, one major) and mild sensory deficit (five cases). The group, however, was small and it is difficult to compare these results with those of other series.

RHIZOTOMY

METHODS

The technique for rhizotomy using the posterior fossa approach is the same as that for microvascular decompression, and has been well described by Burchiel (1987). The whole or part of the sensory division is sectioned, taking care to avoid the motor root (Adams *et al.*, 1982). The amount and site of the section is dependent on the distribution of pain (Adams *et al.*, 1982). Swanson and Farhar (1982) described a combined microvascular decompression procedure with removal of only a few fascicles of portico major to prevent sensory loss.

RESULTS

Recurrence rates
The results of sensory rhizotomy performed through the posterior fossa are comparable to those of microvascular decompression (Burchiel *et al.*, 1981; Zorman and Wilson, 1984). At follow-up of less than 5 years, 96-98% of patients are free of pain (Adams *et al.*, 1982; Piatt and Wilkins, 1984); however, eight patients followed for a mean of 8.5 years showed four (50%) major and one (13%) minor recurrences. Bederson and Wilson (1989) suggested that there is a trend for a higher recurrence rate following rhizotomy than microvascular decompression.

Complications
Mortality (Burchiel *et al.*, 1988) and complication rates are similar to those for microvascular decompression (Zorman and Wilson, 1984; Bederson and Wilson, 1989). The major complication is sensory but this is often not as severe as would be expected (Hussein *et al.*, 1982; Zorman and Wilson, 1984). Mingrino and Salar (1981) showed that 44% of patients had loss of touch sensation after partial sensory rhizotomy. Loss of corneal reflex is more likely if more than 50% of the nerve is sectioned (Adams *et al.*, 1982) and can occur in up to 2% of patients (Bederson and Wilson, 1989). Painful facial dyaesthesia and anaesthesia dolorosa are also more likely after complete section and occur in approximately 8% of patients (Adams *et al.*, 1982; Bederson and Wilson, 1989).

Hearing loss is less common after rhizotomy than following microvascular decompression (Bederson and Wilson, 1989).

SUBTEMPORAL APPROACH

In 1925 Frazier described the procedure of subtotal section of the sensory root by the subtemporal extradural approach. Since the development of procedures on the posterior fossa, few neurosurgeons now use this technique (Burchiel, 1987a). Peet and Schneider (1952) reported on 553 patients and had an operative mortality rate of 1.6% and significant complications in 26%. Moderate to severe keratitis was found in 15% of patients and 8% required tarsorraphy. Up to 6% had facial palsies, some of which were immediate and others delayed; many resolved. Although the data are incomplete a recurrence rate of 5.4% was noted.

Taarnhoj (1982) has reported on 230 patients who had undergone this procedure. Sixty per cent of the patients remained free of pain, 38% had a recurrence and 2% no relief from this approach. The recurrence rate was 20%. There were three (1.3%) deaths.

CURRENT STATUS

The advantages and disadvantages of microvascular decompression are summarized in the Table 9.3. There is no doubt that surgery on the posterior fossa carries the highest risk of mortality in the hands of inexperienced neurosurgeons and yet, at the same time, although not offering a permanent cure, this approach appears to give the longest interval for freedom of pain. However, there are extremely few long-term reports on prospective controlled trials, despite thousands of procedures having been carried out. As mentioned in Chapter 8, many of the analyses are poorly done and have not been subjected to good statistical analysis.

It is therefore argued that this operation should never be performed as other alternatives are available that do not have the risk of mortality (Morley, 1985). Trigeminal neuralgia is not usually a life-threatening condition and suicide is rare owing to the wide availability of surgery and drugs. However, trigeminal neuralgia can severely affect a patient's quality of life and this must be considered. There has been one suicide in our unit, in a patient with bilateral trigeminal neuralgia who underwent bilateral radiofrequency thermocoagulation with

Table 9.3   Advantages and disadvantages of microvascular decompression

Advantages	Disadvantages
Longer lasting than other procedures	Up to 1% mortality rate
Preservation of nerve function	Severe neurological morbidity in up to 1%
No loss of touch sensation	Cranial nerve damage, especially eighth nerve
No anaesthesia dolorosa	Craniotomy needs experienced neurosurgeon
	Expensive
	Possible only on medically fit patients

severe sensory loss, but I have not seen a single reference to suicide in the modern literature. This is probably because few neurosurgeons carry out long-term follow-up on all their patients and very few have reported on psychological postoperative morbidity.

All other procedures have a lower mortality rate, although deaths do occur as in any branch of surgery. Rosser and Kind (1978) in their assessment of quality of life state that there are differences between disability and distress, and these factors need to be considered. On the other hand, Jannetta (1985) has argued that the procedure should be performed as the treatment of choice as it treats the cause of disease. Opinion, however, still remains divided on aetiology (see Chapter 4), and compression of the trigeminal nerve cannot be the only cause as it is not found in all patients and recurrences do occur after decompression, especially in the long term.

Apart from mortality, morbidity from posterior fossa surgery extends beyond the trigeminal nerve. The initial morbidity may be as high as 60%, with persisting morbidity as high as 30%, although this may represent only minor complications (Breeze and Ignelzi, 1982). When I interviewed over 60 patients after posterior fossa surgery, they said that it took them around 6 months to get back to their usual way of life. Cranial nerve morbidity is the most persistent problem and hearing is most frequently affected. Rhizotomy causes fewer eighth nerve problems but more fifth nerve problems than microvascular decompression (Bederson and Wilson, 1989).

The greatest advantage of microvascular decompression is the preservation of sensation. Many patients do not actively complain about loss of touch sensation after surgery, but it may nevertheless affect their lives. However, when asked in a questionnaire if the sensory changes after radiofrequency thermocoagulation affected their quality of life, 18% said they did considerably and 45% slightly (Zakrzewska, 1990). There have been no formal studies attempting to weigh up the relative importance of these complications in relation to patients' quality of life and their relationship to pain. It remains difficult to advise patients on the choice of operation with such a paucity of scientific data.

Recurrence rates after posterior fossa surgery are much lower than those for any other surgery, but have not been validated scientifically. The procedure has, however, to be performed by a neurosurgeon experienced in microsurgical techniques with excellent anaesthetic support and so is expensive compared with other procedures.

Unfortunately, without carefully controlled trials using independent observers with random allocation of patients, it is difficult to decide which is the best treatment (Loeser, 1993). My own attempts to do this were successful only in so far as I independently assessed three different groups of patients, but I was unable to determine who was allocated to which group (Zakrzewska and Thomas, 1993). As more pressure is put on clinicians to carry out both process and outcome audit, so these shortfalls will become more apparent, and only those units that set and follow careful standards and report on complications will gain more patients.

10

Management of Complications after Surgery for Trigeminal Neuralgia

INTRODUCTION

This chapter tries to address some of the problems that occur after patients have undergone surgery. Some of the complications that patients develop are more challenging to manage than newly diagnosed severe trigeminal neuralgia.

Compared with the enormous literature on surgical management of trigeminal neuralgia there are remarkably few papers dealing with postoperative complications (Sweet and Poletti, 1988). Those papers that deal more exclusively with complications tend to give guidelines on how to prevent them, but not on how to cope with them if they do occur. Jannetta and Bissonette (1985) have written a chapter entitled 'Management of the failed patient with trigeminal neuralgia' but concentrate exclusively on those with recurrence. Severe dysaesthesia and anaesthesia dolorosa are excluded on the basis that they are 'not relieved of their pain by procedures we can perform'. I would argue that it is the responsibility of the surgeons to manage the complications that their surgery has produced.

It is important for clinicians to accept that patients with trigeminal neuralgia are never totally cured and will need long-term follow-up. It is preferable for patients to be followed up in the same centre and not to seek care elsewhere.

Patients are often informed about outcome and complications based on published literature and yet these may not be a true reflection of what happens in practice (Sweet and Poletti, 1988). Now that audit is carried out fairly regularly in British National Health Service hospitals, it should be possible to give patients information on outcome data based on procedures carried out at the local hospital.

Sweet and Poletti (1988) were concerned by this lack of knowledge on postoperative complications and wrote to 200 neurosurgeons asking them to send in data. The results from 140 respondent neurosurgeons are quoted frequently in this chapter, as this survey gives a better indication of outcome after surgery than the literature. The board of the American Association of Neurological Surgeons has now set up an anonymous database for the collection of data on postoperative complications. The results will be circulated to the profession, with advice on how some of them can be avoided. It will, hopefully, also enable new methods to be developed. Formal audit on long- and short-term complications and recurrence should be carried out routinely in all neurosurgical units. This should be done prospectively and by independent observers, as carried out by North and colleagues (1990).

We also found that surveying our patients by postal questionnaire yielded more data on complications than noted in outpatient clinics (Zakrzewska and Thomas, 1993). Patients with complications either will not tell their surgeons for fear of upsetting them (Rawlinson, 1983) or go to other centres (Jannetta and Bissonette, 1985).

RECURRENCE OF TRIGEMINAL NEURALGIA

Every patient should be warned that recurrence is possible after surgery. Some patients fail to obtain any relief after surgery. These are not true recurrences and many are a result of technical failures. Many patients will undergo repeat surgery and do well whereas others never obtain relief and probably have a so-called 'atypical trigeminal neuralgia'.

Some recurrences occur very early, especially after peripheral surgery, whereas others occur many years later (Burchiel *et al.*, 1988). Some surgeons prefer to ensure long-term pain relief at the risk of more immediate complications, whereas others argue that recurrences are easier to manage than some of the complications, especially anaesthesia dolorosa (Siegfried, 1981; Lunsford and Apfelbaum, 1985). It is important that the patient is involved in this decision-making process.

ASSESSMENT OF A RECURRENCE

When a patient returns in pain, after being rendered totally pain-free, it is essential to establish whether the pain is a true recurrence or another form of facial pain. A history needs to be taken with as much care as at first presentation and the McGill Pain Questionnaire should be repeated (Zakrzewska and Thomas, 1993). The character of the pain may change and the pain may be less severe. The site of the pain, especially after peripheral treatment, may have changed and a careful note of trigger areas needs to be included. Many patients return as soon as the pain recurs; others first try previous medication. If the medication provides relief, this is fairly diagnostic of recurrence.

It is worthwhile assessing the circumstances in which the recurrence occurred. Stress plays an important role and must be looked for as it is as likely to bring on a recurrence as it was to have affected the initial attack (Harris, 1926). Other psychological and behavioural assessments should be repeated. Only after these careful assessments will it become apparent whether there has been a true recurrence of trigeminal neuralgia or whether some other type of facial pain has intervened or been unmasked (van Loveren *et al.*, 1982; Zakrzewska and Thomas, 1993).

A review of the patient's medical history is essential as this may affect the choice of treatment. Many patients are elderly; their medical status may have changed sufficiently for some treatment options to be no longer viable.

Special note must be taken of any postoperative complications the patient may have experienced. Not only must the signs and symptoms be elicited, but also their effect on the patient's quality of life. These effects can sometimes be the determining factor as to which, if any, operation is decided on in the future. We have found that patients with classical trigeminal neuralgia were more likely to request a repeat radiofrequency thermocoagulation procedure than those who had 'atypical trigeminal neuralgia' (Jassim, 1994).

If the recurrence is mild most surgeons advocate the use of drugs in the first instance. It is well recognized that some patients have transient recurrences, which either settle spontaneously or after a short course of medication. It is, therefore, important to establish whether the recurrence is transient or permanent and this can be done only by a trial of medication. If, however, the pain persists and the medication causes too many side-effects, surgery needs to be considered. As with primary surgery, all patients must be given a choice based on adequate information. In general recurrence rates after repeat operation are very similar but there are very few large series to prove this statistically. Recurrence rates after patients have previously had different surgery are variable: some patients show no difference from the new patients, whereas in other series they have done less well. Various prognostic factors have been put forward, especially by surgeons performing microvascular decompression, and these were discussed in Chapters 8 and 9.

RECURRENCE AFTER PERIPHERAL SURGERY

If pain recurrence is in a different branch from the previously treated one, most clinicians prefer to carry out further peripheral surgery. Migration of pain can occur in up to 38% of patients who have had cryotherapy (Zakrzewska and Nally, 1988). In some instances patients may continue to have repeated peripheral surgery for many years in order to remain pain-free (Quinn, 1965; Freemont and Millac, 1981; Zakrzewska and Nally, 1988).

Few reports give details of recurrence rates after repeated surgery, but they can be variable (Zakrzewska and Nally, 1988).

If the pain becomes more extensive and involves more branches and divisions, peripheral surgery is no longer appropriate and other types of operation need to be considered.

RECURRENCE AFTER SURGERY AT THE GASSERIAN GANGLION

Although it appeared at first that injection of retrogasserian glycerol would be as effective as radiofrequency thermocoagulation, long-term results have shown this not to be the case.

Many of the recurrences after retrogasserian glycerol are managed by further surgery. A few surgeons go on immediately to do posterior fossa surgery (Fujimaki *et al.*, 1990); others do so only with a proportion of patients (Burchiel, 1987; North *et al.*, 1990; Slettebo *et al.*, 1993). Most surgeons will repeat a glycerol injection and, if that fails a second time, proceed to either radiofrequency thermocoagulation or posterior fossa surgery (Burchiel *et al.*, 1981; Lunsford and Apfelbaum, 1985; Rappaport, 1986; Young, 1989; North *et al.*, 1990).

A similar trend is seen in patients who have had radiofrequency thermocoagulation. Of 181 patients who had a recurrence of pain after radiofrequency thermocoagulation, Broggi *et al.* (1990) performed 160 successful repeat radiofrequency thermocoagulations (11 patients had to have between three and five repeat procedures before relief was obtained). Six patients opted for other types of surgery and 15 refused further surgery.

Some patients may opt for peripheral surgery such as neurectomy or alcohol blocks if the pain is localized (Onofrio, 1975; Burchiel *et al.*, 1981; Ferguson *et al.*, 1981), whereas others choose to have only medical therapy (Onofrio, 1975; Siegfried, 1981; Hitchcock *et al.*, 1983).

Microcompression of the gasserian ganglion is also followed by recurrences. Lichtor and Mullan (1990) estimated that 15% of patients who live for over 10 years will ultimately require intracranial surgery, even after repeated decompressions.

RECURRENCE AFTER POSTERIOR FOSSA SURGERY

Some neurosurgeons do not repeat posterior fossa procedures, whereas others will do repeat surgery if the patient is healthy and has an estimated 5-year life survival (Jannetta and Bissonette, 1985). Only a small proportion of patients with recurrences end up having repeat posterior fossa surgery. Many patients are managed with medication (Apfelbaum, 1977; Burchiel *et al.*, 1981; Breeze and Ignelzi, 1982; Taarnhoj, 1982; Pollack *et al.*, 1988). Some patients are offered more peripheral surgery, neurectomy, radiofrequency thermocoagulation or retrogasserian glycerol injection (Taarnhoj, 1982; Pollack *et al.*, 1988). The rest of the patients have repeat microvascular decompression or partial rhizotomy (Apfelbaum, 1977; Burchiel *et al.*, 1981; Taarnhoj, 1982).

When repeating posterior fossa surgery it is important to review the initial operative findings and response to treatment. A decision has to be made as to whether to perform microvascular decompression or rhizotomy (partial or complete). Most neurosurgeons perform a rhizotomy, especially if no compression is seen, whereas others prefer to carry out repeat microvascular decompression (Taarnhoj, 1982; Jannetta and Bissonette, 1985).

The same or a new incision is made and the procedure is identical, except that adhesions must be looked for carefully. The trigeminal nerve is usually more difficult to find and needs to be identified carefully and inspected along its entire length (Jannetta and Bissonette, 1985).

Jannetta and Bissonette (1985) compared their first findings with the second findings and found new compressions as a result of elongation of vessels, venous recollateralization and atrophy of muscle implants, thus allowing further compression. One cyst and one tumour were found, and only one patient had no evidence of recompression. Recurrences do occur after reoperation, and some may obtain no relief after the second operation (Jannetta and Bissonette, 1985). Too few repeat microvascular decompressions have been done for long-term evaluation, but Taarnhoj (1982) has reported ten recurrences after a second posterior fossa procedure. However, no mention is made as to how they were managed.

Complications appear to be similar to those after primary surgery. If the trigeminal neuralgia is unmanageable medically or by other surgery, tractotomy can be performed (Rohrer and Burchiel, 1993).

TRACTOTOMY AND THE DORSAL ROOT ENTRY ZONE OPERATION

Sjoqvist in 1938 performed the first nine bulbar trigeminal tractotomies after seeing a patient with a bulbar infarct who had complete facial analgesia and thermoanalgesia but preservation of touch sensation (Sweet, 1985). The procedure, however, results in clumsiness and ataxia, and was modified by numerous surgeons in the light of increased knowledge of the organization of the trigeminal nucleus.

Nashold thus developed the dorsal root entry zone (DREZ) operation, which aims to lesion the secondary neurons buried in the nucleus caudalis (Bernard *et al.*, 1987). The nucleus caudalis is destroyed by a special thermal radiofrequency electrode, which affects all three divisions. Ipsilateral analgesia and thermoanalgesia extends over the whole face, oral cavity and pharynx, resulting in loss of the gag reflex. Most patients also develop ataxia, which lasts for several months (Nashold and Rossitch, 1990).

Tractotomy can be performed as an open or closed procedure under general anaesthesia using stereotactic techniques, and the former has been well described by Burchiel (1987a). Pain relief is obtained at the expense of dense analgesia of the face.

ABNORMAL SENSATIONS

Relief from severe trigeminal neuralgia often results in dense analgesia. Some procedures are more likely than others to produce profound analgesia. However, loss of light touch sensation does not always result in distressing dysaesthesia, and other psychological and physical factors may need to be considered (Lichtor and Mullan, 1990).

Firmer decompression in microcompression of the ganglion (Lichtor and Mullan, 1990) and higher temperatures in radiofrequency thermocoagulation (Latchaw *et al.*, 1981; Broggi *et al.*, 1990) result in more loss of touch sensation but lower recurrence rates. The use of a curved needle for radiofrequency thermocoagulation has also reduced the frequency of sensory loss (Tobler *et al.*, 1983). In most procedures there is a link between recurrence rates and the degree of loss of sensation.

Patients who have had a severe attack of herpes simplex after operation are more likely to develop postoperative dysaesthesia (Lunsford, 1990).

Dysaesthesias have been labelled as marked or mild but there are no universal diagnostic criteria. Anaesthesia dolorosa is the most severe form of dysaesthesia. Moderate dysaesthesia can, if necessary, be managed with non-narcotic analgesics or anxiolytics (Guidetti *et al.*, 1979; Sweet, 1988). Most clinicians try to manage more marked dysaesthesia with tricyclic antidepressants (Meglio and Cioni, 1989; Broggi *et al.*, 1990).

Anaesthesia dolorosa is recognized to be an extremely difficult condition to manage; it occurs most commonly in patients who have had radiofrequency thermocoagulation (see Table 8.3) or rhizotomy. The condition develops weeks or months after surgery, and progresses over several years, after which time it is static. It is a continuous burning, stinging, stabbing or aching pain localized to the anaesthetic part of the face, most commonly around the eye and mouth. Its constant nature causes the patient more distress than the initial severe trigeminal neuralgia. Changes in temperature, especially cold, aggravate the pain and there appears to be no relief. The pain becomes chronic, and is affected by various psychological and behavioural factors, as discussed in Chapter 3.

In the literature on trigeminal neuralgia there are few guidelines on how to manage these patients, possibly related to the unknown aetiology of anaesthesia dolorosa and lack of response to medical therapy. The DREZ operation developed by Nashold is now a method of treatment. In a report of three patients, one had an excellent result, one a good result and the third was considered a failure (Nashold and Rossitch, 1990).

Stimulators can be put in the gasserian ganglion, thalamus, internal capsule (Hosobuch *et al.*, 1973) and, if successful, can be replaced with a neuropacemaker (Meglio and Cioni, 1989). I have no experience of these devices and have not met any patients who have had them.

I have treated these patients with a variety of tricyclic antidepressants. Response is very variable. Patients may benefit from cognitive behavioural therapy, as this helps the patient accept the disability and develop a positive attitude toward it. Constant reassurance is necessary.

OTHER FACIAL PAINS

Many authors allude to groups of patients who do not have typical trigeminal neuralgia. There is a continuous background dull ache or burning sensation between attacks of paroxysmal pain, and this is often termed atypical trigeminal neuralgia (Hakanson, 1981; Latchaw *et al.*, 1981; Szapiro *et al.*, 1985; Burchiel *et al.*, 1988; Sweet, 1988). All have noticed that this group of patients do less well with surgical treatment, and Sweet and Wespic (1974) even observed that patients 'complain more of their pain or even a new pain even in the presence of analgesia'. I have seen patients who complain of other types of facial pain, which are present before operation if looked for carefully but are unmasked by the surgical procedure which abolishes the sharp, shooting pain (Jassim, 1994). Loeser (1984) postulates that this pain occurs in patients who have previously had classical trigeminal neuralgia but who, after surgery, which in most instances is a denervating procedure, develop symptoms as a result of the surgery. I have patients who have developed other types of facial pain even when no surgery has been carried out. This could be psychogenic pain, related to the fear of recurrent attacks and inability to affect a permanent cure.

Tricyclic antidepressant drugs and psychological or behavioural support play an important role in trying to control these other types of facial pain.

These instances of postoperative facial pain highlight the importance of taking a good history, and the need for the development of definitive objective measurements. Great care must be taken to avoid surgical procedures in patients who do not have classical trigeminal neuralgia. I stress to patients that surgery will eliminate only a sharp, shooting pain and no other type of dull, burning pain. If patients go ahead and have surgery, their expectations will be realistic and they are more likely to accept any residual pain that may remain.

ORAL PROBLEMS

Patients who have had peripheral procedures intraorally are at risk of developing complications such as those encountered in any minor surgical procedure, e.g. infection, bleeding (Zakrzewska and Nally, 1988). Most problems are transient and require analgesics or a short course of antibiotics such as metronidazole. After intraoral surgery there may be some alteration in the soft tissue morphology, which can result in poorly fitting dentures; adjustments are normally easy to make.

After radiofrequency thermocoagulation many patients develop transient unilateral paresis of the muscles of mastication. This can make eating extremely difficult, especially as it is inevitably associated with sensory loss. Patients cannot masticate well on the affected side and food dribbles out of the corner of the mouth. In my postoperative survey of patients, up to 34% of patients had problems with eating (Zakrzewska, 1990). Patients who wear dentures find it very difficult to control them, and this adds to the eating difficulty (Zakrzewska, 1990). Patients need reassurance that this is only temporary and that they should wait for an improvement in the paresis before obtaining new dentures. Only a small proportion have long-term problems.

The sensory loss also affects the oral cavity and patients need be aware of this. Cheek biting is common. Patients may not be aware of developing dental problems as they experience little or no pain. It is important to stress to patients that they continue to attend a dentist on a regular basis. This can sometimes be difficult as many patients ascribe the initial attack of trigeminal neuralgia to dental treatment and are reluctant to undergo further treatment in case the problem recurs.

EYE PROBLEMS

Eye problems do occur in patients who have reduced or no corneal sensation after surgery. Despite the large numbers of patients who have no or reduced corneal sensation, relatively few develop problems. Lewis *et al.* (1982) postulated that this is because touch and the larger myelinated fibres are preserved, and so good corneal nutrition is ensured.

Corneal reflexes must be checked as soon as possible after surgery so the eye can be protected immediately if the reflex is absent. Patients should be issued with protective glasses before they leave hospital. Careful instructions must be given about daily inspection of the eye. Any problems such as redness or increased lacrimation should be referred immediately for an ophthalmological opinion.

In the literature there are few patients recorded who have lost an eye as a result of corneal ulceration (Sweet and Wepsic, 1974; Broggi *et al.*, 1990). A very small proportion may require tarsorrhaphy (Onofrio, 1975; Hitchcock *et al.*, 1983; Broggi *et al.*, 1990). Of 197 patients with loss of corneal reflex after radiofrequency thermocoagulation, only five required tarsorrhaphy (Broggi *et al.*, 1990).

AUDITORY PROBLEMS

These occur mainly in patients who have undergone posterior fossa surgery. Minimal retraction during surgery can reduce the number who develop problems (Fritz *et al.*, 1988). Little can be done for patients who develop hearing loss, so it is important that they are warned of this complication before surgery and that patients with contralateral deafness do not have microvascular decompression. In Sweet and Poletti's survey (1988), several hundred hearing losses were recorded.

Patients who have undergone radiofrequency thermocoagulation may complain of tinnitus or blowing noises, as a result of paresis of the tensor tympani. In most patients this effect is transient, and they can be reassured that it will gradually disappear.

OTHER COMPLICATIONS

Meningitis—aseptic or rarely bacterial—occurs mainly after posterior fossa surgery (Sweet and Poletti, 1988; Young, 1988) but has also been recorded after radiofrequency thermocoagulation (Sweet and Poletti, 1988). If an organism is cultured, the appropriate antibiotics can be prescribed. If all cultures are negative, then steroids are used (Lunsford and Apfelbaum, 1985; Lunsford, 1990).

After radiofrequency thermocoagulation, arterial subarachnoid haemorrhages have occurred from the placement of the needle electrode and so it is essential that patients are screened carefully for bleeding tendencies before surgery and that the procedure is stopped immediately a bleed is suspected (Sweet and Poletti, 1988). Subcranial bleeding around the zygoma occurs more commonly after microcompression owing to the use of larger needles (Mullan and Lichtor, 1983).

Blood pressure monitoring is essential during procedures at the level of the gasserian ganglion as changes in the blood pressure can result in myocardial infarction, bradycardia and even asystole (Sweet and Poletti, 1988; Sweet, 1990). Drugs should be available to counteract these changes (Mullan and Lichtor, 1983; Sweet and Poletti, 1988).

CONCLUSION

Complications after surgery are common, but most are minor and transient. However, no one surgical technique (apart from peripheral procedures) is free of major complications. If complications develop, appropriate treatments must be given which, in many instances, may need to be only in terms of explanation and reassurance.

11

How Do You Manage a Patient With Trigeminal Neuralgia?

INTRODUCTION

The vast amount of literature on the management of trigeminal neuralgia is ample proof that there is no one universally accepted method of treatment for this intriguing condition. We still do not know whether trigeminal neuralgia is a disease or a symptom of some sort of as yet unrecognized condition. Until the aetiology is established there will continue to be an array of different treatments available for this chronic pain condition. As there is no one perfect treatment, all clinicians must be prepared to advise on a wide variety of treatments (Lichtor and Mullan, 1990).

A recent survey carried out among 159 British consultants with an interest in treating neurogenic pain showed remarkably wide divergence of opinion. Ninety-nine consultants agreed that anticonvulsants should be used. Other treatments in order of popularity were: neurolytic somatic block, 59; antidepressants, 55; simple analgesics, 37; somatic nerve block, 33; rhizotomy, 32; neurectomy, 28; sympathetic nerve block, 21; and opioids and cordotomy were proposed by a few (Davies et al., 1993). It is therefore important that more emphasis is placed on mutual decision-making between patient and clinician (Tew and van Loveren, 1988). Standards of care need to be established which should lead to improved results both in terms of pain relief and quality of life.

In attempting to advise patients the clinician should consider some of the following questions posed by Jannetta and Bissonette (1985):

1. What has been the true effect of a certain form of therapy for a specific syndrome?
2. Do subgroups exist where the rates of success or failure may vary, depending upon specific or general characteristics of the population being treated?

3. Is one form of treatment to be preferred over another in these various subgroups?
4. Is it ethical, indeed is it moral, to subject all or certain patients to a specific form of treatment?
5. What is the risk of temporary or permanent morbidity or death with a given procedure?
6. Is a procedure that offers better quality of survival and a greater chance for permanent cure but that may carry a higher risk of morbidity or mortality justified?
7. Are the risks of a specific operative procedure higher or lower if it is a repeat operation?
8. Under what circumstances is a surgeon justified in trying an operation he or she has not performed before?
9. Finally, when an operation has failed, what are the results of the various techniques that can be utilized?

These are difficult questions and some of the answers need to be supplied by the patients themselves once they have been fully informed.

ESTABLISHING THE DIAGNOSIS AND TREATMENT PLANS/SUPPORT

The key to management of trigeminal neuralgia lies in the diagnosis. The treatment for trigeminal neuralgia is markedly different from that of other forms of facial pain, and so extreme care must be taken to ensure the diagnosis is correct.

The making of the diagnosis lies not only in eliciting a good clinical history and examination as described in Chapter 2, but also in performing detailed pain, psychological, behavioural and personality assessments, as discussed in Chapter 3.

INFORMING THE PATIENT OF THE DIAGNOSIS

Once the diagnosis is established the clinician is ready for the first step in the management of this condition, which is to tell the patient the diagnosis. This is as important as anything else that may be done for the patient in the future and yet is so frequently neglected. How much information we give our patients and how we communicate this needs to be assessed for each patient.

In their book *How to Break Bad News*, Buckman and Kason (1992) describe six steps that enable the breaking of bad news to be beneficial both to the patient and clinician. These are summarized in Table 11.1.

The first step, 'Getting Started', ensures that the physical and emotional needs of the patient are met. The interview should take place in a quiet room

Table 11.1   Steps in giving out news about trigeminal neuralgia (Buckman and Kason, 1992)

1.	SET THE SCENE Ensure physical surroundings correct Establish where interview is to take place Establish who is to be present Establish patient's well-being and mood
2.	FIND OUT HOW MUCH THE PATIENT KNOWS
3.	FIND OUT HOW MUCH THE PATIENT WANTS TO KNOW

4.	INFORM THE PATIENT
	Decide on agenda
	   Diagnosis
	   Treatment options
	   Prognosis
	   Support
	Start from the patient's knowledge
	Educate
	   Small chunks
	   Plain English
	   Check patient understands
	   Clarify points
	   Listen to patient's agenda

5.	RESPOND TO PATIENT'S FEELINGS Identify and acknowledge reactions
6.	PLANNING AND FOLLOW-UP Organise next treatment Ensure patient aware of contract for support and follow-up Summarize

where the patient feels the clinician has time to sit and talk. Other visitors such as students or junior staff may be present if the patient is agreeable. A nurse should be present if possible as she or he may need to reinforce the information at a later time. It is important that both clinician and patient are comfortable and ready for this two-way interview. Enquiring about the patient's general physical state not only allows the patient to talk but enables the clinician to gauge the patient's mental state.

Step 2 involves establishing how much the patient knows and understands of his/her condition. The patient may deny having any knowledge about the disease either to see whether the new information supplied tallies with previous experience or for emotional reasons. In assessing the patient's knowledge the clinician will take into account the style of the statements (knowledge of medical terms) and the patient's emotional state, both through verbal and non-verbal communication. By this stage the patient should be aware that the clinician is listening and interested in the patient.

Step 3 is one that is often forgotten and yet Buckmann and Kason (1992) consider it pivotal to the course of the interview. The clinician needs to know how much the patient wants to know at the time; this is often dependent on his/her rapport with the patient (Lloyd, 1991). Some patients want to know everything, others, especially the elderly, only want some information. It is important that patients realize that, even though they do not want all the information at the present time, the lines of communication remain open.

Once the clinician has this knowledge, then information about the condition or only its treatment and general management may be given. The clinician has been given an invitation and can now proceed to step 4, which is 'Sharing the information'. The first part involves divulging the information and the second is listening to the patient's reaction to it. The clinician needs to be clear about the information to be imparted. In the case of trigeminal neuralgia, the patient needs to be told of the diagnosis and the wide variety of treatments available. Each treatment should indicate some measure of the prognosis. Whichever treatment the patient chooses, the clinician must stress that support will be given and that there is sometimes no simple answer.

The patient's knowledge must be used as the starting point at this stage. This ensures continuity and reinforces that the clinician was listening to the patient and that his or her views are being taken into account. It is crucial to give the information in small chunks of non-medical language and assume that at best only 50% of the information will be retained. The interview should be broken up at intervals to check that the patient understands all the information and, if not, to clarify at this stage. Any written information is very useful at this point; I use a simple diagram to explain various surgical procedures (Fig. 11.1). It is important to listen carefully to the patient's own agenda; the clinician should take the lead from the patient and blend it in with his/her own.

This then merges imperceptibly into step 5, 'Responding to the patient's feeling'. This is the step at which the clinician's experience and ability to concentrate on the patient is invaluable. The response of most patients to a diagnosis

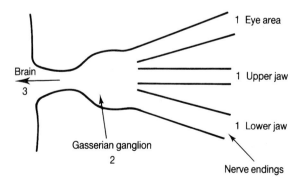

Figure 11.1 Diagram used with patients to explain the sites of different surgical procedures.

of trigeminal neuralgia is within the bounds of social acceptability, although conflicts may arise if the patient has had different information. Reactions to the diagnosis can include disbelief, shock, fear and anxiety. Many patients feel anger, which can be directed towards clinicians. Fear is a common finding among patients with trigeminal neuralgia as they are unable to predict when the next attack of pain will occur and whether they will be able to cope with it. I often find that patients are angry with their dental surgeon, either for not recognizing the condition or for having provoked it by dental treatment. It is crucial to emphasize that the aetiology of the condition is unknown and, although dental treatment may play a role, it is not the cause. Patients may also feel relief that they now know the diagnosis but this may result in overdependence or even seduction of the clinician in the form of lavish gifts in order to receive special care.

The final stage is that of planning and follow-through. Although it is important to empathize with the patient, the clinician must also offer a treatment plan. This is not based just on the clinician's viewpoint but also on the understanding of the patient's problems. It is crucial to offer the patient support in terms of coping strategies and support groups.

This stage must end with a summary that shows the clinician has been listening and is aware of the issues. It should end with what Buckman and Kason (1992) call 'a contract', by which the patient knows that he or she has a future and will be seen again. If a referral is to be made, it is important that the patient knows he or she can communicate with the original clinician if necessary.

The relatives or other significant others may wish to be involved. The patient, however, must first give consent to the imparting of this information. I find it extremely helpful to discuss everything with the significant other; the same six steps should be used with them.

I think it is important for the patient to realize that, although the condition is serious, it is not fatal, although it is unrealistic to expect a 'cure' in all patients. If patients are reassured inappropriately they will later lose confidence in the clinician (Kessel, 1979). Clinicians therefore need to learn counselling skills, which are increasingly important in the management of chronic illness. Many patients' complaints that end up in the courts are due to poor communication and lack of counselling skills.

Counselling is done in a wide variety of ways and several forms may be combined. These skills have been developed particularly in the management of patients with cancer, and have been well summarized by Fallowfield (1988).

The commonest form of counselling, and the one most often used by untrained counsellors, is directive counselling where the counsellor directs the behaviour of the patient wanting help. The counsellor may provide help in understanding the disease and in decision-making. This informative counselling is needed for many patients with trigeminal neuralgia who have to decide which treatment to choose. Some patients develop negative thinking and coping strategies, and confrontational counselling will enable the patient to recognize these features and help develop positive feedback. Some patients need to have a sense of control, and catalytic counselling will enable them to establish achievable goals to which they can strive. Supportive counselling provides the patient with empathy and real concern for their fears and needs.

Fallowfield (1988) has stressed that counsellors must not be volunteers and fellow sufferers, as their emotions can be projected on to the patient and result in their own emotional burn-out. Counsellors, therefore, provide a very different role from self-help groups, which by their very nature comprise fellow sufferers. Patients can also be offered further help through support or self-help groups.

SUPPORT AND SELF-HELP GROUPS

These types of groups are becoming increasingly important in health-care provision, as shown by a recent historical review of them in the USA (Borkman, 1990). Support and self-help groups are often considered to be one and the same thing, but there is a marked difference between them.

Self-help groups have clear educational and supportive aims that focus on personal growth, whereas support groups are there to help members emotionally and educationally through an external crisis and can be led by people who are not members (Rootes and Aanes, 1992). Rootes and Aanes (1992) put forward seven criteria that self-help groups should aim towards. They should focus on a single life-disrupting event and their primary purpose should be to support a personal change and to educate. The membership must be voluntary and a member leader must be known to all participants. The leader must be a fellow sufferer and not a professional. The group must maintain anonymity and confidentiality and be non-profit-making. Patients become aware that they are not alone, and this acceptance and understanding gives patients a sense of hope.

For the group to be effective, all members must be prepared to share their experiences honestly, accept responsibility for themselves and be committed to personal change. This personal commitment to change is pivotal. Participating in such groups may reduce disease-related stress, change patient behaviour, and improve relationships with other family members and the patient's doctor (Trojan, 1989).

It is important that self-help groups have input from professionals, but this must be indirect and non-authoritarian. The professional has to change from being a provider to a partner with self-help groups (Stewart, 1990). Professionals therefore need to understand the role of these groups.

Surveys have been undertaken to assess the value of such groups (Trojan, 1989). One of patients with ankylosing spondylitis, which used as a control patients who did not attend a self-help group, showed marked differences in psychological variables between the two groups (Barlow *et al.*, 1992). Self-help group participants showed less reliance on medical personnel and derived significant social support from fellow members. Compliance with treatment was also increased in this group. Other workers have had similar results (Trojan, 1989; Kelleher, 1990).

Self-help groups may play an increasingly important role in the management of patients who have incurable, progressive, unpredictable and difficult-to-diagnose conditions, as patients often feel that they have exhausted professional knowledge (Barlow *et al.*, 1992).

Self-help groups and the gathering of information by the patient can also be seen as an adaptive function. It allows the patient to displace the needs of an incurable condition to an activity (Buckman and Kason, 1992).

Patients with trigeminal neuralgia may benefit not just from a support group but also from a self-help group. Such a group could give patients some control over the pain and help them to develop coping strategies.

At present I am aware of only one fully organized support group for patients with trigeminal neuralgia, the Trigeminal Neuralgia Association, which is based in the USA (further details are given in the Appendix). This nationwide non-profit-making organization is run by patients with trigeminal neuralgia with a very extensive medical advisory board. Its major goals, as set out in a leaflet, are:

1. To provide information, mutual aid, support and encouragement.
2. To reduce the isolation of those affected by the disorder.
3. To increase awareness and understanding of the problem.
4. To serve as a resource and information centre to centralize current trigeminal neuralgia data.
5. To facilitate and promote research on trigeminal neuralgia.

The group also aims to set up local mutual support groups which may in the future become self-help groups.

It is important to ensure that only patients with trigeminal neuralgia join the group, and the Association has therefore suggested that all would-be participants should first be seen by a specialist who would confirm the diagnosis.

In view of the lack of specialized groups, patients may find it useful to form groups that include patients with any type of pain. These groups are fairly common and may be of benefit; they can be found through local pain clinics. The Appendix includes details of such groups, e.g. SHIP (Self-Help In Pain) which is based in England and has a regular newsletter, but many others do exist.

INFORMATION LEAFLETS

Adequate information about the illness, treatments and prognosis can alleviate much psychological distress related to a disease. Nowadays patients wish to be more fully informed and the profession has to respond to this (Lloyd, 1991). Information leaflets also reinforce the message that the patient is not alone and that others have a similar condition. There are leaflets written about trigeminal neuralgia (McConaghy, 1994, and see Appendix), and many neurosurgeons have their own information leaflets (Tew and van Loveren, 1988; Rovit, 1990) Inevitably the information will to some extent be biased by the person writing the leaflet, but it can act as a prompt for patients to ask more questions. Difficulties arise with patients who are unable to read or understand what they are reading owing to poor knowledge of the language, low intelligence or dementia.

Although information may be available, how one uses it to the best advantage for any particular patient still remains difficult. Medical therapy results in side-effects, especially in large doses and in the elderly, and patients need to be aware of this. Recurrence rates are not the only issues that must be stressed and complications can be important—if not more significant—in the long term. Nugent (1981) argued that if patients were to be given a full list of complications after microvascular decompression, fewer would undergo the procedure. A well-informed patient is also more likely to accept the side-effects of treatment (Tew and van Loveren, 1988).

MEDICAL MANAGEMENT

All new patients are initially treated medically as response to treatment is, in part, diagnostic. If the patient responds to treatment, the clinician can be fairly confident that the correct diagnosis has been made.

The decision then has to be made as to whether to remain on medical therapy or to consider surgery. If surgery is indicated, its timing needs to be determined.

Some neurosurgeons argue that early surgical treatment arrests the progression of the condition and ensures that surgery is carried out on a medically fit younger patient, which theoretically carries less risk of mortality and significant morbidity (Bederson and Wilson, 1989).

In practice, I find that those patients who are poorly controlled medically because they have been treated by less experienced clinicians and who are referred directly to a neurosurgeon rather than a neurologist tend to have surgery earlier in the course of their condition.

Many patients remain on medication for many years. Poor pain control and intolerance to the drugs are the main reasons for surgery.

There is an increasing number of drugs available, as discussed fully in Chapter 6. A thorough understanding of the mechanism of action of these drugs is crucial if good pain control with minimal side-effects is to be achieved. Patients must be carefully taught how to use the drugs and should be encouraged to keep pain diaries (see Chapter 5) until they learn how to control the pain. Severe haematological and biochemical reactions do occur, but are relatively rare. Most of the side-effects are those reported by the patients and affecting the quality of life. Side-effects are often insidious and patients are aware of them only once they have stopped the medication (Rovit, 1990).

SURGICAL MANAGEMENT

There is currently no ideal procedure and, in selecting one type, the advantages and disadvantages need to be weighed up as summarized in tables in Chapters 8 and 9. The ideal procedure should provide immediate pain relief, have a low recurrence rate, be free of risks and side-effects, easy to perform and repeatable (Illingworth, 1986).

Although different neurosurgical procedures have been compared within the same units there has to date been no single randomized controlled trial to evaluate the effectiveness of a variety of different procedures using the same outcome criteria in several centres. Thousands of procedures have been reported but few have been meticulously evaluated by an independent observer (Lichtor and Mullan, 1990; North *et al.*, 1990; Zakrzewska and Thomas, 1993). Sweet and Poletti (1988), after their survey of neurosurgeons, suggested that a central database be set up so that all surgeons in the USA could send in details anonymously of procedures performed and complications ensuing.

Surgical protocols for the management of patients with trigeminal neuralgia should be established so that prospective multicentre long-term evaluations can be made. There should be mutually agreed definitions for numbness, paraesthesia, hyperaesthesia, etc., and how these can be subjectively and objectively evaluated (Lichtor and Mullan, 1990).

Some measure of patient satisfaction after different forms of surgery is necessary if outcomes are to be compared. Apfelbaum (1977), in the conclusion of a report, mentioned a patient questionnaire which suggested that patients were less keen to have repeat radiofrequency thermocoagulation than microvascular decompression. We, on the other hand, have found all our patients to be equally satisfied with the form of surgery they had undergone (Zakrzewska and Thomas, 1993). It is recognized that patients' assessment of results will also be extremely biased and have a strong emotional overlay, but, despite this, they should be included in any analysis of results (Lichtor and Mullan, 1990).

FACTORS TO BE EVALUATED IN ASSESSING OUTCOME

Pain relief and recurrence rates
It is appreciated that surgical evaluations are difficult to carry out as surgeons vary considerably in the surgical procedures they will perform. Surgeons are influenced by the ease of performance of a procedure, their own experience and their ethical views. Morley (1985) has argued that there is no place for microvascular decompression and has advocated peripheral techniques or procedures at the level of the gasserian ganglion. Jannetta (1985), on the other hand, advocates microvascular decompression for the majority of his patients.

Longitudinal studies on younger patients treated by different neurosurgeons but in the same unit should also be included as they provide data as to what is done to and for the patient in the long term (Jannetta and Bissonette, 1985).

All procedures provide pain relief, although it can be delayed, as seen most frequently with glycerol injections into the gasserian ganglion.

Recurrence rates are highest in patients undergoing peripheral procedures, and some neurosurgeons argue that their use is therefore limited (Illingworth, 1986). Others suggest that peripheral techniques can be extremely useful but arrangements must be in place to deal with the recurrences. Patients must be aware that they can contact their clinician easily and that further surgery is available (Morley, 1985).

Recurrences do occur after microvascular decompression, although from available data the time interval appears to be much longer. All procedures performed at the level of the gasserian ganglion have similar recurrence rates, although it is generally considered highest for glycerol injections.

The more peripheral the procedure, the easier it is to perform a repeat procedure. Some patients accept repeat procedures whereas others want some other type of surgery.

Mortality

There is no mortality associated with peripheral procedures. Isolated deaths have occurred in patients undergoing surgery at the level of the gasserian ganglion, but there is a 1% mortality rate associated with microvascular decompression. This mortality rate is lower among experienced neurosurgeons (Sweet, 1990). It has been argued that a 1% mortality risk is too high a price to pay for the relief of pain from a condition that is, in itself, not fatal (Morley, 1985).

Complications

Morbidity, like mortality, is increased as the surgery becomes more complex. Morbidity after peripheral techniques is extremely low and confined to the area of surgery. After gasserian ganglion surgery there are few complications outside the trigeminal nerve territory, whereas hearing loss is common after posterior fossa surgery. Sensory loss and anaesthesia dolorosa can be extremely unpleasant for patients undergoing radiofrequency thermocoagulation of the gasserian ganglion. Other techniques used at this level have been developed to reduce this side-effect.

PSYCHOLOGICAL MANAGEMENT

Severe and intractable chronic pain leads to psychological and behavioural disturbances, as discussed in Chapter 3. At present, extremely few assessments have been carried out on patients with trigeminal neuralgia and no treatment protocols incorporating psychological and behavioural methods have been proposed. Some patients, however, may be helped more by referral to a psychiatrist or psychologist than to a neurosurgeon, particularly if the pain is atypical and triggered by psychological factors.

Among other factors, fear and anxiety need to be allayed as this can lead to a reduction in pain. Depression may also be present in patients with severe trigeminal neuralgia (Zakrzewska and Thomas, 1993). Many patients benefit from the use of psychotropic medications such as tricyclic antidepressants (Merskey, 1983).

In other chronic pain problems, behavioural and cognitive therapies have helped to restore patients to normal function in spite of pain and hence have improved the quality of life (Chapman *et al.*, 1981; Linton, 1982; Weisenberg and Caspi, 1989). In patients with temporomandibular joint dysfunction the illness behaviour questionnaire has proved a good screening instrument to identify patients who do better with psychological treatment rather than aggressive surgical management (Speculand *et al.*, 1983).

Some of these techniques involve the development of coping strategies which have been shown to benefit patients with pain (Crook *et al.*, 1984). Coping is broadly defined as cognitive and behavioural responses to stressful events that tax the person's capacity to adjust (Lazarus *et al.*, 1974). Patients must first appreciate that stress is present, assess it and then choose a coping strategy. Coping strategies can include relaxation techniques, problem solving, stress management, cognitive restructuring, behavioural and imaginal rehearsal, self-monitoring, self-reinstruction and self-reinforcement of effort to change (Weisenberg and Caspi, 1989). If incorrect coping strategies are adopted, adverse effects may occur and so they need to be carefully monitored (Weisenberg and Caspi, 1989).

In patients with chronic pain, learning to cope with stress is not sufficient and they need to alter their attitudes and behaviour towards anxiety, avoidance and withdrawal (Crook *et al.*, 1984). A limited number of patients may benefit from techniques that include hypnotherapy, biofeedback and operant conditioning (Merskey, 1983). Many patients with trigeminal neuralgia restrict their social activities during severe episodes of pain. It is sometimes useful to determine what these activities are and whether the patient is keen to return to them. Returning to these activities can be used as a treatment goal (Fordyce, 1983).

Psychological and behavioural therapies are equally important in patients who have had surgery and/or developed complications.

All patients with trigeminal neuralgia could benefit from psychological treatment in addition to medical or surgical management, as it gives them an opportunity to be in control of the pain. It is often the lack of control and feeling of powerlessness that leads patients to react with anger and anxiety to their condition (Weisenberg and Caspi, 1989; Buckman and Kason, 1992).

TREATMENT OPTIONS

In the two algorithms shown in Figs 11.2 and 11.3, I have attempted to present my personal views. The reasons for my choices are summarized at the end of Chapters 6–9 under Current status. Other authors use different criteria for for-

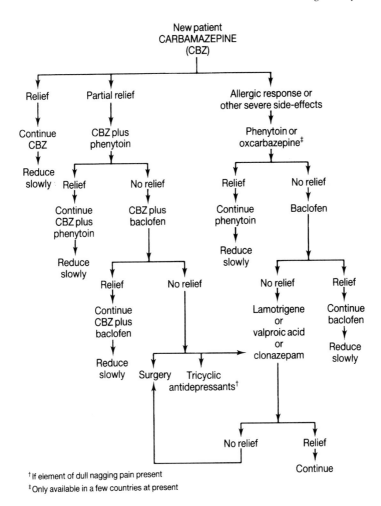

Figure 11.2   Medical management of a patient with trigeminal neuralgia.

mulating their algorithms, which in part are based on their own familiarity with the various techniques (Lunsford and Apfelbaum, 1985; Burchiel, 1987a; Fromm and Terrence, 1987).

I have put patients into two broad categories, dependent on age. Patients over the age of 65 years, especially if medically unfit, are not often eligible for posterior fossa surgery. The age and fitness of the patient also affect the choice of drugs and type of surgery. A fit younger patient with the potential for a long life is likely to request a procedure that offers more long-term pain relief than an elderly medically compromised patient.

The severity of the pain and its effect on the quality of life of an individual are of critical importance. Patients will make widely different choices dependent on this factor alone, and yet it is crucial for the clinician also to assess the effect of

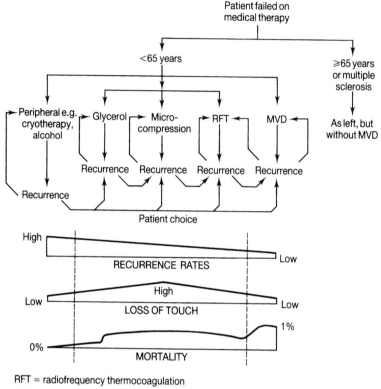

RFT = radiofrequency thermocoagulation
MVD = microvascular decompression

Figure 11.3 Surgical management of patient with trigeminal neuralgia. MVD, microvascular decompression; RFT, radiofrequency thermocoagulation.

treatment and complications on that individual's quality of life. The various treatment options should be discussed frequently so that, during an acute severe attack, patients are not suddenly faced for the first time with the need to make a quick decision. Patients need to have the confidence of knowing that there is always someone at hand to help them in a crisis (Morley, 1985).

CONCLUSION

Signicant others should be taken into consideration as they are often as involved as the patients themselves. This is especially important in the management of elderly patients. In the final analysis, the most important goal is to achieve pain control with no mortality and minimum morbidity for, as John Dryden put it:

> The happiness mankind can gain
> is not in the pleasure, but in the relief from pain.

Appendix: Useful Addresses

Trigeminal Neuralgia Association
PO Box 340
Barnegat Light
New Jersey 08006
USA

Telephone: 609-361-1014

For information about pain clinics in the UK and the services they offer:

The Pain Clinic Directory
College of Health
St Margaret's House
21 Old Ford Road
London E2 9PL

SHIP (Self-Help In Pain/Pain Wise UK)
Co-ordinator: Ms Rosalie Everatt RGN
33 Kingsdown Park
Tankerton
Kent CT5 2DT
UK

Telephone: (01227) 264677, 277886

American Chronic Pain Association
PO Box 850
Racklin
California 95677
USA

Telephone: 916-632-0922
(Over 500 chapters in the USA and Canada)

Leaflets on trigeminal neuralgia and facial pain:

Dr Joanna Zakrzewska
Department of Oral Medicine
Eastman Dental Hospital
256 Gray's Inn Road
London WC1X 8LD
UK

Telephone: (0171) 915 1172
Facsimile: (0171) 915 1105

Pain Information Pack (contains leaflets on trigeminal neuralgia and facial pain):

The Pain Relief Foundation
Pain Research Institute
Rice Lane
Liverpool L9 1AE
UK

Telephone: (0151) 523 1486
Facsimile: (0151) 521 6155

References

Abbott M and Killeffer FA (1970) Symptomatic trigeminal neuralgia. *Bull Los Angeles Neurol Soc* **35**, 1.

Adams CBT (1989) Microvascular decompression: an alternative view and hypothesis. *J Neurosurg* **57**, 1–12.

Adams CBT, Kaye AH and Teddy PJ (1982) The treatment of trigeminal neuralgia by posterior fossa microsurgery. *J Neurol Neurosurg Psychiatry* **45**, 1020–1026.

Agerberg G and Bergenholz A (1989) Craniomandibular disorders in adult populations of West Bothnia, Sweden. *Acta Odontol Scand* **47**, 129–140.

Agerberg G and Carlsson GE (1972) Functional disorder of the masticatory system. I. Distribution of symptoms according to age and sex judged from investigation by questionnaire. *Acta Odontol Scand* **30**, 597–613.

Ameli NO (1965) Avicenna and trigeminal neuralgia. *J Neurol Sci* **2**, 105–107.

Amoils SP (1967) The Joule Thomson Cryoprobe. *Arch Ophthalmol* **78**, 201–207.

Andrasik F and Holroyd KA (1980) Reliability and concurrent validity of headache questionnaires data. *Headache* **20**, 44–46.

André (1756) *Observations Pratiques sur les Maladies de l'Urethre*. Paris: Delaguette.

Apfelbaum RI (1977) A comparison of percutaneous radiofrequency trigeminal neurolysis and microvascular decompression of the trigeminal nerve for the treatment of tic douloureux. *Neurosurgery* **1**, 16–21.

Apfelbaum RI (1983) Surgery for tic douloureux. *Clin Neurosurg* **31**, 351–368.

Apfelbaum RI (1984) Surgery for tic douloureux. *Clin Neurosurg* **31**, 667–683.

Apfelbaum RI (1988) Surgical management of disorders of the lower cranial nerves. In: Schmidek HH and Sweet WH (eds) *Operative Neurosurgical Techniques, Indications, Methods and Results*, Vol 2, pp 1097–1109. Philadelphia: WB Saunders.

Arias MJ (1986) Percutaneous retrogasserian glycerol rhizotomies for trigeminal neuralgia. A prospective study of 100 cases. *Neurosurgery* **65**, 32–36.

Arnott J (1848) On severe cold or congelation as a remedy of disease. *London Medical Gazette* NS7, 936–938.

Arnott J (1849) *Practical illustrations of the treatment of the principal varieties of headache by the local application of benumbing cold; with remarks on the remedial and anaesthetic uses of congelation in diseases of the skin and surgical operations*. London: J Churchill.

Arnott J (1851) *On neuralgic, reumatic and other painful affections: with notices of improved modes of treatment*. London: J Churchill.

Aylard PR, Gooding JH, McKenna PJ and Snaith RP (1987) A validation study of three anxiety and depression self-assessment scales. *J Psychosom Res* **31**, 261–268.

Bahl FH, Ozuna J and Ritchie DL (1991) Interaction between calcium channel blockers and the antiepileptic drugs carbamazepine and phenytoin. *Neurology* **41**, 740–742.

Baker KA, Taylor JW and Lilly GE (1985) Treatment of trigeminal neuralgia: use of baclofen in combination with carbamazepine. *Clin Pharm* **4**, 93–96.

Balbi A, Sottofattori E, Mezzei M and Sannita WG (1991) Study of bioequivalence of magnesium and sodium valproates. *J Pharm Biomed Anal* **9**, 317–321.

Barba, D. and Alksne JF (1984) Success of microvascular decompression with and without prior surgical therapy for trigeminal neuralgia. *J Neurosurg* **60**, 104–107.

Barlow JH, Macey SJ and Struthers G (1992) Psychological factors and self-help in ankylosing spondylitis patients. *Clin Rheumatol* **11**, 220–225.

Barnard D (1986) Cryosurgery of the nerve. In: Bradley PF (ed) *Cryosurgery of the Maxillo-facial Region*, Vol II, pp 93–118. Florida: CRC Press.

Barnard D (1989) Cryoanalgesia in the management of paroxysmal trigeminal neuralgia. *Hospital Dentistry and Oral and Maxillo-Facial Surgery* **1**, 58–60.

Barnard D, Lloyd J and Evans CJ (1981) Cryoanalgesia in the management of chronic facial pain. *J Maxillofac Surg* **9**, 101–102.

Barnard JDW, Lloyd JW and Glynn CJ (1978) Cryosurgery in the management of intractable facial pain. *Br J Oral Surg* **16**, 135–142.

Beck AT, Ward CH, Mendelson M *et al.* (1961) An inventory for measuring depression. *Arch Gen Psychiatry* **4**, 561–571.

Beck DW, Olson JJ and Urig ES (1986) Percutaneous retrogasserian glycerol rhizotomies for treatment of trigeminal neuralgia. *Neurosurgery* **65**, 28–31.

Bederson JB and Wilson CB (1989) Evaluation of microvascular decompression and partial sensory rhizotomy in 252 cases of trigeminal neuralgia. *J Neurosurg* **71**, 359–367.

Belber CJ and Rak RA (1987) Balloon compression rhizolysis in the surgical management of trigeminal neuralgia. *Neurosurgery* **20**, 908–913.

Bell C (1829) On the nerves of the face; second part. *Philos Trans R Soc Lond* **119**, 317–330.

Bennett MH and Jannetta PJ (1983) Evoked potentials in trigeminal neuralgia. *Neurosurgery* **13**, 242–247.

Bennett MH and Lunsford LD (1984) Percutaneous retrogasserian glycerol rhizotomy for tic douloureux. Part 2: Results and implications of trigeminal evoked potential studies. *Neurosurgery* **14**, 431–435.

Benoldi D, Mirizzi S, Zucchi A and Allegra F (1991) Prevention of post-herpetic neuralgia. Evaluation of treatment with oral prednisone, oral acylovir and radiotherapy. *Int J Dermatol* **30**, 288–290.

Beppu S, Sato Y, Amemiya Y and Tode I (1992) Practical application of meridian acupuncture treatment for trigeminal neuralgia. *Anaesthesia and Pain Control in Dentistry* **1**, 103–108.

Beran R (1993) Cross-reactive skin eruption with both carbamazepine and oxcarbazepine. *Epilepsia* **34**, 163–165.

Bergenheim AT, Hariz MI and Laitinen LV (1991) Selectivity of retrogasserian glycerol rhizotomy in the treatment of trigeminal neuralgia. *Stereotact Funct Neurosurg* **56**, 159–165.

Bergner M, Bobbitt RA, Carter W and Gilson B (1981) The Sickness Impact Profile: development and final revision of a health status measure. *Med Care* **19**, 787–805.

Bergouignan M (1942) Cures heureuses de neuralgies essentielles par le diphenyl-hydantionate de soude. *Rev Laryngol Otol Rhinol* **63**, 34–41.

Bernard EJ Jr, Nashold BS Jr, Caputi F and Moosy JJ (1987) Nucleus caudalis DREZ lesions for facial pain. *Br J Neurosurg* **1**, 81–92.

Bertilsson L (1978) Clinical pharmacokinetics of carbamazepine. *Clin Pharmacokinet* **3**, 128–143.

Bertilsson L and Tomson T (1986) Clinical pharmacokinetics and pharmacological effects of carbamazepine and carbamazepine-10,11-epoxide. *Clin Pharmacokinet* **11**, 177–198.

Betts T, Goodwin G, Withers RM and Yuen AWC (1991) Human safety of lamotrigine. *Epilepsia* **32**, (Suppl. 2), S17–S21.

Biltz H (1908) Uber die Konstitution der Einwirkungspradukte von substitut Hornstoffen auf Benzil und uber einige neue Methoden zur Darstellung der 5,5-Diphenylhydantoin. *Berl Dtsch Chem Ges* **41**, 1379.

Bittar GT and Graff-Radford SB (1992) A retrospective study of patients with cluster headache. *Oral Med Oral Surg Oral Pathol* **73**, 519–525.

Bittar, GT and Graff-Radford, SB (1993) The effects of streptomycin/lidocaine block on trigeminal neuralgia: a double blind crossover placebo controlled study. *Headache* **33**, 155–160.

Bjerring P, Arendt-Nielsen L and Soderberg U (1990) Argon laser induced cutaneous sensory and pain thresholds in post-herpetic neuralgia. Quantitive modulation by topical capsaicin. *Acta Derm Venereol* **70**, 121–125.

Black RG (1974) A laboratory model for trigeminal neuralgia. *Adv Neurol* **4**, 651.

Blair GAS and Gordon DS (1973) Trigeminal neuralgia and dental malocclusions. *BMJ* **4**, 38–40.

Blau JN (1993) Behaviour during a cluster headache. *Lancet* **342**, 723–725.

Blom S (1962) Trigeminal neuralgia. Its treatment with a new anticonvulsant drug (G32883). *Lancet* **i**, 839–840.

Bochner F, Hooper WD, Tyrer JH and Eadie MJ (1972) The effect of dosage increments on blood phenytoin concentrations. *J Neurol Neurosurg Psychiatry* **35**, 873–876.

Bogucki A (1990) Studies on nitroglycerin and histamine provoked cluster headache attacks. *Cephalalgia* **10**, 71–75.

Bond MR (1979) *Pain. Its Nature, Analysis and Treatment.* Edinburgh: Churchill Livingstone.

Bonica JJ (1974) Organization and function of a pain clinic. *Adv Neurol* **4**, 433–443.

Bonica JJ (1990) *The Management of Pain*, 2nd edn. Philadelphia: Lea and Febiger.

Borkman T (1990) Self-help groups at the turning point: emerging egalitatian alliances with the format health-care system? *Am J Commun Psychiatry* **18**, 321–332.

Boston K, Pearce SA and Richardson PH (1989) The Pain Cognitions Questionnaire. *J Psychosom Res* **34**(1), 103–110.

Boucheret RK (1971) Herpes zoster ophthalmicus with trochlear nerve involvement, after alcohol injection into the gasserian ganglion. *Br J Ophthalmol* **55**, 761.

Bowsher D (1992) Acute herpes zoster and postherpetic neuralgia: effects of acyclovir and outcome of treatment with amitriptyline. *Br J Gen Pract* **42**, 244–246.

Bracco, D (1980) Historical developments. In: Marcel RJ (ed) *Handbook of Cryosurgery*, pp 3–14. New York: Marcel Dekker.

Braham J and Saia A (1960) Phenytoin in the treatment of trigeminal and other neuralgias. *Lancet* **ii**, 892–893.

Brandt F and Wittkamp P (1983) Spatresultate der thermokoagulation im ganglion gasseri beim tic douloureux. *Neurochirurgia* **26**, 133–135.

Breeze R and Ignelzi RJ (1982) Microvascular decompression for trigeminal neuralgia. Results with special reference to the late recurrence rate. *J Neurosurg* **57**, 487–490.

Bremerich A, Claeys T, Kovacs B and Cesteleyn L (1991) Somato-sensory evoked potentials in facial pain diagnosis. *Acta Stomatol Belg* **88**, 117–121.

Brewis M, Poskanzer DC, Rolland C and Miller H (1966) Neurological disease in an English city. *Acta Neurol Scand* **42** (Suppl. 24): 1–89.

Brisman R (1987) Trigeminal neuralgia and multiple sclerosis. *Arch Neurol* **44**, 379–381.

Brody DS (1980) Physicians' recognition of behavioral, psychological, and social aspects of medical care. *Arch Intern Med* **140**, 1286–1289.

Broggi G, Franzini A, Lasio G et al. (1990) Long-term results of percutaneous retrogasserian thermorhizotomy for 'essential' trigeminal neuralgia: considerations in 1000 consecutive patients. *Neurosurgery* **26**, 783–786.

Broggi G, Franzini A, Giorgi C, Servello D and Brock S (1993) Trigeminal neuralgia: new surgical strategies. *Acta Neurochir* **58** (Suppl.), 171–173.

Brown JA and Pruel MC (1988) Trigeminal depressor response during percutaneous microcompression of the trigeminal ganglion for trigeminal neuralgia. *Neurosurgery* **23**, 745–748.

Browne TR and Penry JK (1973) Benzodiazepines in the treatment of epilesy. *Epilepsia* **15**, 277–310.

Bruyn GW (1986) Glossopharyngeal neuralgia. In: Clifford Rose F (ed) *Handbook of Clinical Neurology. Headache*, Vol 4,(48) pp 459–473. Amsterdam: Elsevier Science.

Buckman R and Kason Y (1992) *How to Break Bad News*. London: MacMillan.

Burchiel K (1993) Is trigeminal neuralgia a neuropathic pain? *Am Pain Soc J* **2**(1) 12–16.

Burchiel KJ (1980) Abnormal impulse generation in focally demyelinated trigeminal roots. *J Neurosurg* **53**, 674–683.

Burchiel KJ (1987a) Surgical treatment of trigeminal neuralgia: major operative procedures. In: Fromm GH (ed) *The Medical and Surgical Management of Trigeminal Neuralgia*, pp 101–120. New York: Futura.

Burchiel KJ (1987b) Surgical treatment of trigeminal neuralgia: minor operative procedures. In: Fromm GH (ed) *The Medical and Surgical Management of Trigeminal Neuralgia*, pp 71–99. New York: Futura.

Burchiel KJ (1988) Percutaneous retrogasserian glycerol rhizolysis in the management of trigeminal neuralgia. *J Neurosurg* **69**, 361–366.

Burchiel KJ, Steege TD, Howe JF and Loeser JD (1981) Comparison of percutaneous radiofrequency gangliolysis and microvascular decompression for the surgical management of tic douloureux. *Neurosurgery* **9**, 111–118.

Burchiel KJ, Clarke H, Haglund M and Loeser JD (1988) Long term efficacy of microvascular decompression in trigeminal neuralgia. *J Neurosurg* **69**, 35–38.

Burton BS (1882) On the propyl derivatives and decomposition products of ethylacetoacetate. *Am Chem J* **3**, 385–395.

Bussone G, Leone M and Peccarisi C *et al.* (1990) Double blind comparison of lithium and verapamil in cluster headache prophylaxis. *Headache* **30**, 411–417.

Caccia MR (1975) Clonazepam in facial neuralgia and cluster headaches. Clinical and electrophysiological study. *Eur Neurol* **13**, 560–563.

Calvin WH, Loeser JD and Howe JF (1977). A neurophysiological theory for the pain mechanism of tic douloureux. *Pain* **3**, 147–154.

Campbell RL, Trentacosti CD, Eschenroeder TA and Harkins S (1990) An evaluation of sensory changes and pain relief in trigeminal neuralgia following intracranial microvascular decompression and / or trigeminal glycerol rhizotomy. *J Oral Maxillofac Surg* **48**, 1057–1062.

Carlsson AM (1983) Assessment of chronic pain. I. Aspects of the reliability of the visual analogue scale. *Pain* **16**, 87.

Carraz G, Darbon M, Lebreton S and Beriel H (1964a) Proprietes pharmacodynamiques de l'acide *n*-dipropylacetique et de ses derives. Quantrieme memoire: le *n*-dipropyl acetamide. *Therapy* **19**, 469–475.

Carraz G, Farr R, Chateau R and Bonnin J (1964b) First clinical trials of the antiepiletic activity of *n*-dipropylacetic acid. *Ann Med Psychol* **122**, 577–584.

Carter BL, Garnett WR, Pellock JM *et al.* (1981) Effect of antacids on phenytoin bioavailability. *Ther Drug Monit* **3**, 333–340.

Cawson RA (1991) *Essentials of Dental Surgery and Pathology*. Edinburgh: Churchill Livingstone.

Chakravorty BG (1966) Association of trigeminal neuralgia with multiple sclerosis. *Arch Neurol* **14**, 95–99.

Chandra B (1976) The use of clonazepam in the treatment of tic douloureux (a preliminary report). *Proc Aust Assoc Neurol* **13**, 119–122.

Chapman SL, Brena SF and Bradford LA (1981) Treatment outcome in a chronic pain rehabilitation program. *Pain*, **11**, 255–168.

Chen ACN and Treede RD (1985) The McGill Pain Questionnaire in the assessment of phasic and tonic experimental pain: behavioural evaluation of the 'pain inhibiting pain' effect. *Pain* **22**, 67–79.

Chinitz A, Seelinger DF and Greenhouse AH (1966) Anticonvulsant therapy in trigeminal neuralgia. *Am J Med Sci* **252**, 62–67.

Choi CR, Kang SK and Rha HK (1982) Percutaneous stereotactic thermocoagulation for trigeminal neuralgia. *App Neurophysiol* **45**, 512–515.

Choudhury BK, Pahari S, Acharyya A, Goswami A and Bhattacharyya MK (1991) Percutaneous retrogasserian radiofrequency thermal rhizotomy for trigeminal neuralgia. *J Indian Med Assoc* **89**, 294–296.

Clark A and Fallowfield, LJ (1986) Quality of life measurements in patients with malignant disease: a review. *J R Soc Med* **79**, 165–169.

Cobb CA, III and Fung D (1983) Quantitative analysis of lesion parameters in radiofrequency trigeminal rhizotomy. *J Neurosurg* **58**, 388–391.

Connor JA (1985) Neural pacemakers and rhythmicity. *Annu Rev Physiol* **47**, 17–28.

Conrad P (1985) The meaning of medications: another look at compliance. *Soc Sci Med* **20**, 29–37.

Cooper, IS and Lee, AS (1961) Cryothalamectomy—hypothermic congelation: a technical advance in basal ganglia surgery. Preliminary report. *J Am Geriatr Soc* **9**, 714–718.

Cooper, IS, Grissman, F and Johnson, R (1962) A complete system for cryogenic surgery. *St Barnabas Hosp Med Bull* **1**, 11–16.

Court JE and Kase CS (1976) Treatment of tic douloureux with a new anticonvulsant (clonazepam). *J Neurol Neurosurg Psychiatry* **39**, 297–299.

Craig KD and Prkachin KM (1983) Nonverbal measures of pain. In: Melzack R (ed) *Pain Measurement and Assessment*, pp 173–179. New York: Raven Press.

Crawford P, Chadwick DJ, Martin C *et al.* (1990) The interaction of phenytoin and carbamazepine with combined oral contraceptive steroids. *Br J Clin Pharmacol* **30**, 892–896.

Crook J, Rideout E and Browne G (1984) The prevalence of pain complaints in a general population. *Pain* **18**, 299–314.

Crowley JJ, Cusack BJ, Jue SG *et al.* (1987) Cigarette smoking and theophylline metabolism: effect of phenytoin. *Clin Pharmacol Ther* **42**, 334–340.

Cushing H (1920) The major trigeminal neuralgias and their surgical treatment based on experiences with 332 gasserian operations. The varieties of facial neuralgia. *Am J Med Sci* **160**, 157–185.

Dahle L, von Essen C, Kourtopoulos H *et al.* (1989) Microvascular decompression for trigeminal neuralgia. *Acta Neurochir* **99**, 109–112.

Dalton MJ, Powell JR, Messenheimer JA and Clark J (1986) Cimetidine and carbamazepine: a complex drug interaction. *Epilepsia* **27**, 553–558.

Dam M, Ekberg R, Loyning Y *et al.* (1989) A double-blind study comparing oxcarbazepine and carbamazepine in patients with newly diagnosed, previously untreated epilepsy. *Epilepsy Res* **3**, 70–76.

Dandy WE (1925) Section of the sensory root of the trigeminal nerve at the pons. *Bull John Hopkins Hosp* **36**, 105–106.

Dandy WE (1934) Concerning the cause of trigeminal neuralgia. *Am J Surg* **24**, 447–455.

Daniels DL, Pech P, Pojunas K *et al.* (1986) Trigeminal nerve: anatomic correlation with MR imaging. *Radiology* **159**, 577.

Darlow LA, Brooks ML and Quinn PD (1992) Magnetic resonance imaging in the diagnosis of trigeminal neuralgia. *J Oral Maxillofac Surg* **50**, 621–626.

Daut RL, Cleeland CS and Flanery RC (1983) Development of the Wisconsion Brief Pain Questionnaire to assess pain in cancer and other diseases. *Pain* **17**, 197.

Davies HT, Crombie IK and Macrea WA (1993) Balanced views on neurogenic pain. *Pain* **54**, 341–346.

Davies MS (1970) Corneal anaesthesia after alcohol injection of the trigeminal sensory root. Examination of 100 anaesthetic corneae. *Br J Ophthalmol* **54**(9), 577–586.

De La Porte C, Verlooy J, Veekmans G *et al.* (1990) Consequences and complications of glycerol injection in the cavum of Meckel: a series of 120 consecutive injections. *Stereotact Funct Neurosurg* **5455**, 73–75.

de Lange EE, Jidvoye GJ and Joormolen JHC (1986) Arterial compression of fifth cranial nerve causing trigeminal neuralgia. *Radiology* **158**, 721–727.

Dechant KL and Clissold SP (1992) Sumatripan. A review of its pharmacodynamic and pharmacokinetic properties, and therapeutic efficacy in the acute treatment of migraine and cluster headaches. *Drugs* **43**, 776–798.

Degenaar JJ (1979) Some philosophical considerations on pain. *Pain* **7**, 281–304.

Devor M, Goorin-Lippermann R and Angelides K (1993) Na⁺ channel immunolocalization in peripheral mammalian axons and changes following nerve injury and neuroma formation. *J Neurosci* **13**, 1976–1992.

Dickinson RG, Hooper WD, Dunstan PR and Eadie MJ (1989) First dose and steady-state pharmacokinetics of oxcarbazepine and its 10-hydroxy metabolite. *Eur J Pharmacol* **37**, 69–74.

Dieckmann G, Veras G and Sogabe K (1987) Retrogasserian glycerol injection or percutaneous stimulation in the treatment of typical and atypical trigeminal pain. *Neurol Res* **9**, 48–49.

Dill WA, Kargenko A, Wolff LM and Glazko AJ (1956) Studies on 5,5-phenylhydantoin (Dilantin) in animals and man. *J Pharmacol Exp Ther* **118**, 270–279.

Dixon JS and Bird HA (1981) Reproducibility along a 10 cm vertical visual analogue scale. *Ann Rheum Dis* **40**, 87–89.

Dorland's Illustrated Medical Dictionary, 25th edn. (1974) Philadelphia: WB Saunders.

Dreifuss FE and Langer DH (1987) Hepatic considerations in the use of anticonvulsant drugs. *Epilepsia* **28**, (Suppl. 2), S23–S29.

Dreifuss FE, Santilli N, Langer DH *et al.* (1987) Valproic acid hepatitis fatalities: a retrospective review. *Neurology* **37**, 379–385.

Dubner R (1993) Neuropathic pain. New understanding leads to new treatments. *Am Pain Soc J* **2**(1), 8–11.

Dubner R and Bennett GJ (1983) Spinal and trigeminal mechanisms of nociception. *Annu Rev Neurosci* **6**, 381–418.

Dubner R, Sharav Y, Gracely RH and Price DD (1987) Idiopathic trigeminal neuralgia: sensory features and pain mechanisms. *Pain* **31**, 23–33.

Duncan JS, Patsalos PN and Shorvon SD (1991) Effects of discontinuation of phenytoin, carbamazepine, and valproate on concomitant antiepileptic medication. *Epilepsia* **32**, 101–115.

Dworkin SF and LeResche L (ed) (1992) Research diagnostic criteria for temporomandibular disorders: review, criteria, examination and specification, critique. *Journal of Craniomandibular Disorders: Facial and Oral Pain*, **6**(4), 301–355.

Dworkin SF, Huggins KH, LeResche L *et al.* (1990a) Epidemiology of signs and symptoms in temporomandibular disorders: clinical signs in cases and controls. *J Am Dental Assoc* **120**, 273–281.

Dworkin SF, LeResche L, DeRouen T and Von Korff M (1990b) Assessing clinical signs of temporo-mandibular disorders: reliability of clinical examiners. *J Prosthet Dent* **63**, 574–579.

Dworkin RH, Hartstein G, Rosner HL *et al.* (1992) A high-risk method for studying psychosocial antecedents of chronic pain: the prospective investigation of herpes zoster. *J Abnorm Psychol* **101**, 200–205.

Editorial (1988) Diagnostic criteria. *Cephalalgia* **8**, 67–69.

Edwards LC, Pearce SA, Turner-Stokes L and Jones A (1992) The pain beliefs questionnaire: an investigation of beliefs in the causes and consequences of pain. *Pain* **51**, 267–272.

Eichelbaum M, Ekbom K, Bertilsson L *et al.* (1975) Plasma kinetics of carbamazepine and its epoxide metabolite in man after single and multiple doses. *Eur J Clin Pharmacol* **8**, 337–341.

Eichelbaum M, Kothe KW, Hoffman F and von Unruh GE (1979) Kinetics and metabolism during combined antiepileptic therapy. *Clin Pharmacol Ther* **26**, 366–371.

Ekbom K (1970) A clinical comparison of cluster headache and migraine. *Acta Neurol Scand* **46**, (Suppl. 41) 1–48.

Elpick M (1989) Clinical issues in the use of carbamazepine in psychiatry: a review. *Psychol Med* **19**, 591–604.

Elyas AA, Patsalos PN, Agbato OA *et al.* (1986) Factors influencing simultaneous concentrations of total and free carbamazepine and carbamazepine-10,11-epoxide in serum of children with epilepsy. *Ther Drug Monit* **8**, 288–292.

Epstein LH and Abel GG (1977) Analysis of biofeedback training effects for tension headache patients. *Behav Ther* **8**, 37–47.

Esmann V and Wildenhoff KE (1980) Idoxuridine in herpes zoster. *Lancet* **ii**, 474.

Esposito S, Delitala A, Bruni P *et al.* (1985) Therapeutic protocol in the treatment of trigeminal neuralgia. *App Neurophysiol* **48**, 271–273.

Eversole LR, Stone CE, Matheson D and Kaplan H (1985) Psychometric profiles and facial pain. *Oral Surg Oral Med Oral Pathol* **60**, 269–274.

Eysenck HS and Eysenck SRG (1969) *Manual of the Eysenck Personality Inventory*. London: University of London Press.

Faigle JW and Menge GP (1990) Pharmacokinetic and metabolic features of oxcarbazepine and their clinical significance: comparison with carbamazepine. *Int Clin Psychopharmacol* **5** (Suppl. 1), 73–82.

Fallowfield LJ (1988) Counselling for patients with cancer. *BMJ* **297**, 727–728.

Farago F (1987) Trigeminal neuralgia: its treatment with two new carbamazepine analogues. *Eur Neurol* **26**, 73–83.

Fardy MJ and Patton DWP (1994) Complications associated with peripheral alcohol injections in the management of trigeminal neuralgia. *Br J Oral Maxillofac Surg* **32**, 387–391.

Fardy MJ, Zakrzewska JM and Patton DW (1994) Peripheral surgical techniques for the management of trigeminal neuralgia—alcohol and glycerol injections. *Acta Neurochir* **129**(3–4), 181–185.

Feinmann C (1985) Pain relief by antidepressants: possible modes of action. *Pain* **23**, 1–8.

Feinmann C (1993) The long-term outcome of facial pain treatment. *J Psychosom Res* **37**, 381–387.

Feinmann C and Harris M (1984) Psychogenic facial pain. Part 1: The clinical presentation. *Br Dent J* **156**, 165–168.

Feinmann C and Peatfield R (1993) Orofacial neuralgia. Diagnosis and treatment guidelines. *Drugs* **46**, 263–268.

Feinmann C, Harris M and Cawley R (1984) Psychogenic facial pain: presentation and treatment. *BMJ* **288**, 436–538.

Feldman KF, Dorhofer G, Faigle JW and Imof P (1981) Pharmacokinetics and metabolism of GP47 779, the main human metabolite of oxcarbazepine (GP47 680) in animals and healthy volunteers. In: Dam M, Gram L and Penry JK (eds) *Advances in Epileptology: XIIth Epilepsy International Symposium*, pp 89–96. New York: Raven Press.

Ferguson GG, Brett DC, Peerless SJ, Barr HWK and Girvin JP (1981) Trigeminal neuralgia: a comparison of the results of percutaneous rhizotomy and microvascular decompression. *J Can Sci Neurolog* **8**, 207–213.

Fields HL (1987) *Pain*. Maidenhead: McGraw-Hill.

Fields HL (ed) (1990) *Pain Syndromes in Neurology*. London: Butterworths.

Fishman B, Pasternak S, Wallenstein S, Houde RW, Holland J and Foley KM (1986) The Memorial Pain Assessment Card: a valid instrument for evaluation of cancer pain. *Am Soc Clin Oncol* **5**, 239 (abstract 935).

Flor H, Kerns RD and Turk DC (1987) The role of spouse reinforcement, perceived pain, and activity levels of chronic pain patients. *J Psychosom Res* **31**, 251–259.

Fordyce WE (1976) *Behavioral Methods for Chronic Pain and Illness*. St Louis: Mosby CV.

Fordyce WE (1983) The validity of pain behavior measurement. In: Melzack R (ed) *Pain Measurement and Assessment*, pp 145–153. New York: Raven Press.

Fothergill J (1773) Of a painful affection of the face. Medical observations and inquiries. *Soc Physicians Lond* **5**, 129–142.

Fraioli B, Esposito V, Ferrante L *et al.* (1989a) Microsurgical treatment of glossopharyngeal neuralgia: case reports. *Neurosurgery* **25**, 630–632.

Fraioli B, Esposito V, Guidetti B *et al.* (1989b) Treatment of trigeminal neuralgia by thermocoagulation, glycerolization and percutaneous compression of the gasserian ganglion and/or retrogasserian rootlets: long-term results and therapeutic protocol. *Neurosurgery* **24**, 239–245.

Frank FT, Gaist A, Fabrizi F *et al.* (1985) Resultats de la thermocoagulation percutanee selective du ganglion de Gasser dans la nevralgie faciale essentielle. Synthese des resultats obtenus chez 939 patients traités. *Neurochirurgie* **31**, 179–182.

Frazier CH (1925) Subtotal resection of sensory root for the relief of major trigeminal neuralgia. *Arch Neurol Psychiatry* **73**, 378–384.

Frazier CH and Russell EC (1924) Neuralgia of the face: an analysis of 754 cases with relation to pain and other sensory phenomena before and after operation. *Arch Neurol Psychiatr* **11**, 557–563.

Freemont AJ and Millac P (1981) The place of peripheral neurectomy in the management of trigeminal neuralgia. *Postgrad Med J* **57**, 75–76.

Fritz W, Schafer J and Klein HH (1988) Hearing loss after microvascular decompression for trigeminal neuralgia. *J Neurosurg* **69**, 367–370.

Fromm GH (1987) Etiology and pathogenesis of trigeminal neuralgia. In: Fromm GH (ed.) *The Medical and Surgical Management of Trigeminal Neuralgia*. New York: Futura.

Fromm GH (1991) Pathophysiology of trigeminal neuralgia. In: Fromm GH and Sessle BJ (eds) *Trigeminal Neuralgia: Current Concepts Regarding Pathogenesis and Treatment*, pp 105–130. Boston: Butterworth–Heinemann.

Fromm GH and Sessle BJ (1991) Summary and conclusions. In: Fromm GH and Sessle BJ (eds) *Trigeminal Neuralgia, Current Concepts Regarding Pathogenesis and Treatment*, pp 205–221. Boston: Butterworth–Heinemann.

Fromm GH and Terrence CF (1987a) Comparison of L-baclofen and racemic baclofen in trigeminal neuralgia. *Neurology* **37**, 1725–1728.

Fromm GH and Terrence CF (1987b) Medical treatment of trigeminal neuralgia. In: Fromm GH (ed) *The Medical and Surgical Management of Trigeminal Neuralgia*, pp 61–70. New York: Futura.

Fromm GH, Terrence CF, Chattha AS and Glass JD (1980) Baclofen in trigeminal neuralgia: its effect on the spinal trigeminal nucleus: a pilot study. *Arch Neurol* **37**, 768–771.

Fromm GH, Chattha AS, Terrence CF and Glass JD (1981) Role of inhibitory mechanisms in trigeminal neuralgia. *Neurology* **31**, 683–687.

Fromm GH, Terrence CF and Maroon JC (1984a) Trigeminal neuralgia: current concepts regarding etiology and pathogenesis. *Arch Neurol* **41**, 1204–1207.

Fromm GH, Terrence CF and Chattha AS (1984b) Baclofen in the treatment of trigeminal neuralgia: double-blind study and long-term follow up. *Ann Neurol* **15**, 240–244.

Fromm GH, Graff-Radford SB, Terrence CF and Sweet WH (1990) Pre-trigeminal neuralgia. *Neurology* **40**, 1493–1495.

Fromm GH, Nakata M and Kondo T (1991) Differential action of amitriptyline on neurons in the trigeminal nucleus. *Neurology* **41**, 1932–1936.

Fromm GH, Sato K and Nakata M (1992) The action of GABA-B antagonists in the trigeminal nucleus of the rat. *Neuropharmacology* **31**, 475–480.

Fromm GH, Aumentado D and Terrence CF (1993) A clinical and experimental investigation of the effects of tizanidine in trigeminal neuralgia. *Pain* **53**, 265–271.

Fujimaki T, Fukushima T and Miyazaki S (1990) Percutaneous retrograsserian glycerol injection in the management of trigeminal neuralgia: long-term follow-up results. *J Neurosurg* **73**, 212–216.

Fusco BM and Alessandri M (1992) Analgesic effect of capsaicin in idiopathic trigeminal neuralgia. *Anesth Analg* **74**, 375–377.

Gabai IJ and Spierings EL (1989) Prophylactic treatment of cluster headaches with verapamil. *Headache* **29**(3) 167–168.

Gardner WJ and Miklos MV (1959) Response of trigeminal neuralgia to decompression of sensory root. Discussion of cause of trigeminal neuralgia. *JAMA* **170**, 1773–1776.

Gardner WS (1962) Concerning the mechanism of trigeminal neuralgia and hemifacial spasm. *J Neurosurg* **19**, 947–958.

Gelber BR, Gogela LJ and Pierson EW (1989) Posterior fossa partial trigeminal rhizotomy: an alternative to microvascular decompression. *Nebraska Med J* **74**, 105–108.

Gillham RA, Williams N, Weidmann K *et al.* (1988) Concentration–effect relationship with carbamazepine and its epoxide on psychomotor and cognitive function in epileptic patients. *J Neurol Neurosurg Psychiatry* **51**, 929–933.

Gilman JT, Alvarez LA and Duchowny M (1993) Carbamazepine toxicity resulting from generic substitution. *Neurology* **43**, 2696–2697.

Ginwalla MSN (1961) Surgical treatment of trigeminal neuralgia of the third division. *Oral Surg Oral Med Oral Pathol* **14**, 1300–1304.

Glaser MA (1928) Atypical facial neuralgia so called. A critical analysis of 143 cases. *Arch Neurol Psychiatry* **20**, 537–557.

Goggin T, Gough H, Bissessar A *et al.* (1987) A comparative study of the relative effects of anticonvulsant drugs and dietary folate on the red cell folate status of patients with epilepsy. *Q J Med* **65**, 911–919.

Goldberg DP (1972) *The Detection of Psychiatric Illness by Questionnaire.* Oxford: Oxford University Press.

Goldberg DP and Hillier VF (1979) A scaled version of the General Health Questionnaire. *Psychol Med* **9**, 139–145.

Gordon A and Hitchcock ER (1983) Illness behaviour and personality in intractable facial pain syndromes. *Pain* **17**, 267–276.

Goss AN (1984) Peripheral cryoneurotomy in the treatment of trigeminal neuralgia. *Aust Dent J* **29**, 222–224.

Goulden KJ, Dooley JM, Camfield PR and Fraser AD (1987) Clinical valproate toxicity induced by acetylsalicylate. *Neurology* **37**, 1393–1394.

Goya T, Wakisaka S and Kinoshita K (1990) Microvascular decompression for trigeminal neuralgia with special reference to delayed recurrence. *Neurol Med Chir (Tokyo)* **30**, 462–467.

Gracely RH (1980) Psychophysical assessment of human pain. In: Bonica JJ and Albe-Fessard D (eds) *Advances in Pain Research and Therapy 3,* p 805. New York: Raven Press.

Gracely RH and Dubner R (1981) Pain assessment in humans — a reply to Hall. *Pain* **11**, 109–120.

Gram L and Jensen PK (1989) Carbamazepine. Toxicity. In: Levy RH, Dreifuss FE, Mattson RH, Meldrum BS and Penry JK (eds) *Antiepileptic Drugs,* pp 555–565. New York: Raven Press.

Grant FC (1922) Alcoholic injection of second and third divisions of trigeminal nerve. Clinical results with more exact technic. *JAMA* **78**, 1780–1781.

Grant FC (1936) Alcohol injection in the treatment of major trigeminal neuralgia. *JAMA* **107**, 771–774.

Grantham EG and Segerberg LH (1952) An evaluation of palliative surgical procedures in trigeminal neuralgia. *J Neurosurg* **9**, 390–394.

Gregg JM and Small EW (1986) Surgical management of trigeminal pain with radiofrequency lesions of peripheral nerves. *J Oral Maxillofac Surg* **44**, 122–125.

Gregg JM, Banerjee T, Ghia JN and Campbell R (1978) Radiofrequency thermoneurolysis of peripheral nerves for control of trigeminal neuralgia. *Pain* **5**, 231–248.

Grimaldi R, Lecchini S, Crema F and Perucca E (1984) In vivo plasma protein binding interaction between valproic acid and naproxen. *Eur J Drug Metab Pharmacokinet* **9**, 359–363.

Grushka M and Sessle BJ (1984) Applicability of the McGill Pain Questionnaire to the differentiation of 'toothache' pain. *Pain* **19**, 49–57.

Grushka M, Sessle BJ and Miller R (1987) Pain and personality profiles in burning mouth syndrome. *Pain* **28**, 155–167.

Guidetti B, Fraioli B and Refice GM (1979) Modern trends in surgical treatment of trigeminal neuralgia. *J Maxillofac Surg* **7** (4), 315–319.

Hakanson S (1978) Transoral trigeminal cisternography. *Surg Neurol* **10**, 137–144.

Hakanson S (1981) Trigeminal neuralgia treated by the injection of glycerol into the trigeminal cistern. *Neurosurgery* **9**, 638–646.

Hakanson S (1984) Tic douloureux treated by the injection of glycerol into the retrogasserian subarachnoid space. Long term results. *Acta Neurochir Suppl* **33**, 471–472.

Hall EH, Tezezhalmy GT and Pelleu GB (1986) A set of descriptors for the diagnosis of dental pain syndromes. *Oral Surg Oral Med Oral Patho* **61**, 153–157.

Hamilton, M (1960) A rating scale for depression. *J Neurol Neurosurg Psychiatry* **23**, 56–62.

Hamilton, M (1987) Assessment of psychopathology. In Hindmarch I and Stonier PD (eds) *Human Psychopharmacology Measures and Methods*, Vol 1, pp 1–17. Chichester: John Wiley.

Hampf G, Bowsher D, Wells C and Miles J (1990) Sensory and autonomic measurements in idiopathic trigeminal neuralgia before and after radiofrequency thermocoagulation: differentiation from some other causes of facial pain. *Pain* **40**, 241–248.

Hanakita J and Kondo A (1988) Serious complications of microvascular decompression operations for trigeminal neuralgia and hemifacial spasm. *Neurosurgery* **22**, 348–352.

Hanks GW, Trueman T, Lloyd JW *et al.* (1985) Depression and anxiety in pain clinic patients. Rapid assessment by microcomputer. *Anaesthesia* **40**, 676–679.

Hannerz J and Greitz D (1992) MRI of intracranial arteries in nitroglycerin induced cluster headache attacks. *Headache* **32**, 485–488.

Hardebo JE (1993) Subcutaneous sumatriptan in cluster headache: a time study of the effect on pain and autonominc symptoms. *Headache* **33**, 18–21.

Hardman FG (1967) Oral surgical management of trigeminal neuralgia. In: *Transactions of the Congress of the International Association of Oral Surgery*, pp 171–176. Copenhagen: Munksgaard.

Hardy DG and Rhoton AL (1978) Microsurgical relationship of the superior cerebellar artery and the trigeminal nerve. *J Neurosurg* **49**, 669–678.

Hardy PAJ and Bowsher DR (1989) Contact thermography in idiopathic trigeminal neuralgia and other facial pains. *Br J Neurosurg* **3**, 399–402.

Hardy RW (1977) Percutaneous gasserian thermocoagulation in the treatment of trigeminal neuralgia. *Cleveland Clinic Quarterly* **44**, 113–117.

Hariz MI and Laitinen LV (1986) Mesures quantitatives pre et post-operatoires de la sensibilite faciale dans le tic douloureux. *Neurochirurgie* **32**, 433–439.

Harris M and Feinmann C (1990) Psychosomatic disorders. In: Jones JH and Mason DK (eds) *Oral Manifestations of Systemic Disease*, 2nd edn, pp 30–60. London: Baillière Tindall.

Harris M, Feinmann C, Wise M and Treasure F (1993) Temporomandibular joint and orofacial pain: clinical and medicolegal management problems. *Br Dent J* **174**, 129–136.

Harris W (1912) Alcohol injection of the Gasserian ganglion for trigeminal neuralgia. *Lancet* **i**, 218–221.

Harris W (1926) Chronic paroxysmal trigeminal neuralgia. In: *Neuritis and Neuralgia*, pp 150–222. Oxford: Oxford University Press.

Harris W (1940) An analysis of 1433 cases of paroxysmal trigeminal neuralgia (trigeminal-tic) and the end results of Gasserian alcohol injection. *Brain* **63**, 209–224.

Harris W (1950) Rare forms of paroxysmal trigeminal neuralgia and their relation to disseminated sclerosis. *BMJ* **2**, 1015–1019.

Harris W and Wright AD (1932) Treatment of clonic facial spasm (a) by alcohol injection (b) by nerve anastomosis. *Lancet* **i**, 657–662.

Hartel F (1912) Die Lietungsanasthesie und injektionsbehandlung des ganglion gasseri und der trigeminusstamme. *Arch Klin Chir* **100**, 193–292.

Hartley F (1892) Intracranial neurectomy of the second and third division of the fifth nerve: a new method. *NY Med J* **55**, 317–319.

Hartley R, Aleksandrowicz J, Ng PC *et al.* (1990) Breakthrough seizures with generic carbamazepine: a consequence of poorer bioavailability? *Br J Clin Pract* **44**, 270–273.

Hassenbusch SJ, Kunkel RS, Kosmorsky GS *et al.* (1991) Trigeminal cisternal injection of glycerol for the treatment of chronic intractable cluster headaches. *Neurosurgery* **29**, 504–508.

Hathaway SR and McKinley JC (1967) *The Minnesota Multiphasic Personality Inventory Manual*. New York: Psychological Corporation.

Heaton RK, Ghetto CJ, Lehman AW *et al.* (1982) A standardized evaluation of psychosocial factors in chronic pain. *Pain* **12**, 165–174.

Henderson WR (1967) Trigeminal neuralgia: the pain and its treatment. *BMJ* **1**, 7–15.

Hering R and Kuritzky A (1989) Sodium valproate in the treatment of cluster headache: an open clinical trial. *Cephalalgia* **9**, 195–198.

Herring R, Komizki A and Bachar M (1982) Baclofen in trigeminal neuritis. *Harefuah* **102**, 63–64.

Hippocrates (1978) *Hippocratic Writings*, pp 223–224. Translated by Chadwick J, Mann WN, Lonie IM and Withington ET. Lloyd GER (ed) Penguin Books.

Hitchcock E, Teixeira M and Pinto J (1983) Percutaneous trigeminal radiofrequency rhizotomy. *J R Coll Surg Edinb* **28**, 74–79.

Hooper WD, Dubetz DK, Bochner F *et al.* (1975) Plasma protein binding of carbamazepine. *Clin Pharmacol Ther* **17**, 433–440.

Horowitz M, Wilner N and Alvarez W (1979) Impact of event scale: a measure of subjective stress. *Psychosom Med* **41**, 209–218.

Horrax G and Poppen JL (1935) Trigeminal neuralgia. *Surg Gynecol Obstet* **61**, 394–402.

Horsley V, Taylor J and Coleman WS (1891) Remarks on the various surgical procedures devised for the relief or cure of trigeminal neuralgia (tic douloureux). *BMJ* **2**, 1139–1143, 1191–1193, 1249–1252.

Hosobuchi Y, Adams JE and Ruskin B (1973) Chronic thalamic stimulation of the control of facial anesthesia dolorosa. *Arch Neurol* **29**, 158.

Houtkooper MA, Lammertsma A, Meyer JWA *et al.* (1987) Oxcarbazepine (GP47 680): a possible alternative to carbamazepine. *Epilepsia* **28**, 693–698.

Howe JF, Loeser JD and Black RG (1976) Percutaneous radiofrequency trigeminal gangliolysis in the treatment of tic douloureux. *West J Med* **124**, 351–356.

Hu JW, Dostrovsky JO and Sessle BJ (1981) Functional properties of neurons in cat trigeminal subnucleus caudalis (medullary dorsal horn). I. Responses to oro-facial noxious and non-noxious stimuli and projections to thalamus and subnucleus oralis. *J Neurophysiol* **45**, 173–192.

Hunt JR (1907) Unherpetic inflammations of the geniculate ganglion: a new syndrome and its complications. *J Nerv Ment Dis* **34**, 73–96.

Hunt S (1988) Measuring health in clinical care and clinical trials. In: Teeling-Smith G (ed) *Measuring Health: A Practical Approach*, pp 7–23. London: John Wiley.

Hunt S, McEwan J and McKenna SP (1986) *Measuring Health Status*. London: Croom Helm.

Hunter M (1983) The headache scale: a new approach to the assessment of headache pain based on pain descriptors. *Pain* **16**, 361–373.

Hussein M, Wilson LA and Illingworth R (1982) Patterns of sensory loss following fractional posterior fossa Vth nerve section for trigeminal neuralgia. *J Neurol Neurosurg Psychiatry* **45**, 786.

Hutchins LG, Jarnsberger HR, Hardin CW *et al.* (1989) The radiological assessment of trigeminal neuropathy. *Am J Neuroradiol* **10**, 1031–1038.

Iannone A, Baker AB and Morrell F (1958) Dilantin in the treatment of trigeminal neuralgia. *Neurology* **8**, 126–128.

Illingworth R (1986) Trigeminal neuralgia: surgical aspects. In: Vinken PJ, Bruyn GW and Klawans (eds) *Handbook of Clinical Neurology* Vol 4, pp 449–458. Amsterdam: Elsevier Science.

Illingworth RD (1989) Posterior fossa approach for trigeminal neuralgia. In: Symon L, Thomas DGT and Clark K (eds) *Rob & Smith's Operative Surgery. Neurosurgery*, pp 443–452. London: Butterworth.

International Association for the Study of Pain (1986) Classification of chronic pain. Descriptions of chronic pain syndromes and definitions of pain terms. *Pain* (Suppl. 3), S49–57.

International Association for the Study of Pain (1994) *Classification of Chronic Pain*. Meriskey and Bogduk (eds). Amsterdam: Elsevier Science.

International Headache Society (1988) Classification and diagnostic criteria for headache disorders, cranial neuralgias and facial pain. *Cephalagia* **8**(7), 67–69.

Iragui VS, Wiederhold WC and Romine JS (1986). Evoked potentials in trigeminal neuralgia associated with multiple sclerosis. *Arch Neurol* **43**, 444–446.

Ischia S, Luzzani A and Polati E (1990) Retrogasserian glycerol injection: a retrospective study of 112 patients. *Clin J Pain* **6**, 291–296.

Jaeger R (1957) Permanent relief of tic douloureux by gasserian injection of hot water. *Arch Neurol Psychiatry* **77**, 1–7.

Jaeger R (1959) The results of injecting hot water into the Gasserian ganglion for the relief of tic douloureux. *J Neurosurg* **16**, 656–663.

Jannetta PJ (1967) Arterial compression of the trigeminal nerve at the pons in patients with trigeminal neuralgia. *J Neurosurg Suppl* **36**, 159–162.

Jannetta PJ (1976) Microsurgical approach to the trigeminal nerve for tic douloureux. In: Krayenbuhl HA (ed) *Progress in Neurological Surgery*, Vol 7, pp 180–200 Basel: Kanger.

Jannetta PJ (1977) Treatment of trigeminal neuralgia by suboccipital and transtentorial cranial operations. *Clin Neurosurg* **24**, 538–549.

Jannetta PJ (1981) Vascular decompression in trigeminal neuralgia. In: Samii M and Jannetta PJ (eds) *The Cranial Nerves*, pp 332–340. Berlin: Springer.

Jannetta PJ (1985) Microsurgical management of trigeminal neuralgia. *Arch Neurol* **42**, 800.

Jannetta PJ (1990) Microvascular decompression of the trigeminal nerve root entry zone. In: Rovit RL, Murali R and Jannetta PT (eds) *Trigeminal Neuralgia*, pp 201–222. Baltimore: Williams and Wilkins.

Jannetta PJ and Bennett MH (1981) The pathophysiology of trigeminal neuralgia. In: Samii M and Jannetta PJ (eds) *The Cranial Nerves*, pp 312–315. Berlin: Springer Verlag.

Jannetta PJ and Bissonette DJ (1985) Management of the failed patient with trigeminal neuralgia. *Clin Neurosurg* **32**, 334–347.

Jassim SA (1994) *Patients' Assessment of Outcome After Radiofrequency Thermocoagulation for Management of Trigeminal Neuralgia*. MSc Dissertation. University of London.

Jawad S, Yuen WC, Peck AW *et al.* (1987) Lamotrigine: single-dose pharmacokinetics and initial one week experience in refractory epilepsy. *Epilepsy Res* **1**, 194–201.

Jefferson A (1963) Trigeminal root and ganglion injections using phenol and glycerine for the relief of trigeminal neuralgia. *J Neurol Neurosurg Psychiatry* **26**, 345–352.

Jefferson A (1966) Trigeminal neuralgia: trigeminal root and ganglion injections using phenol in glycerin. In: Knighton RS and Dumke PR (eds) *Pain. Henry Ford Hospital International Symposium*, pp 365–371. Boston: Little Brown.

Jensen NO, Dam M and Jackobsen K (1986) Oxcarbazepine in patients hypersensitive to carbamazepine. *Ir J Med Sci* **155**, 297.

Jensen PK, Moller A, Gram L *et al.* (1990) Pharmacokinetic comparison of two carbamazepine slow-release formulations. *Acta Neurol Scand* **82**, 135–137.

Jenson TS, Rasmussen P and Reske-Nelson E (1982) Association of trigeminal neuralgia with multiple sclerosis: clinical and pathological features. *Acta Neurol Scand* **65**, 182–189.

Jerome A, Holroyd KA, Theofanous AG *et al.* (1988) Cluster headache pains vs. other vascular headache pain: differences revealed with two approaches to the McGill Pain Questionnaire. *Pain* **34**, 35–42.

Johnson, ES, Ratcliffe DM and Wilkinson M (1985) Naproxen sodium in the treatment of migraine. *Cephalalgia* **5**, 5–10.

Juniper RP (1991) Trigeminal neuralgia—treatment of the third division by radiologically controlled cryoblockade of the inferior dental nerve at the mandibular lingula. *Br J Oral Maxillofac Surg* **29**, 154–158.

Kanpolat Y and Onol B (1980) Experimental percutaneous approach to the trigeminal ganglion in dogs with histopathological evaluation of radiofrequency lesions. *Acta Neurochir Wien* **1980** (Suppl), 363–366.

Kaplan SA, Alexander K, Jack ML *et al.* (1974) Pharmacokinetic profiles of clonazepam in dog and humans and flunitrazepam in dog. *J Pharm Sci* **63**, 527–532.

Katusic S, Beard CM, Bergstralh E and Kurland LT (1990) Incidence and clinical features of trigeminal neuralgia. *Ann Neurol* **27**, 89–95.

Keefe FJ and Beckham JC (1990) Behavioral assessment of chronic orofacial pain. *Anesth Prog* **37**, 76–81.

Keefe FJ, Kopel S and Gordon SB (1978) *A Practical Guide to Behavioral Assessment*. New York: Springer.

Keele KD (1948) The pain chart. *Lancet* **ii**, 6–8.

Kehler CH, Brodsky JB, Samuels SI, Britt RH and Silverberg GD (1982) Blood pressure response during percutaneous rhizotomy for trigeminal neuralgia. *Neurosurgery.* **10**(2), 200–202.

Kelleher DJ (1990) Do self-help groups help? *Int Disability Stud* **12**, 66–69.

Kellner R (1986) *Somatization and Hypochondriasis*. New York: Praeger.

Kerns RD, Turk DC and Rudy TE (1985) The West Haven–Yale Multidimensional Pain Inventory (WHYMPI). *Pain* **23**, 345–356.

Kerr FWL (1963) The etiology of trigeminal neuralgia. *Arch Neurol* **8**, 15–25.

Kessel N (1979) Reassurance. *Lancet* **i**, 1128–1133.

Khanna JN and Galinde JS (1985) Trigeminal neuralgia. Report of 140 cases. *Int J Oral Surg* **14**, 325–332.

Killian JM and Fromm GH (1968) Carbamazepine in the treatment of neuralgia. Use and side effects. *Arch Neurol* **19**, 129–136.

Kiluk KI, Knighton RS and Newman JD (1968) The treatment of trigeminal neuralgia and other facial pain with carbamazepine. *Mich Med* **67**, 1066–1069.

Kinney RK, Gatchel RJ, Ellis E and Holt C (1992) Major psychological disorders in chronic TMD patients: implications for successful management. *J Am Dent Assoc* **123**(10), 49–54.

Kirkpatrick DB (1989) Familial trigeminal neuralgia — a case report. *Neurosurgery* **24**, 758–761.

Kirschner M (1933) Die Punktionstechnik und die Elektrokoagulation des Ganglion Gasseri. Über 'gezielte' Operationen. *Arch Klin Chir* **176**, 581–620.

Kirschner M (1931) Zur electrochirurgie. *Arch Klin Chir* **167**, 761–768.

Kishore-Kumar R, Max MB, Schafer SC *et al.* (1990) Desipramine relieves post-herpetic neuralgia. *Clin Pharmacol Ther* **47**, 305–312.

Klepac RK, Dowling J, Rokke P, Dodge L and Schafer L (1981) Interview vs. paper and pencil administration of the McGill Pain Questionnaire. *Pain* **11**, 241.

Klun B (1992) Microvascular decompression and partial sensory rhizotomy in the treatment of trigeminal neuralgia: personal experience with 220 patients. *Neurosurgery* **30**, 49–52.

Kolluri S and Heros RC (1984) Microvascular decompression for trigeminal neuralgia. A five year follow-up study. *Surg Neurol* **22**, 235–240.

Krabbe AA (1986) Cluster headaches — a review. *Acta Neurol Scand* **74**, 1–9.

Krause F (1892) Resktion des Trigeminus innerhalb der Schadelhohle. *Arch Klin Chir* **44**, 821–832.

Kremer EF, Atkinson JH and Ignelzi RJ (1980) Measurement of pain: patient preference does not confound pain measurement. *Pain* **10**, 241.

Kremer EF, Atkinson JH and Kremer AM (1983) The language of pain: affective descriptors of pain are a better predictor of psychological disturbance than pattern of sensory and affective descriptors. *Pain* **16**, 185–192.

Kudrow L (1980) *Cluster Headache: Mechanisms and Management*. New York: Oxford Press.

Kugelberg E and Lindblom U (1959) The mechanism of the pain in trigeminal neuralgia. *J Neurol Neurosurg Psychiatr* **22**, 36–43.

Kurland LT (1958) Descriptive epidemiology of selected neurologic and myopathic disorders with particular reference to a survey in Rochester, Minnesota. *J Chron Dis* **8**, 378–418.

Kytta J and Rosenberg PH (1988) Comparison of propofol and methohexitone anaesthesia for thermocoagulation therapy of trigeminal neuralgia. *Anaesthesia* **43**(Suppl), 50–53.

Lahr MB (1985) Hyponatremia during carbamazepine therapy. *Clin Pharmacol Ther* **37**, 693–696.

Lambert PA and Venaud G (1987) Utilisation du valpromide en therapeutique psychiatrique. *L'Encephale* **13**, 367–373.

Lance JW, Fine RO and Curran DA (1963) An evaluation of methysergide in the prevention of migraine and other vascular headaches. *Med J Aust* **i**, 814–818.

Langmayr JJ and Russegger L (1992) Surgical treatment of glossopharyngeal neuralgia. *Wien Med Wochenschr* **142**(13), 281–283.

Larkin JG, McKee PJW, Forrest G *et al.* (1991) Lack of enzyme induction with oxcarbazepine (600 mg daily) in healthy subjects. *Br J Clin Pharmacol* **31**, 65–71.

Larrey DJ (1829) *Clinique chirurgical exercée particulierement dans les camps et les hopitaux militaires depuis 1792 jusqu'en 1829*. Paris: Gabon and JB Ballière.

Larson AG and Marcer D (1984) The who and why of pain: analysis by social class. *BMJ* **288**, 883–886.

Larssen LE and Previc TS (1970) Somatosensory responses to mechanical stimulation as recorded in the human electroencephalograph. *Clin Neurophysiol* **28**, 162–172.

Latchaw JP, Hardy RW, Forsythe SB and Cook AF (1981) Trigeminal neuralgia treated by radiofrequency coagulation. *J Neurosurg* **59**, 479–484.

Lazar ML (1978) Trigeminal neuralgia: recent advances in management. *Texas Med* **74**, 45–48.

Lazar ML (1980) Current treatment of tic douloureux. *Oral Surg* **50**, 504–508.

Lazarus RS, Averill JR and Opton EM (1974) The psychology of coping. Issues of research and assessment. In: Coelko CV, Hamberg DA and Adams JE (eds) *Coping and Adaptation*, pp 249–315. New York: Basic Books.

Lechin F, van der Dijs B, Lechin ME *et al.* (1989) Pimozide therapy for trigeminal neuralgia. *Arch Neurol* **46**, 960–963.

Lennon MC, Dohrenwend BP, Zautra AJ and Marbach JJ (1990) Coping and adaptation to facial pain in contrast to other stressful life events. *J Pers Soc Psychol* **59**, 1040–1050.

LeResche L and Dworkin SF (1984) Facial expression accompanying pain. *Soc Sci Med* **19**, 1325–1330.

Levi R, Edman GV, Ekbom K and Waldenlind E (1992a) Episodic cluster headache. I: Personality and some neuropsychological characteristics in male patients. *Headache* **32** (3), 119–125.

Levi R, Edman GV, Ekbom K and Waldenlind E (1992b) Episodic cluster headache. II: High tobacco and alcohol consumption in males. *Headache* **32**, 184–187.

Levine M, Jones MW and Sheppard I (1985) Differential effects of cimetidine on serum concentrations of carbamazepine and phenytoin. *Neurology* **35**, 562–565.

Lewis RA, Keltner JL and Cobb CA (1982) Corneal anesthesia after percutaneous radiofrequency trigeminal rhizotomy. A retrospective study. *Arch Ophthalmol* **100**, 301–303.

Lewy FH and Grant FC (1938) Physiopathologic and pathoanatomic aspects of major trigeminal neuralgia. *Arch Neurol Psychiatry* **40**, 1126–1134.

Lichtor T and Mullan JF (1990) A 10-year follow-up review of percutaneous microcompression of the trigeminal ganglion. *J Neurosurg* **72**, 49–54.

Lindstrom P and Lindblom V (1987) The analgesic effect of tocainide in trigeminal neuralgia. *Pain* **28**, 45–50.

Linton SJ (1982) A critical review of behavioural treatment for chronic benign pain other than headache. *Br J Clin Psychol* **21**, 321–337.

Lipton JA and Marbach JJ (1983) Components of the response to pain and variables influencing the response in three groups of facial pain patients. *Pain* **16**, 343–359.

Littler BO (1984) Alcohol blockade of the inferior dental nerve under radiographic control in the management of trigeminal neuralgia. *Oral Surg Oral Med Oral Pathol* **57**, 132–135.

Lloyd GG (1991) *Textbook of General Hospital Psychiatry.* Edinburgh: Churchill Livingstone.

Lloyd JW, Barnard JDW and Glynn CJ (1976) Cryoanalgesia. A new approach to pain relief. *Lancet* **ii**, 932–934.

Lobato RD, Rivas JJ, Sarabia R and Lamas E (1990) Percutaneous microcompression of the gasserian ganglion for trigeminal neuralgia. *J Neurosurg* **72**, 546–553.

Locke J (1789) Letters to Dr Mapletoft (1677), nos 9–12. *The European magazine and London review* **15**, 185–186; 273–274.

Loeser JD (1977) The management of tic douloureux. *Pain* **3**, 155–162.

Loeser JD (1984) Tic douloureux and atypical facial pain. In: Wall PD and Melzack R (eds) *Textbook of Pain*, pp 426–434. Edinburgh: Churchill Livingstone.

Loeser JD (1990) Cranial neuralgias. In: Bonica JJ (ed) *The Management of Pain*, pp 676–686. Philadelphia: Lee and Febiger.

Loeser JD (1993) True believer, with questions. *Am Pain Soc J* **2**, 231–233.

Loeser JD (1994) Tic douloureux and atypical facial pain. In: Wall PD and Melzack R (eds) *Textbook of Pain*, 3rd edn, pp 699–711. Edinburgh: Churchill Livingstone.

Loeser JD, Calvin WH and Howe JF (1983) Pathophysiology of trigeminal neuralgia. *Clin Neurosurg* **24**, 527–537.

Loiseau P, Yuen W, Duche B *et al.* (1990) A randomised, double-blind, placebo-controlled, crossover, add-on trial of lamotrigine in patients with treatment resistant partial seizures. *Epilepsy Res* **7**, 136–145.

Lowe SS, Meurer M, Ingram GS and Thomas DGT (1983) Anaesthesia for trigeminal nerve thermocoagulation. *Anaesthesia* **38**, 152–154.

Lunsford LD (1990) Percutaneous retrogasserian glycerol rhizotomy. In: Rovit RL, Murali R and Jannetta PJ (ed) *Trigeminal Neuralgia*, pp 145–164. Baltimore: Williams and Wilkins.

Lunsford LD and Apfelbaum RI (1985) Choice of surgical therapeutic modalities for treatment of trigeminal neuralgia: microvascular decompression, percutaneous retrogasserian thermal or glycerol rhizotomy. *Clin Neurosurg* **32**, 319–333.

Lunsford LD and Bennett MH (1984) Percutaneous retrogasserian glycerol rhizotomy for tic douloureux: Part I. *Neurosurgery* **14**, 424–430.

MacCosbe PE and Toomey K (1983) Interaction of phenytoin and folic acid. *Clin Pharm* **2**, 362–369.

Macphee GJA, Butler E and Brodie MJ (1987) Intradose and circadian variation in circulating carbamazepine and its epoxide in epileptic patients: a consequence of autoinduction of metabolism. *Epilepsia* **28**, 286–294.

Mairs AP and Stewart TJ (1990) Surgical treatment of glossopharyngeal neuralgia via the pharyngeal approach. *J Laryngol Otol* **104**, 12–16.

Marbach JJ and Lund P (1981) Depression, anhedonia and anxiety in temporomandibular joint and other facial pain syndrones. *Pain* **11**, 73–84.

Markham JW (1973) Sudden loss of vision following alcohol block of the infra-orbital nerve. *J Neurosurg* **38**, 655–657.

Mason DA (1972) Peripheral neurectomy in the treatment of trigeminal neuralgia of the second and third divisions. *J Oral Surg* **30**, 113–120.

Mason WE, Kollros P and Jannetta PJ (1991) Trigeminal neuralgia and its treatment in a 13-month-old child: a review and case report. *J Craniomandibular Disord: Fac Oral Pain* **5**, 213–216.

Maxwell RE (1990) Clinical diagnosis of trigeminal neuralgia and differential diagnosis of facial pain. In: Rovit RL, Murali R and Jannetta PJ (eds) *Trigeminal Neuralgia*, pp 53–78. Baltimore: Williams & Wilkins.

Mayer ML, James MH, Russell RJ, Kelly JS and Pasternak CA (1986) Changes in excitability induced by herpes simplex virus in rat dorsal root ganglion neurons. *J Neurosci* **6**, 391–402.

McArdle MJ (1970) Atypical facial neuralgia in trigeminal neuralgia. In: Hassler R and Walker AE (eds) *Pathogenesis and Pathophysiology*, pp 35–42. Stuttgart: Georg Thieme Verlag.

McConaghy DJ (1994) Trigeminal neuralgia: A personal review and nursing implications. *J Neurosci Nurs* **26**(2), 85–89.

McCreary C, Turner J and Dawson E (1981) Principal dimensions of the pain experience and psychological disturbance in chronic low back pain patients. *Pain* **11**, 85–92.

McGlone F and Wells C (1991) Peroperative monitoring during percutaneous thermocoagulation of the gasserian ganglion for the treatment of trigeminal neuralgia. *Br J Neurosurg* **5**, 39–42.

McGovern B, Geer VR, LaRaia PJ *et al.* (1984) Possible interaction between amiodarone and phenytoin. *Ann Intern Med* **101**, 650–651.

McKee PJW, Blacklaw J, Butler E *et al.* (1991) Monotherapy with conventional and controlled-release carbamazepine: a double-blind double-dummy comparison in epileptic patients. *Br J Clin Pharmacol* **32**, 99–104.

McKee PJW, Blacklaw J, Butler E *et al.* (1992) Variability and clinical relevance of the interaction between sodium valproate and carbamazepine in epileptic patients. *Epilepsy Res* **11**, 193–198.

McKee PJW, Blacklaw J, Forrest G *et al.* (1994) A double-blind, placebo-controlled interaction study between oxcarbazepine and carbamazepine, sodium valproate and phenytoin in epileptic patients. *Br J Clin Pharmacol* **37**, 37–92.

McKinney MW, Londeen TF, Turner SP and Levitt SR (1990) Chronic TN disorder and non TN disorder pain: a comparison of behavioral and psychological characteristics. *Cranio* **8**, 40–46.

McQuay HJ, Carroll D, Moxon A, Glynn CJ and Moore RA (1990) Benzydamine cream for the treatment of post-herpetic neuralgia: minimum duration of treatment periods in a cross-over trial. *Pain* **40**, 131–135.

Mechanic D (1962) The concept of illness behaviour. *J Chron Dis* **15**, 189–194.

Meglio M and Cioni B (1989) Percutaneous procedures for trigeminal neuralgia: microcompression versus radiofrequency thermocoagulation. Personal experience. *Pain* **38**, 9–16.

Melikian AP, Straughn AB, Slywka GWA *et al.* (1977) Bioavailability of 11 phenytoin products. *J Pharmacokinet Biopharm* **5**, 133–146.

Melzack R (1975) The McGill Pain Questionnaire: major properties and scoring methods. *Pain* **1**, 277–299.

Melzack R (1986) Neurophysiological foundations of pain. In: Sternbach RA (ed) *The Psychology of Pain*, 2nd edn, pp 1–24. New York: Raven Press

Melzack R (1987) The short-form McGill Pain Questionnaire. *Pain* **30**, 191–197.

Melzack R and Wall PD (1965) Pain mechanisms: a new theory. *Science* **15**, 971–979.

Melzack R, Terrence C, Fromm G and Amsel R (1986) Trigeminal neuralgia and atypical facial pain: use of the McGill Pain Questionnaire for discrimination and diagnosis. *Pain* **27**, 297–302.

Merritt HH and Putnam TJ (1938) A new series of anticonvulsant drugs tested by experiments on animals. *Arch Neurol Psychiatry* **39**, 1003–1015.

Merskey H (1983) The psychological treatment of pain. In: Swerdlow M (ed) *Relief of Intractable Pain*, pp 25–63. Amsterdam: Elsevier Science.

Merskey H (1986) Psychiatry and pain. In: Sternbach RA (ed) *The Psychology of Pain*, 2nd edn, pp 97–120. New York: Raven Press.

Mikati M, Bassett N and Schachter S (1992) Double-blind randomised study comparing brand-name and generic phenytoin monotherapy. *Epilepsia* **33**, 359–365.

Miles TS and Hribar D (1981) Recovery of function after cryosurgical lesions of peripheral nerves in rats. *Neurosci Lett* **24**, 285–288.

Miller RR, Porter J and Greenblatt DJ (1979) Clinical importance of the interaction of phenytoin and isoniazid: a report from the Boston Collaborative Drug Serveillance Program. *Chest* **75**, 356–358.

Mingrino S and Salar G (1981) Alteration in sensibility in trigeminal neuralgia before and after selective section of the root by posterior approach. In: Samii M and Jannetta PJ (eds) *Cranial Nerves*, pp 347–351. Berlin: Springer.

Miserococchi G, Cabrini G, Motti ED *et al.* (1989) Percutaneous selective thermorhizotomy in the treatment of 'essential' trigeminal neuralgia. The importance of lesion selectivity. *J Neurol Sci* 33, 179–182.

Mitchell RG (1980) Pre-trigeminal neuralgia. *Br Dent J* 149, 167–170.

Mittal B and Thomas DGT (1986) Controlled thermocoagulation in trigeminal neuralgia. *J Neurol Neurosurg Psychiatry* 49, 932–936.

Mock D, Frydman W and Gordon AS (1985) Atypical facial pain: A retrospective study. *Oral Surg* 59, 472–474.

Mongini F, Caselli C, Macri V and Tetti C (1990) Thermographic findings in cranio-facial pain. *Headache* 30, 497–504.

Montgomery SA and Asberg M (1979) A new depression scale designed to be sensitive to change. *Br J Psychiatry* 134, 382–389.

Moosa RC, McFadyen ML, Miller R and Rubin J (1993) Carbamazepine and its metabolites in neuralgias: concentrations affect relationships. *Eur J Clin Pharmacol* 45, 197–301.

Moraci A, Buonaiuto A, Punzo A *et al.* (1992) Trigeminal neuralgia treated by percutaneous thermocoagulation. Comparative analysis of percutaneous thermocoagulation and other surgical techniques. *Neurochirurgia* 35, 48–53.

Morgenlander JC and Wilkins RH (1990) Surgical treatment of cluster headache. *J Neurosurg* 72, 866–871.

Morley TP (1985) Case against microvascular decompression in the treatment of trigeminal neuralgia. *Arch Neurol* 42, 801–802.

Morselli PL (1989) Carbamazepine absorption, distribution and excretion. In: Levy RH, Dreifuss FE, Mattson RH, Meldrum BS and Penry JK (eds) *Antiepileptic Drugs*, pp 473–490. New York: Raven Press.

Mullan S (1990) Percutaneous microcompression of the trigeminal ganglion. In: Rovit RL, Murali R and Jannetta PJ (eds) *Trigeminal Neuralgia*, pp 137–144. Baltimore: Williams and Wilkins.

Mullan S and Lichtor T (1983) Percutaneous microcompression of the trigeminal ganglion for trigeminal neuralgia. *J Neurosurg* 59, 1007–1012.

Mumford JM (1976) *Toothache and Orofacial Pain*, 2nd edn. Edinburgh: Churchill Livingstone.

Mumford JM and Miles JB (1977) Thermography and orofacial pain. *Acta Thermographica* 2, 155–161.

Musolino R, Gallitto G, Morgante L *et al.* (1980) The antiepileptic properties of *n*-dipropylacetamide. *Acta Neurol* 2, 107–114.

Nally FF, Flint SR, Bennett SD and Talhi FS (1984) The role of cryotherapy in the management of paroxysmal trigeminal neuralgia. An analysis of 112 patients. *J Ir Coll Physicians Surg* 13, 184–192.

Nashold BS and Rossitch E (1990) Anaesthesia dolorosa and the DREZ operation. In: Rovit RL, Murali R and Jannetta PT (eds) *Trigeminal Neuralgia*, pp 223–237. Baltimore: Williams and Wilkins.

Nielsen AC and Williams TA (1980) Depression in ambulatory medical patients: prevalence by self-report questionnaire and recognition by non-psychiatric physicians. *Arch Gen Psychiatry* 37, 999.

Noach EL and van Rees H (1964) Intestinal distribution of intravenously administered phenytoin in the rat. *Arch Int Pharmacol Ther* 150, 52–61.

North RB, Kidd DH, Piantadosi S and Carson BS (1990) Percutaneous retrogasserian glycerol rhizotomy. Predictors of success and failure in treatment of trigeminal neuralgia. *J Neurosurg* 72, 851–856.

Nugent GR (1981) Comments on an article by Burchiel *et al. Neurosurgery* 9, 118–119.

Nugent GR (1982) Technique and results of 800 percutaneous radiofrequency thermocoagulations for trigeminal neuralgia. *App Neurophysiol* 45, 504–507.

Nugent GR and Berry B (1974) Trigeminal neuralgia treated by differential percutaneous radiofrequency coagulation of the gasserian ganglion. *J Neurosurg* 40, 517–523.

Nurmikko T, Wells C and Bowsher D (1991) Pain and allodynia in postherpetic neuralgia: role of somatic and sympathetic nervous systems. *Acta Neurol Scand* 84, 146–152.

Nurmikko TJ (1991) Altered cutaneous sensation in trigeminal neuralgia. *Arch Neurol* 48, 523–527.

Ohnhaus EE and Adler R (1975) Methodological problems in the measurement of pain: a comparison between the verbal rating scale and the visual analogue scale. *Pain* 1, 379.

Olafson RA, Rushton JG and Sayres GP (1966) Trigeminal neuralgia in a patient with multiple sclerosis. *J Neurosurg* **24**, 755–759.

Olesen J (1986) Role of calcium entry blockers in the prophylaxis of migraine. *Eur Neurol* **25** (Suppl. 1), 72–79.

Olpe HR, Demieville H and Baltzer V (1978) The biological activity of D- and L-baclofen (Lioresal). *Eur J Pharmacol* **52**, 133–136.

Onofrio BM (1975) Radiofrequency percutaneous gasserian ganglion lesions. Results in 140 patients with trigeminal pain. *J Neurosurg* **42**, 132–139.

Parmer BJ, Shah KH and Gandhi IC (1989) Baclofen in trigeminal neuralgia — a clinical trial. *Int J Dent Res* **1**, 109–113.

Patrick D (1981) Standardisation of comparative health status measures: using scales developed in America in English-speaking country. In: Sudman S (ed) *Health Survey Research Methods*, 3rd biennial conference, Hyattsville, Maryland. 81 pp.

Patrick HT (1914) The symptomatology of trifacial neuralgia. *JAMA* **58**, 1519–1525.

Patsalos PN (1990) A comparative pharmacokinetic study of conventional and chewable carbamazepine in epileptic patients. *Br J Clin Pharmacol* **29**, 574–577.

Patsalos PN (1994) Phenobarbitone to gabapentin: a guide to 82 years of anti-epileptic drug pharmacokinetic interactions. *Seizure* **3**, 167–170.

Patsalos PN and Duncan JS (1993) Antiepileptic drugs. A review of clinically significant drug interactions. *Drug Safety* **9**, 156–184.

Patsalos PN and Duncan JS (1994) New antiepileptic drugs. A review of their current status and clinical potential. *CNS Drugs* **2**, 40–77.

Patsalos PN and Lascelles PT (1977a) Effect of sodium valproate on plasma protein binding of diphenylhydantoin. *J Neurol Neurosurg Psychiatry* **50**, 570–575.

Patsalos PN and Lascelles PT (1977b) In vitro hydroxylation of diphenylhydantoin and its inhibition by other commonly used antiepileptic drugs. *Biochem Pharmacol* **26**, 1929–1933.

Patsalos PN and Sander JWAS (1994) Newer antiepileptic drugs. Towards an improved risk–benefit ratio. *Drug Safety* **11**, 37–67.

Patsalos PN, Stephenson TJ, Krishna S *et al.* (1985) Side-effects induced by carbamazepine-10,11-epoxide. *Lancet* **ii**, 496.

Patsalos PN, Duncan JS and Shorvon SD (1988) Effect of removal of individual antiepileptic drugs on antipyrine kinetics in patients taking polytherapy. *Br J Clin Pharmacol* **26**, 253–259.

Patsalos PN, Elyas AA and Zakrzewska JM (1990a) Protein binding of oxcarbazepine and its primary active metabolite, 10-hydroxycarbazepine, in patients with trigeminal neuralgia. *Eur J Clin Pharmacol* **39**, 413–415.

Patsalos PN, Russell-Jones D, Finnerty G *et al.* (1990b) The efficacy and tolerability of chewable carbamazepine compared to conventional carbamazepine in patients with epilepsy. *Epilepsy Res* **5**, 235–239.

Patsalos PN, Zakrzewska JM and Elyas AA (1990c) Dose-dependent enzyme induction by oxcarbazepine? *Eur J Clin Pharmacol* **39**, 187–188.

Pearce I, Frank GJ and Pearce JMS (1983) Ibuprofen compared with paracetamol in migraine. *Practitioner* **227**, 465–467.

Peatfield RC, Fozard JR and Clifford-Rose F (1986) Drug treatment of migraine. In: Clifford-Rose F (ed) *Handbook of Clinical Neurology*, Vol. 4 (48). Headache, pp 173–216. New York: Elsevier Science.

Peet MM and Schneider RC (1952) Trigeminal neuralgia. A review of six hundred and eighty nine cases with a follow up study on sixty five per cent of the group. *J Neurosurg* **9**, 367–377.

Peikert A, Hentrich M and Ochs G (1991) Topical 0.025% capsaicin in chronic post-herpetic neuralgia: efficacy, predictors of response and long-term course. *J Neurol* **238**, 452–456.

Peiris JB, Perera GLS, Devendra SV and Lionel NDW (1980) Sodium valproate in trigeminal neuralgia. *Med J Aust* **2**, 278.

Penman J (1968) Trigeminal neuralgia. In: Vinken PJ and Bruyn GW (eds) *Handbook of Clinical Neurology*, pp 296–325. Amsterdam: Elsevier Science.

Perkin GD and Illingworth RD (1989) The association of hemifacial spasm and facial pain. *J Neurol Neurosurg Psychiatry* **52**, 662–665.

Peto R, Pike MC, Armitage P *et al.* (1977) Design and analysis of randomized clinical trials requiring prolonged observation of each patient. II. Analysis and examples. *Br J Cancer* **35**, 1–39.

Petri R (1970) Results of trigeminal rhizotomy. In: Hassler and Walker (eds) *Trigeminal Neuralgia Pathogenesis and Pathophysiology*, pp 22–25. Verlag.

Pfaffenrath VM, Pollmann W and Keeser W (1993) Atypical facial pain — application of the IHS criteria in a clinical sample. *Cephalalgia* **13** (Suppl. 12), 84–88.

Phillips JG and Whitlock RIH (1976) The effect of an alcoholic injection for facial pain. *Br J Oral Surg* **14**, 173–178.

Piatt JH and Wilkins RH (1984) Treatment of tic douloureux and hemifacial spasm by posterior fossa exploration: therapeutic implications of various neurovascular relationships. *Neurosurgery* **14**, 462–471.

Pilowsky I and Bond M (1969) Pain and its management in malignant disease: elucidation of staff–patient transactions. *Psychosom Med* **31**, 400–404.

Pilowsky I and Spence ND (1975) Patterns of illness behaviour of patients with intractable pain. *J Psychosom Res* **19**, 279–287.

Pilowsky I and Spence ND (1976) Pain and illness behaviour: a comparative study. *J Psychosom Res* **20**, 131–134.

Pisani F, Fazio A, Oteri G and Di Perri R (1981) Dipropylacetic acid plasma levels: diurnal fluctuations during chronic treatment with dipropylacetamide. *Ther Drug Monit* **3**, 297–301.

Pisani F, Fazio A and Oteri G *et al.* (1986) Carbamazepine–viloxazine interaction in patients with epilepsy. *J Neurol Neurosurg Psychiatry* **49**, 1142–1145.

Pisani F, Fazio A and Oteri G *et al.* (1988) Effect of valpromide on the pharmacokinetics of carbamazepine-10,11-epoxide. *Br J Clin Pharmacol* **25**, 611–613.

Politis C, Adriaensen H, Bossuyt M and Fossion E (1988) The management of trigeminal neuralgia with cryotherapy. *Acta Stomatol Belg* **85**, 197–205.

Pollack IF, Jannetta PJ and Bissonette DJ (1988) Bilateral trigeminal neuralgia: a 14-year experience with microvascular decompression. *J Neurosurg* **68**, 559–565.

Poppen JL (1960) *An Atlas of Neurosurgical Techniques*. Philadelphia WB Saunders.

Posner J, Holdich T and Crome P (1991) Comparison of lamotrigine pharmacokinetics in young and elderly healthy volunteers. *J Pharm Med* **1**, 121–128.

Pujol M (1787) *Essai sur la maladie de la face, nommée tic douloureux; avec quelques réflexions sur le raptus caninus de Coelius Aurelianus*. Paris: Théophile Barrois.

Putman TJ and Hampton AO (1936) A technique of injection into the Gasserian ganglion under roentgenographic control. *Arch Neurol Psychiatr* **35**, 92–98.

Quinn JH (1965) Repetitive peripheral neurectomies for neuralgia of second and third divisions of trigeminal nerve. *J Oral Surg* **23**, 600–608.

Rambeck B, Salke-Treumann A, May T and Boenigt HE (1990) Valproic acid-induced carbamazepine-10,11-epoxide toxicity in children and adolescents. *Eur Neurol* **30**, 79–83.

Ramsey RE, Pellock JM, Garnett WR *et al.* (1991) Pharmacokinetics and safety of lamotrigine (Lamictal) in patients with epilepsy. *Epilepsy Res* **10**, 191–200.

Rappaport ZH (1986) Percutaneous retrogasserian glycerol injection for trigeminal neuralgia: one year follow-up. *The Pain Clinic* **1**, 57–61.

Rappaport ZH and Devor M (1994). Trigeminal neuralgia: the role of self sustaining discharge in the trigeminal ganglion. *Pain* **56**, 127–138.

Rappaport ZH and Gomori JM (1988) Recurrent trigeminal cistern glycerol injections for tic douloureux. *Acta Neurochir* **90**, 31–34.

Rasmussen P (1991) Facial pain IV: A prospective study of 1052 patients with a view of: precipitation factors, associated symptoms, objective psychiatric and neurological symptoms. *Acta Neurochir* **108**, 100–109.

Rasmussen P and Rushede J (1970) Facial pain treated with carbamazepine (Tegretol). *Acta Neurol Scand* **46**, 385–408.

Ratner EJ, Person P, Kleinman DJ *et al.* (1979) Jawbone cavities and trigeminal and atypical facial neuralgias. *Oral Surg Oral Med Oral Pathol* **48**, 3–20.

Rawlinson E (1983) Quality of life after treatment for laryngeal cancer: the patient's viewpoint. *Can J Radiography Radiother Nucl Med* **14**, 125–127.

Reading AE (1983) The McGill Pain Questionnaire: an appraisal. In: Melzack R (ed) *Pain Measurement and Assessment*, pp 55–61. New York: Raven Press.

Reading AE (1984) Testing pain mechanisms in persons in pain. In: Wall PD and Melzack R (eds) *Textbook of Pain*, pp 195–204. Edinburgh: Churchill Livingstone.

Reading AE and Newton JR (1978) A card sort method of pain assessment. *J Psychosom Res* **22**, 265–276.

Reinikainen KJ, Keranen T, Halonen T *et al.* (1987) Comparison of oxcarbazepine and carbamazepine: a double-blind study. *Epilepsy Res* **1**, 284–289.

Remillard G (1994) Oxcarbazepine and intractable trigeminal neuralgia. *Epilepsia* **35**, (Suppl. 3), S28–S29.

Remmer H, Hirschmann J and Greiner J (1969) Die Bedeutung von Kumulation und Elimination fur die Dosierung von Phenytoin (Diphenylhydantoin) *Dtsch Med Wochenschr* **94**, 1265–1272.

Rengachary S, Watanabe IS, Singer P and Bopp WJ (1983) Effect of glycerol on peripheral nerve: an experimental study. *Neurosurgery* **13**, 681–688.

Reunanen M, Heinonen EH, Nyman L and Anttila M (1992) Comparative bioavailability of carbamazepine from slow-release preparations. *Epilepsy Res* **11**, 61–66.

Rhoton AL, Maniscalco JE, Hoagland HV and Chorvat BD (1977) Percutaneous stereotaxic radiofrequency lesions for trigeminal neuralgia. *J Fla Med Assoc* **64**, 488–493.

Richards P, Shawdon J and Illingworth R (1983) Operative findings on microsurgical exploration of the cerebello-pontine angle in trigeminal neuralgia. *J Neurol Neurosurg Psychiatr* **46**, 1098–1101.

Richardson MF and Straka JA (1973) Alcohol block of the mandibular nerve. Report of a complication. *J Natl Med Assoc* **65**, 63.

Richens A and Dunlop A (1975) Serum phenytoin levels in the management of epilepsy. *Lancet* **ii**, 247–248.

Roberts AM, Person P, Chandran NB and Hori JM (1984) Further observations on dental parameters of trigeminal and atypical facial neuralgias. *Oral Surg Oral Med Oral Pathol* **58**, 121–129.

Robertson DR and George CF (1990) Treatment of postherpetic neuralgia in the elderly. *Br Med Bull* **46**, 113–123.

Rockliff BW and Davis EH (1966) Controlled sequential trials of carbamazepine in trigeminal neuralgia. *Arch Neurol* **15**, 129–136.

Rohrer DC and Burchiel KM (1993) Trigeminal neuralgia and other trigeminal dysfunction syndromes. In: Barrow DL (ed) *Surgery of the Cranial Nerves of the Posterior Fossa*, pp 201–219. American Association Neurological Surgeons. Springfield, Illinois.

Romano JM and Turner JA (1985) Chronic pain and depression. Does the evidence support a relationship? *Psychol Bull* **97**, 18–34.

Rootes LE and Aanes DL (1992) A conceptual framework for understanding self-help groups. *Hosp Commun Psychiatry* **43**, 379–381.

Rosser R and Kind P (1978) A scale of valuations of states of illness: is there a social concensus? *Int J Epidemiol* **7**, 347–358.

Rothman KJ and Monson RR (1973) Epidemiology of trigeminal neuralgia. *J Chron Dis* **26**, 1–12.

Rothman KJ and Wepsic JG (1974) Side of facial pain in trigeminal neuralgia. *J Neurosurg* **40**, 514–516.

Rovit RL (1979) Radiofrequency thermocoagulation of the Gasserian ganglion for the treatment of trigeminal neuralgia. In: Ransohoff J (ed) *Modern Techniques in Surgery. Neurosurgery* Installment 1, pp 12-1–12-14. Mount Kisco, NY: Futura.

Rovit RL (1990) Percutaneous radiofrequency thermocoagulation. In: Rovit RL, Murali R and Jannetta PJ (eds) *Trigeminal Neuralgia*, pp 107–136. Baltimore: Williams and Wilkins.

Rowbotham MC and Fields HL (1989) Post-herpetic neuralgia: the relation of pain complaint, sensory disturbance and skin temperature. *Pain* **39**, 129–144.

Rowbotham MC, Reisner-Keller LA and Fields HL (1991) Both intravenous lidocaine and morphine reduce the pain of postherpetic neuralgia. *Neurology* **41**, 1024–1028.

Rowe AHR (ed) (1989) *A Companion to Dental Studies: Clinical Dentistry*, Vol. 3. Oxford: Blackwell.

Rudy TE, Turk TC, Aacki HS and Curtin AD (1995) An empirical taximetric alternative to traditional classification of temporomandibular disorders. *Pain* (in press)

Ruge D, Brochner R and Davis L (1958) A study of the treatment of 637 patients with trigeminal neuralgia. *J Neurosurg* **15**, 528–536.

Rushton JG and MacDonald HNA (1957) Trigeminal neuralgia. Special considerations of nonsurgical treatment. *JAMA* **165**, 437–440.

Rushton JG and Olafson R (1965) Trigeminal neuralgia associated with disseminated sclerosis: report of 35 cases. *Arch Neurol* **13**, 383–386.

Rushton JG, Srevens JC and Miller RH (1981) Glossopharyngeal (vagoglossopharyngeal) neuralgia. A study of 217 cases. *Arch Neurol* **38**, 201–205.

Russell K, Portenoy RK, Duma C and Foley KM (1986) Acute herpetic and post herpetic neuralgia: clinical review and current management. *Ann Neurol* **20**, 651–661.

Ryle JA (1936) *The Natural History of Disease*. London: Oxford University Press.

Sahni KS, Pieper DR, Anderson R and Baldwin NG (1990) Relation of hypesthesia to the outcome of glycerol rhizolysis for trigeminal neuralgia. *J Neurosurg* **72**, 55–58.

Saini SS (1987) Retrogasserian glycerol injection therapy in trigeminal neuralgia *J Neurol Neurosurg Psychiatry* **50**, 1536–1538.

Salar G, Mingrino S and Iob I (1983) Alterations of facial sensitivity induced by percutaneous thermocoagulation for trigeminal neuralgia. *Surg Neurol* **19**, 126–130.

Salonen L and Hellden L (1990) Prevalence of signs and symptoms of dysfunction in the masticatory system: An epidemiologic study in an adult Swedish population. *Craniomandib Disord Facial Oral Pain* **4**, 241–250.

Salter M, Brooke RI, Merskey H *et al.* (1983) Is the temporo-mandibular pain and dysfunction syndrome a disorder of mind? *Pain* **17**, 151–166.

Sander JWAS and Patsalos PN (1992) An assessment of serum and red blood cell folate concentrations in patients with epilepsy on lamotrigine therapy. *Epilepsy Res* **13**, 89–92.

Sander JWAS, Patsalos PN, Oxley JR *et al.* (1989) A randomised double-blind placebo-controlled add-on trial of lamotrigine in patients with severe epilepsy. *Epilepsy Res* **4**, 222–229.

Sanders M and Henny CP (1992) Results of selective percutaneous controlled radiofrequency lesion for treatment of trigeminal neuralgia in 240 patients. *Clin J Pain* **8**, 23–27.

Savitskaya ON (1980) Comparative effectiveness of anti-epileptic preparations in treatment of patients with neuralgia of the trigeminal nerve. *Zh Nevropatol Psikhiatr* **80**, 530–535.

Sawchuk RJ, Pepin SM, Leppik IE and Gumnit RJ (1982) Rapid and slow release of phenytoin in epileptic patients at steady state: comparative plasma levels and toxicity. *J Pharmacokinet Biopharm* **10**, 356–382.

Schiffman E and Friction JR (1988) Epidemiology of TMJ and craniofacial pain. In: Friction JR, Kroening RJ and Hathaway KM (eds) *TMJ and Craniofacial Pain: Diagnosis and Management*, pp. 1–10. St Louis: IEA Publ.

Schiffman E, Friction JR, Haley D and Shapiro BL (1989) The prevalence and treatment needs of subjects with temporomandibular disorders. *J Am Dent Assoc* **120**, 295–304.

Schoenen J and Maertens de Noordhout A (1994) Headache. In: Wall PD and Melzack R (eds) *Textbook of Pain*, 3rd edn, pp 495–521. Edinburgh: Churchill Livingstone.

Schwarcz JR (1982) Percutaneous thermocontrolled differential retrogasserian rhizotomy for idiopathic trigeminal neuralgia. *Acta Neurochir* **74**, 51–58.

Scott J and Huskisson EC (1976) Graphic representation of pain. *Pain* **2**, 175–184.

Scott J and Huskisson EC (1979a) Accuracy of subjective measurements made with or without previous scores: an important source of error in serial measurements of subjective states. *Ann Rheum Dis* **38**, 558–559.

Scott J and Huskisson EC (1979b) Vertical or horizontal visual analogue scales. *Ann Rheum Dis* **38**, 559–560.

Seltzer Z and Devor M (1979) Ephaptic transmission in chronically damaged peripheral nerves. *Neurology* **29**, 1061–1064.

Semmes RLO and Shen DD (1991) Comparative pharmacodynamics and brain distribution of E-Δ^2-valproate and valproate in rats. *Epilepsia* **32**, 232–241.

Sengupta RP and Stunden RJ (1977) Radiofrequency thermocoagulation of gasserian ganglion and its rootlets for trigeminal neuralgia. *BMJ* **1**, 142–143.

Sens MAA and Higer HP (1991) MRI of trigeminal neuralgia: initial clinical results in patients with vascular compression of the trigeminal nerve. *Neurosurg Rev* **14**, 69–73.

Sessle BJ (1986) Recent developments in pain research: central mechanisms of orofacial pain and its control. *J Endodon* **12**, 435–444.

Sessle BJ (1993) Neural mechanisms implicated in the pathogenesis of trigeminal neuralgia and other neuropathic pain states. *Am Pain Soc J* **2**(1), 17–20.

Sessle BJ and Hu JW (1991) Mechanisms of pain arising from articular tissues. *Can J Physiol Pharmacol* **69**, 617–628.

Shaber EP and Krol AJ (1980) Trigeminal neuralgia—a new treatment concept. *Oral Surg Oral Med Oral Pathol* **49**, 286–293.

Shapiro SA, Goodwin S and Campbell RL (1988) Microvascular decompression for intractable trigeminal neuralgia. *Indiana Med* **81**, 776–778.

Shelden CH, Pudenz RH, Freshwater DB and Crue BL (1955) Compression rather than decompression for trigeminal neuralgia. *J Neurosurg* **12**, 123–126.

Shindler W (1961) 5H-Dibenz[b,f]azepines. *Chem Abstr* **55**, 1671.

Shuhan G, Benren X and Yuhuan Z (1991) Treatment of primary trigeminal neuralgia with acupuncture in 1500 cases. *J Trad Chin Med* **11**(1) 3–6.

Siegfried J (1977) 500 percutaneous thermocoagulations of the gasserian ganglion for trigeminal pain. *Surg Neurol* **8**, 126–131.

Siegfried J (1981) Percutaneous controlled thermocoagulation of gasserian ganglion in trigeminal neuralgia. Experiences with 1000 cases. In: Samii M and Jannetta PJ (eds) *The Cranial Nerves*, pp 322–330. Berlin: Springer.

Sillanpaa M (1981) Carbamazepine. Pharmacology and clinical use. *Acta Neurol Scand* **64** (Suppl. 88), 115–119.

Silverberg GD and Britt RH (1978) Percutaneous radio-frequency rhizotomy in the treatment of trigeminal neuralgia. *West J Med* **129**, 97–100.

Sindou M and Martens P (1993) Microsurgical vascular decompression (MVD) in trigeminal and glossopharyngeal neuralgias. A twenty-year experience. *Acta Neurochir Suppl* **58**, 168–170.

Sindou M, Keravel Y, Abdennebi B and Szapiro J (1987) Treaitment neurochirurgical de la neuralgie trigeminale. Abord direct ou methode percutanee? *Neurochirurgie* **33**, 89–111.

Singh N, Sachdev KK and Brisman R (1982) Trigeminal nerve stimulation: short latency somatosensory evoked potentials. *Neurology* **32**, 97–101.

Sjaastad O (1992) *Cluster Headache Syndrome*. London: WB Saunders.

Sjaastad O and Stensrud P (1969) Appraisal of BC-105 in migraine prophylaxis. *Acta Neurol Scand* **45**, 594–600.

Sjoqvist O (1938) Studies in pain conduction in the trigeminal nerve. A contribution to the surgical treatment of facial pain. *Acta Psychiatrica Neurol Scand Suppl.* **17**, 1–139.

Slettebo H, Hirschberg H and Lindegaard KF (1993) Long-term results after percutaneous retrogasserian glycerol rhizotomy in patients with trigeminal neuralgia. *Acta Neurochir* **122**, 231–235.

Smart HL, Somerville KW, Williams J, et al. (1985) The effect of sucrafate upon phenytoin absorption in man. *Br J Clin Pharmacol* **20**, 238–240.

Smirne S and Scarlato G (1977) Clonazepam in cranial neuralgias. *Med J Aust* **1**, 93–94.

Smith A (1987) QUALMS about QALYs. *Lancet* **i**, 1134–1136.

Smith G and Covino BG (1985) *Acute Pain*. London: Butterworths.

Smith GT (1988) *Measuring Health: A Practical Approach*. Chichester: John Wiley & Sons.

Sobel D, Norman D, Yorke CH and Newton JH (1980) Radiography of trigeminal neuralgia and hemifacial spasm. *Am J Radiol* **135**, 93–95.

Sokolovic M, Todorovic L, Stajcic Z and Petrovic V (1986) Peripheral streptomycin lidocaine injections in the treatment of idiopathic trigeminal neuralgia. A Preliminary Report. *J Maxillofac Surg* **14**, 8–9.

Solomon S and Lipton RB (1988) Atypical facial pain: a review. *Semin Neurol* **8**, 332–338.

Solomon S and Lipton RB (1990) Facial pain. *Neurol Clin* **8**, 913–927.

Sorayal I, Allen E, Halsall GM and Richens A (1991) Bioavailability of phenytoin from six different oral formulations. *J Pharm Med* **1**, 17–22.

Spaziante R, Cappabianca P, Peca C et al. (1988) Subarachnoid hemorrhage and 'normal pressure' hydrocephalus: fatal complications of percutaneous microcompression of the Gasserian ganglion. *Neurosurgery* **22**, 148–151.

Speculand B, Goss AN, Hughes A et al. (1983) Temporo-mandibular joint dysfunction: pain and illness behaviour. *Pain* **17**, 139–150.

Spielberger CD, Gorsuch RL and Luohere RE (1970) *State–Trait Anxiety Inventory*. Palo Alto, CA: Consulting Psychologists Press.

Spiller WG and Frazier CH (1901) The division of the sensory root of the trigeminus for the relief of tic douloureux, an experimental, pathological and clinical study, with preliminary report of one surgical successful case. *Philadelphia Med J* **8**, 1039–1049.

Spincemaille GHJ, Dingemans W and Lodder J (1985) Percutaneous radiofrequency gasserian ganglion coagulation in the treatment of trigeminal neuralgia. *Clin Neurol Neurosurg* **87**, 91–94.

Spoerel WE, Varkey M and Leung CY (1976) Acupuncture in chronic pain. *Am J Clin Med* **4**, 267–279.

Stajcic Z (1989) Peripheral glycerol injections in the treatment of idiopathic trigeminal neuralgia. A preliminary study. *Int Oral Maxillofac Surg* **18**, 255–257.

Stajcic Z (1990) Evidence that the site of action of glycerol in relieving tic douloureux is its actual site of application. *Dtsch Zahnarztl Z* **45**, 44–46.

Stajcic Z, Juniper RP and Todorovic L (1990) Peripheral streptomycin/lidocaine injections versus lidocaine alone in the treatment of idiopathic trigeminal neuralgia. A double blind controlled trial. *J Craniomaxillofac Surg* **18**, 243–246.

Steardo L, Leo A and Marano E (1984) Efficacy of baclofen in trigeminal neuralgia and some other painful conditions. *Eur Neurol* **23**, 51–55.

Steiger HJ (1991) Prognostic factors in the treatment of trigeminal neuralgia. Analysis of a differential therapeutic approach. *Acta Neurochir* **113**, 11–17.

Steinhoff BJ, Stoll KD, Stodieck SRG and Paulus W (1992) Hyponatremic coma under oxcarbamazepine therapy. *Epilepsy Res* **11**, 67–70.

Stender, A and Grumme T (1969) Late results of gangliolysis as a treatment for trigeminal neuralgia. *J Neurosurg* **31**, 21–24.

Steude U (1979) Radiofrequency percutaneous Gasserian ganglion lesions in the treatment of trigeminal neuralgia. *Neurosurg Rev* **2**, 153–157.

Stewart MJ (1990) Professional interface with mutual-aid self-help groups: a review. *Soc Sci Med* **31**, 1143–1158.

Stookey B and Ransohoff J (1959) *Trigeminal Neuralgia. Its History and Treatment.* Springfield IL: Charles C Thomas.

Stow PJ, Glynn CJ and Minor B (1989) EMLA cream in the treatment of post-herpetic neuralgia. Efficacy and pharmocokinetic profile. *Pain* **39**, 301–305.

Sturman RH and O'Brien FH (1969) Non-surgical treatment of tic douloureux with carbamazepine (G32 883). *Headache* **9**, 88–91.

Sumatriptin Cluster Headache Study Group (1991) *New Eng J Med* **325**, 322–326.

Surman OS, Flynn T, Schooley RT *et al.* (1990) A double-blind, placebo controlled study of oral acyclovir in postherpetic neuralgia. *Psychosomatics* **31**, 287–292.

Swanson SE and Farhar SM (1982) Neurovascular decompression with selective partial rhizotomy of the trigeminal nerve for tic douloureux. *Surg Neurol* **18**, 3–6.

Swanston M, Abraham C, Macrae WA *et al.* (1993) Pain assessment with interactive computer animation. *Pain* **53**, 347–351.

Swedlow M (1980) The treatment of 'shooting' pain. *Postgrad Med J* **56**, 159–161.

Swedlow M and Cundill JG (1981) Anticonvulsant drugs used in the treatment of lacerating pain: a comparison. *Anaesthesia* **36**, 1129–1132.

Sweet WH (1985) The history of the development of treatment for trigeminal neuralgia. *Clinical Neurosurg* **32**, 294–318.

Sweet WH (1986) The treatment of trigeminal neuralgia (tic douloureux). *N Engl J Med* **315**, 174–177.

Sweet WH (1988a) Percutaneous methods for the treatment of trigeminal neuralgia and other faciocephalic pain; comparison with microvascular decompression. *Semin Neurol* **8**, 272–279.

Sweet WH (1988b) Retrogasserian glycerol injection as treatment for trigeminal neuralgia. In: Schmidek HH and Sweet WH (eds) *Operative Neurosurgical Techniques*, pp 1129–1137. Orlando: Grune and Stratton.

Sweet WH (1990) Complications of treating trigeminal neuralgia: an analysis of the literature and response to questionnaires. In: Rovit RL, Murali R and Jannetta PJ (eds) *Trigeminal Neuralgia*, pp 251–279. Baltimore: Williams and Wilkins.

Sweet WH and Poletti CE (1988) Complications of percutaneous rhizotomy and microvascular decompression operations for facial pain. In: Schmidek HH and Sweet WH (eds) *Operative Neurosurgical Techniques*, pp 1139–1143. New York: Grune and Stratton.

Sweet WH and Wepsic JG (1974) Controlled thermocoagulation of trigeminal ganglion and rootlets for differential destruction of pain fibres. Part 1: Trigeminal neuralgia. *J Neurosurg* **39**, 143–156.

Sweet WH, Poletti CE and Macon JB (1981) Treatment of trigeminal neuralgia and other facial pains by retrogasserian injection of glycerol. *Neurosurgery* **9**, 647–653.

Sweet WH, Poletti CE and Roberts JT (1985) Dangerous rises in blood pressure upon heating of the trigeminal rootlets: increased bleeding times in patients with trigeminal neuralgia. *Neurosurgery* **17**, 843–844.

Symonds C (1949) Facial pain. *Ann R Coll Surg Engl* **4**, 206–212.

Szapiro J, Sindou M and Szapiro J. (1985) Prognostic factors in microvascular decompression for trigeminal neuralgia. *Neurosurgery* **17**, 920–929.

Taarnhoj P (1952) Decompression of the trigeminal root at the posterior part of the ganglion as treatment in trigeminal neuralgia. Preliminary communication. *J Neurosurg* **9**, 288–290.

Taarnhoj P (1982) Decompression of the posterior trigeminal root in trigeminal neuralgia. A 30-year follow-up review. *J Neurosurg* **57**, 14–17.

Tartara CA, Galimberti CA, Manni R *et al.* (1991) Differential effects of valproic acid and enzyme-inducing anticonvulsants on nimodipine pharmacokinetics in epileptic patients. *Br J Clin Pharmacol* **32**, 335–340.

Tartara CA, Galimberti CA, Manni R *et al.* (1993) The pharmacokinetics of oxcarbazepine and its active metabolite 10-hydroxy-carbazepine in healthy subjects and in epileptic patients treated with phenobarbitone and valproic acid. *Br J Clin Pharmacol* **36**, 366–368.

Tash RR, Sze G and Leslie DR (1989) Trigeminal neuralgia: MR imaging features. *Radiology* **172**, 767.

Tashiro H, Kondo A, Aoyama I *et al.* (1991) Trigeminal neuralgia caused by compression from arteries transfixing the nerve. Report of three cases. *J Neurosurg* **75**, 783–786.

Taylor JC, Brauer S and Espir LE (1981) Long term treatment of trigeminal neuralgia with carbamazepine. *Postgrad Med J* **5**, 16–18.

Terrence CF (1987a) History of trigeminal neuralgia. In: Fromm GH (ed) *The Medical and Surgical Management of Trigeminal Neuralgia*, pp 1–15. New York: Futura.

Terrence CF (1987b) Differential diagnosis of trigeminal neuralgia. In: Fromm GH (ed) *The Medical and Surgical Management of Trigeminal Neuralgia*, pp 43–60. New York: Futura.

Terrence CF, Sax M, Fromm GH *et al.* (1983) Effect of baclofen enantiomorphs on the spinal trigeminal nucleus and steric similarities of carbamazepine. *Pharmacology* **37**, 88–94.

Tew JM and Keller JT (1977) The treatment of trigeminal neuralgia by percutaneous radiofrequency technique. *Clin Neurosurg* **24**, 557–578.

Tew JM and van Loveren H (1988) Percutaneous rhizotomy in the treatment of intractable facial pain (trigeminal, glossopharyngeal, and vagus nerves). In: Schmidek HH and Sweet WH (eds). *Operative Neurosurgical Techniques*, 2nd edn, Vol 2, pp 1111–1123. New York: Grune & Stratton.

Theisohn M and Heimann G (1982) Disposition of the antiepileptic oxcarbazepine and its metabolites in healthy volunteers. *Eur J Clin Pharmacol* **22**, 545–551.

Theobald W and Kunz HA (1963) Zur Pharmacologie des Antiepilepticums 5-Carbomyl-5H-dibenzo[*b,f*]azepin. *Arzneim Forsch Drug Res* **13**, 122–125.

Thoma KH (1969) *Oral Surgery*. St Louis: Mosby.

Thompson M and Bones M (1985) Non traditional analgesics for the management of post herpetic neuralgia. *Clin Pharmacol* **4**, 170–176.

Tobler WD, Tew JM, Cosman E *et al.* (1983) Improved outcome in the treatment of trigeminal neuralgia by percutaneous stereotactic rhizotomy with a new curved tip electrode. *Neurosurgery* **12**, 313–317.

Tomasulo RA (1982) Abberent conduction in human peripheral nerve: ephaptic transmission? *Neurology* **32**, 712–719.

Tomson T and Bertilsson L (1984) Potent therapeutic effect of carbamazepine-10,11-epoxide in trigeminal neuralgia. *Arch Neurol* **41**, 598–601.

Tomson T and Ekbom K (1981) Trigeminal neuralgia: time course of pain in relation to carbamazepine dosage. *Cephalagia* **1**, 91–97.

Tomson T, Tybring G, Bertilsson L *et al.* (1980) Carbamazepine therapy in trigeminal neuralgia: clinical effects in relation to plasma concentration. *Arch Neurol* **37**, 699–703.

Trojan A (1989) Benefits of self-help groups: a survey of 232 members from 65 disease-related groups. *Soc Sci Med* **29**, 225–232.

Trousseau A (1853) De la neuralgie epileptiforme. *Arch Gen Med* **1**, 33–44.

Truelove EL, Sommers EE, LeResche L *et al.* (1992) Clinical diagnostic criteria for TMD. New classification permits multiple diagnoses. *J Am Dent Assoc* **123**, 47–54.

Turk DC, Meinchenbaum D and Genest M (1983) *Pain and Behavioral Medicine*. New York: Guilford Press.

Turk DC, Rudy TE and Salovey P (1985) The McGill Pain Questionnaire reconsidered: confirming factor structure and examining appropriate uses. *Pain* **21**, 385.

Turner JA and Romano JM (1984) Review of prevalence of co-existing chronic pain and depression. In: Benedetti C, Moricca G and Chapman CR (eds) *Advances in Pain Research and Therapy*, Vol 7, pp 123–130. New York: Raven Press.

Turner JA and Romano JM (1990) Psychologic and psychosocial evaluation. In Bonica JJ (ed) *The Management of Pain*, 2nd edn, pp 595–609. Philadelphia: Lea and Febiger.

Tursky B, Jamner LD and Freidman R (1982) The pain perception profile: a psychophysical approach to the assessment of pain report. *Behav Ther* **13**, 376–394.

Tyrer JH, Eadie MJ, Sutherland JM and Hooper WD (1970) An outbreak of anticonvulsant intoxication in an Australian city. *BMJ* **4**, 271–273.

Tyrer SP, Capon M, Peterson DM, Charlton JE and Thompson JW (1989) The detection of psychiatric illness and psychological handicaps in a British pain clinic population. *Pain* **36**, 63–74.

Valsalan NC and Cooper GL (1982). Carbamazepine intoxication caused by interaction with isoniazid. *BMJ* **285**, 261–262.

van de Welde C, Smeets P, Caemaert J and Van de Velde (1989) Transoval cisternograpy and glycerol injection in trigeminal neuralgia. *J Belge Radiologie* **72**, 83–87.

van Heiningen PNM, Eve MD, Oosterhuis B *et al.* (1991) The influence of age on the pharmacokinetics of the antiepileptic agent oxcarbazepine. *Clin Pharmacol Ther* **50**, 410–419.

van Loveren H, Tew JM, Keller JT and Nurre MA (1982) A 10 year experience in the treatment of trigeminal neuralgia: comparison of percutaneous stereotoxic rhizotomy and posterior fossa exploration. *J Neurosurg* **57**, 757–764.

Vilming ST, Lyberg T and Lataste X (1986) Tizanidine in the management of trigeminal neuralgia. *Cephalagia* **6**, 181–182.

von Korff M, Dworkin SF, Le Resche L and Kruger A (1988) An epidemiological comparison of pain complaints. *Pain* **32**, 173–183.

Walker AE (1970) The differential diagnosis of trigeminal neuralgia. In: Hassler R and Walker AE (eds) *Trigeminal Neuralgia. Pathogenesis and Pathophysiology* pp 30–34. Stuttgart, Georg Thieme Verlag.

Wall PD (1984) Introduction. In: Wall PD and Melzack R (eds) *Textbook of Pain*, pp 1–16. Edinburgh: Churchill Livingstone.

Wall PD and Melzack R (1994) *Textbook of Pain*, 3rd edn. Edinburgh: Churchill Livingstone.

Waltz TA, Dalessio DJ, Copeland B and Abbott G (1989) Percutaneous injection of glycerol for the treatment of trigeminal neuralgia. *J Pain* **5**, 195–198.

Wang JK (1985) Cryoanalgesia for painful peripheral nerve lesions. *Pain* **22**, 191–194.

Warner T, Patsalos PN, Prevett M *et al.* (1992) Lamotrigine-induced carbamazepine toxicity: an interaction with carbamazepine-10,11-epoxide. *Epilepsy Res* **11**, 147–150.

Wartenberg R (1958) *Neuritis, Sensory Neuritis and Neuralgia* pp 337–377. New York: Oxford University Press.

Watson CP (1989) Postherpetic neuralgia. *Neurol Clin* **7**, 231–248.

Watson CP, Chipman M, Reed K *et al.* (1992) Amitriptyline versus maprotiline in postherpetic neuralgia: a randomized, double blind, crossover trial. *Pain* **48**, 29–36.

Watson CP, Evans RJ and Watt VR (1988a) Post-herpetic neuralgia and topical capaisin. *Pain* **33**, 333–340.

Watson CPN, Evans RJ, Watt VR and Birkett N (1988b) Post herpetic neuralgia: 208 cases. *Pain* **35**, 289–297.

Watson CP, Watt VR, Chipman M *et al.* (1991) The prognosis with postherpetic neuralgia. *Pain* **46**, 195–199.

Weddington WW and Blazer D (1979) Atypical facial pain and trigeminal neuralgia: a comparison study. *Psychosomatics* **20**, 348–356.

Weidmann MJ (1979) Trigeminal neuralgia. *Med J Aust* **2**, 628–630.

Weisenberg M and Caspi Z (1989) Cultural and educational influences on pain of childbirth. *J Pain Synd Management* **4**, 13–19.

Welty TE, Pickering PR, Hale BC and Arazi R (1992) Loss of seizure control associated with generic substitution of carbamazepine. *Ann Pharmacother* **26**, 775–777.

White JC and Sweet WH (1969) *Pain and the Neurosurgeon. A 40 Year Experience*, pp 123–256. Springfield, IL: Charles C Thomas.

Whittaker DK (1986) History of cryosurgery. In: Bradly P (ed) *Cryosurgery of the Maxillo-facial Region*, Vol 1, pp 1–15. Florida: CRC Press.

Wilkins RH (1988) Surgical therapy for neuralgia: vascular decompression procedures. *Semin Neurol* **8**, 280–285.

Wilkins RH (1990) Historical perspectives. In: Rovit RL, Murali R and Jannetta PT (eds) *Trigeminal Neuralgia*, pp 1–25. Baltimore: Williams and Wilkins.

Wilkinson M (1985) Migraine — the treatment of acute attack. *Scott Med J* **4**, 258–262.

Williams DA and Thorn BE (1989) Empirical assessment of pain beliefs. *Pain* **36**, 351–358.

Williams RC (1988) Toward a set of reliable and valid measures for chronic pain assessment and outcome research. *Pain* **35**, 239–251.

World Health Organization (1978) Definitions of health. From the preamble to the Constitution of the WHO basic documents, 28th edn. p 1. Geneva: WHO.

Wright GA (1907) Note on treatment of trigeminal neuralgia by injection of osmic acid into the Gasserian ganglion. *Lancet* **ii**, 1603–1604.

Yamaki T, Hashi K, Niwa J *et al.* (1992) Results of reoperation for failed microvascular decompression. *Acta Neurchir* **115**, 1–5.

Yau MK, Adam MA, Wargin WA and Lai AA (1992) A single dose and steady-state pharmacokinetic study of lamotrigine in healthy volunteers. *Third International Cleveland Clinic Bethel Symposium, Cleveland, Ohio.*

Yoshimasu F, Kurland LT and Elveback LR (1972) Tic douloureux in Rochester, Minnesota, 1945–1969. *Neurology* **22**, 952–956.

Young RI (1988) Glycerol rhizolysis for the treatment of trigeminal neuralgia. *J Neurosurg* **69**, 39–45.

Yuen A (1992) Safety issues. In: Richens A (ed) *Clinical Update in Lamotrigine: A Novel Antiepileptic Agent*, pp. 69–75. Tunbridge Wells: Wells Medical.

Zaccara G, Messori A and Moroni F (1988) Clinical pharmacokinetics of valproic acid. *Clin Pharmacokinet* **15**, 367–389.

Zakrzewska JM (1990a) *Evaluation of the long-term management of trigeminal neuralgia by carbamazepine, cryotherapy, radiofrequency thermocoagulation and microvascular decompression.* MD thesis, University of Cambridge, UK.

Zakrzewska JM (1990b) Medical management of trigeminal neuralgia. *Br Dent J* **168**, 399–401.

Zakrzewska JM (1991) Cryotherapy for trigeminal neuralgia: a 10 year audit. *Br J Oral Maxillofac Surg* **29**, 1–4.

Zakrzewska JM and Ivanyi L (1988) In vitro lymphocyte proliferation by carbamazepine, carbamazepine-10,11-epoxide, and oxcarbazepine in the diagnosis of drug induced hypersensitivity. *J Allergy Clin Immunol* **82**, 110–115.

Zakrzewska JM and Nally FF (1988) The role of cryotherapy (cryoanalgesia) in the management of paroxysmal trigeminal neuralgia: a six year experience. *Br J Oral Maxillofac Surg* **26**, 18–25.

Zakrzewska JM and Patsalos PN (1989) Oxcarbazepine — a new drug in the management of intractable trigeminal neuralgia. *J Neurol Neurosurg Psychiatry* **52**, 472–476.

Zakrzewska JM and Patsalos PN (1992) Drugs used in the management of trigeminal neuralgia. *Oral Surg Oral Med Oral Pathol* **74**, 439–450.

Zakrzewska JM and Thomas DGT (1993) Patient's assessment of outcome after three surgical procedures for the management of trigeminal neuralgia. *Acta Neurochir* **122**, 225–230.

Zakrzewska JM, Nally FF and Flint SR (1986) Cryotherapy in the management of paroxysmal trigeminal neuralgia. Four year follow up of 39 patients. *J Maxillofacial Surg* **14**, 5–7.

Zhang KW, Zhao YH, Shun ZT and Li PT (1990) Microvascular decompression by retrosigmoid approach for trigeminal neuralgia: experience in 200 patients. *Ann Otol Rhinol Laryngol* **99**, 29–130.

Zielinski JJ and Haidukewych D (1987) Dual effects of carbamazepine–phenytoin interaction. *Ther Drug Monit* **9**, 21–23.

Zigmond AS and Snaith RP (1983) The Hospital Anxiety and Depression Scale. *Acta Psychiatr Scand* **67**, 361–370.

Zorman G and Wilson CB (1984) Outcome following microsurgical vascular decompression or partial sensory rhizotomy in 125 cases of trigeminal neuralgia. *Neurology* **34**, 1362–1365.

Zung WWK (1965) A self-rating depression scale. *Arch Gen Psychiatry* **12**, 63.

Zurak N, Randic B, Poljakovik Z and Voglein S (1989) Intravenous chlormethiazole in the management of primary trigeminal neuralgia resistant to conventional therapy. *J Int Med Res* **17**, 87–92.

Index